*Praise for*

# BADASSES

"Rollicking."

*—Library Journal*

"Richmond captures the 'tude and, more importantly, the love of the physical nature of football that drove the Raiders."

*—Booklist* (starred review)

"Accessible to even casual football fans, *Badasses* is a potent mix of unlikely antiheroes. . . . The takeaway? Rebellion is good."

*—San Francisco Chronicle*

"One of the best football books ever written."

*—San Jose Mercury News*

"Easily the most entertaining football book of 2010."

*—Tampa Tribune*

# BADASSES

## Also by Peter Richmond

*My Father's War: A Son's Journey*

*Fever: The Life and Music of Miss Peggy Lee*

*Ballpark: Camden Yards and the Building of
an American Dream*

*The Glory Game: How the 1958 NFL Championship
Changed Football Forever* (with Frank Gifford)

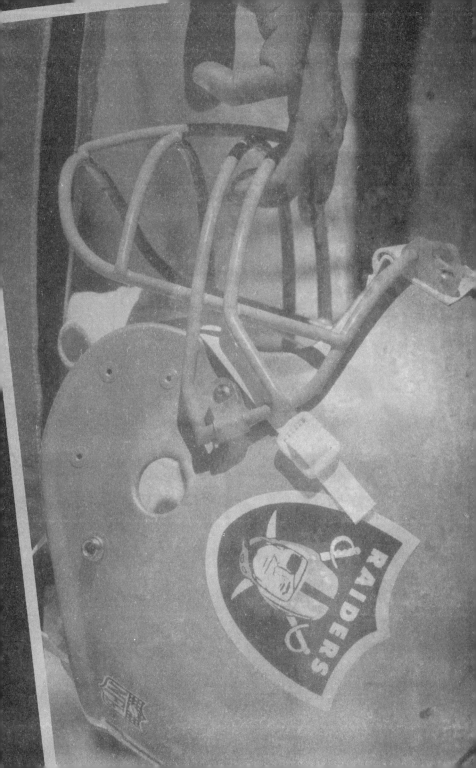

# BADASSES

## THE LEGEND OF SNAKE, FOO, DR. DEATH, AND JOHN MADDEN'S OAKLAND RAIDERS

### PETER RICHMOND

*itbooks*

# *it*books

HarperCollins books may be purchased for educational, business, or sales promotional use. For information please write: Special Markets Department, HarperCollins Publishers, 10 East 53rd Street, New York, NY 10022.

Frontispiece courtesy of Otto Greule/Allsport US

FIRST IT BOOKS PAPERBACK EDITION PUBLISHED 2011.

Designed by William Ruoto

Library of Congress Cataloging-in-Publication Data has been applied for.

ISBN 978-0-06-183431-8 (pbk.)

12  13  14  15    OV/RRD    10  9  8  7  6  5  4

To Maxfield

# Contents

# PART II: BADASS FOOTBALL

# Preface

Could a very good football team be more than just a very good football team? Could it be something more? Could it be legendary—not just Hall of Fame legendary but legendary as in the tales of ancient warriors, half-real and half-mythical, who mattered because they inspired people who needed to believe in figures mightier than their mundane selves?

Could a football team seize the modern imagination because the days of *true* legend have long passed? Because we no longer have myths in sport or in life? Because long gone are the days when, as Ken Stabler put it to me, "you played for the name on the front of the jersey, not the name on the back"?

Or how about this: Could innocent outlaws—"lovable rogues," as Stabler calls the Oakland Raiders of the '70s—who played in a world grown increasingly conventional and downright boring be regarded as something more than just one of the great football teams of all time? Could history judge a collection of weirdly intelligent, proudly individualistic, seamlessly bonded men as something more than just another great sports team? Could they be heroes?

That was the thought that hit me one day. So I ran it by a random Raider from the era—the first Raider I talked to, actually. I asked him whether we could think of the '70s Raiders as heroic, in the you'll-be-hearing-about-them-a-thousand-years-from-now sense. The answer wasn't exactly what I expected.

"You have to go to the Greeks to get the appropriate conception," said defensive lineman Pat Toomay. "The Greeks . . . understood 'heroes' as being capable of anything, from patricide to incest, because of the energy they had to embody to do the admirable things that they did. What the Greeks would see as quintessentially human behavior. Their heroes' nature was exceptional and ambivalent, even aberrant. Their heroes prove to be at once good and bad and accumulate contradictory attributes."

Then Toomay, graduate of Vanderbilt, son of an Air Force general who specialized in Defense Department nuclear strategies, told me that if I wanted to pursue my idea, I should check out Romanian philosopher Mircea Eliade's *The History of Religious Ideas*.

I never did. I was too busy revisiting the golden age of my beloved Raiders, none of whom committed patricide or incest but most of whom lived somewhere outside of the conventional grid. The well-read Toomay, like his black-and-silver brethren, was obviously not your everyday professional football player. He earned a degree in Applied Mathematics. Nor was the Raider linebacker turned state senator who enlivened training camp with trivia games featuring his mastery of animal genetics, nor the linebacker who found he'd been traded during a macroeconomics exam. Nor the defensive tackle who holds a navigational-guidance patent and used to fly his own tiny airplane cross-country to camp. Nor the linebacker who would prefer to discuss the Druids rather than football—and once arrived at practice astride a horse. Nor the center who did a striptease atop the bar of his favorite tavern, nor the fullback who rode his motorcycle through a bar, nor the linebacker who befriended a Hells Angels leader, nor the cornerback who regularly checked into the hospital room along with his motorcycle. Nor the men who arrived fresh from football's faceless, drudging minor leagues and blossomed into black-and-silver stars. Nor the players who would arrive at training camp *early*, so that they could once again plunge back into their unique haven of camaraderie.

But I think I know what Toomay was getting at: that greatness is one thing; legend is another; and myth is still a third. In a low-profile, second-sister town, all three were embodied by a hirsute, off-the-wall football team dressed in black and silver who played football for what Stabler calls "all the right reasons."

How good were John Madden's Badass Oakland Raiders of the '70s? In a modern culture that seems to live by the philosophy "Second place is for losers"—and in this case, first place judged by the number of rings on your fingers—they were not the best. Pittsburgh, Dallas, and Miami all took home more Lombardi trophies in that decade. But in the '70s, no team was so routinely dominant as the Raiders. Or so unusual. Or so damned fun and entertaining to watch playing America's true pastime.

Let's consider some other numbers. After losing the Super Bowl in January of 1968, the Oakland Raiders won seven division titles in the next eight seasons. Between 1970 and 1977, they played in six AFC Championship games. And when quarterback Stabler—the de facto leader, the Badass emblem, the "Snake"—took over for good, in 1973, he led them to five consecutive AFC Championship games, and the Super Bowl XI title to end the '76 season: the Sisyphean myth denied. Their 66 regular-season victories from 1972 to 1977 led the National Football League. By those numbers, numbers that speak of perennial dominance, it's obvious that the Badasses knew how to consistently play the game of football better than anyone out there, year in, year out. They were the ongoing emblem of in-your-face excellence.

The Steelers and Dolphins and Cowboys represented excellence of a very specific kind: simple football excellence. These were football machines, presided over by jut-jawed coaches whose stars seldom made an appearance in the celluloid reel of our imagination.

Pittsburgh and Miami and Dallas never hypnotized *me*, anyway. I was an East Coast college student laboring at the bottom of his class on an Ivy'd campus, chafing against an unseen enemy, against all things privileged and conventional and summer-home-on-Nantucket-ish—smoking my weed in the mornings, barely skimming the textbooks, affecting the archetypal rebel pose. But beneath it all I was truly addicted to nothing but professional football, the game that evokes a primal instinct, a pull to our species' need for team warfare, where a clan must work as one. The sport where strategy is sublimated by sheer physical will. And I was magnetically drawn to the guys whose hair flapped out of their helmets, whose mustaches and beards and eyeblack loomed like warrior makeup behind the face guards, whose delightfully pink-faced coach, unencumbered by coat and tie, waved his arms on the sideline at the officials like a blow-up doll gone amok. ("Holy shit," John Madden told me, of the surprise he'd feel when he'd see himself on film after games. "I know I got pissed, but I didn't think I got *that* pissed.")

Mostly, I was drawn to athletes who retained their individuality, strutted it, while playing a team sport, and to me, this furnished a magical high all its own. I hadn't a clue what I'd do with my life, that I'd end up actually writing about the world they inhabited, but I did know, like Madden did when he gave up thoughts of law school to follow his true bliss, that it would not be part of a vocation involving a coat and tie, and that whatever path I pursued would have to include professional football—played by outlaws.

In the '70s, I reveled not just in those countless Raider victories but in the certainty that if this particular band of brothers could excel, that as long as professional football could include a prime-time team whose image, style, and attitude ran entirely counter to the mainstream product, then Big Football didn't have to be like Big Business or conventional society. The game could be played with obvious joy. Badass football, with its implicit message that rebellion was *good*, could indeed rule the professional landscape, no matter the number of rings it would earn. Better yet, played by iconoclasts and madmen, it could inspire.

Of course, the Raiders of the '70s themselves have their own ranking system for their historic excellence: "Number one—of all time," the savage safety George Atkinson told me, his tones as sharp and confident as the way he played his gnarly game. "Come on, man, I'm ranking us number one. Without a doubt."

But let's put quantifiable measures of success aside for a moment and focus on what made the Raiders so distinct: they arrived just in time to keep the dream of happy revolution alive. As Greil Marcus eloquently suggested in *Lipstick Traces: A Secret History of the 20th Century*, as the '70s unscrolled, a grateful mainstream culture, capitalistic at heart, sighed in relief at having survived the threatening chaos of the '60s, said relief reflected in the titles of songs like the Rolling Stones' "Soul Survivor" and the Bee Gees' "Stayin' Alive." But it was the Grateful Dead's "Touch of Grey" that spoke of a vestigial need for the endurance of the enlivening anarchy of the '60s and its belief that the kids were not only all right but had always *been* right: "I will get by, I will survive."

Survival for mainstream American culture in the '70s, relief that the psychedelic nation hadn't swamped the two-cars-in-every-garage '50s ideals, meant going back to something like real, ordered, structured life. But what was that real life in America in the '70s? It was a tepid, unadventurous, light footprint of a decade that would transition us away from the mostly innocent mayhem of the '60s into the "greed is good" '80s.

For those of us who bemoaned the vanishing of the '60s, the new decade was a dispiriting time when the layering of the plastic tunes of Captain & Tennille and The Carpenters erased the snaggled, buoyant legacies of Hendrix and Joplin and, on the football field, an era when generals replaced coaches. When Don Shula and Chuck Noll and Bud Grant and Tom Landry's steely, businesslike, humorless faces emerged to replace Brooklynite Lombardi's grinning/scowling, gap-toothed smile, Giants coach Allie Sherman's nervous, trench-coated, sideline-cigarette prowls, and Baltimore's little bulldog Weeb Ewbank's odd, oval truck driver's face, the game seemed to lose some of its muddy, giddy humanity.

As I watched these woolly Raiders play their unconventional game beneath a late-afternoon California sun that refused to set when the East had gone dark, I found my true heroes on a football team that not only played the game with a delicious violence and a tangible edge but promised that the metaphoric revolution of the previous decade was alive and weirdly thriving, on the last stage you'd ever expect to see it: a professional football field.

In the Badass Raiders, I saw a vestige of the wildly anarchic good times of the '60s grafted onto a team playing the dark sport that had entranced me since childhood. Sunday afternoons and Monday nights, my Raiders gave every rebel a cause, assured us that being out of the ordinary could be a guiding philosophy of life.

On one level, the game of football is structured and symmetrical; there is no room for tactical error. But reduced to its essence—its *eidos*, if we're still dwelling in ancient Greece, where shoulder-length-haired Spartan phalanxes marched against each other, dueling and killing at an ancient line of scrimmage—isn't this game nothing but loosely structured, balletic mayhem? Mayhem certainly flowed through the blood of the mercenary, sometimes brutal athletes who first played professional football a half century before these Raiders. Viewed as outcasts by sporting society, decried at the time as the lowliest athletic dregs, the professional pioneers were considered defilers of the decorum of the college game. "Real" football was being played in the East and Midwest for nothing but raccoon-coated campus pride. In the national headlines, across the radio waves, football's stars were clean-cut university thoroughbreds. The pro game was an aberration, impure and unruly and unholy.

Only as the game evolved for television's eye—and Madison Avenue began to recognize the marketability of these remarkably tough athletes' elemental, beautiful brutality—did the veneer of respectability begin to dawn in the professional ranks and the sport began to morph from mud-and-blood lunchpail head-butting into Pure Entertainment: the modern NFL, where now, in the words of Raider tight end Raymond Chester, "players are independent contractors. They are each mini–sports corporations."

But in Oakland, there were only two contractors and no corporations. The Raiders were an organism unto themselves, sneering at all others. They were nothing but the product of two men, Al Davis and John Madden: "Al" and "John" to the players, who considered them family in an organization where no one stood on ceremony.

The managing general partner, a magnetic magnate with an indefinable, oft-sinister allure, the ultimate Badass, wanted more than to transform the game, to win at all costs. This was a man who sensed from the very start that he was destined for a singular place in history, and this aura enwrapped him like a coat of armor. Davis wanted to turn football convention on its head. A man who carried himself like a king, he welcomed the game's outcasts into his fold—black and white men both, at a time when this was far from routine—and loved them, as long as they committed themselves to winning for the family, for the cult. A mystical, mysterious figure, a give-a-fuck icon, he suggested to those of us who both loved the game and questioned Nixonian authority that it was not only OK to be yourself, and sketch your own blueprint, but that this was the only path to follow.

The coach? A precocious, next-door-neighbor guy, a leader the likes of whom we'd never seen and never will again: a semi-neurotic, highly sympathetic everyman who roamed the sideline looking like a fan who'd wandered onto the field. A guy unsaddled by any trace of put-on seriousness. John Madden treated his players as peers—not above or beyond them, just *of* them. The man obviously enjoyed what he was doing; he was unique in a fraternity where frowning was the de rigueur expression. He seemed to revel in being part of a *game*, not an industry. He was having fun.

For the most part, though, the Badasses played for their brothers. More than anything, this was their motivation: to not let down their teammates, teammates whom they truly did love. We are, after all, innately social animals. We are encoded to blend with our tribe, and no tribe blended with each other as the Raiders did, as well as with their wild, passionate fans and their entire downtrodden civic community—all the while reassuring us that going against the grain could not only survive as a way of life but also inspire respect, even delight.

And what happens when these outcasts and eccentrics start to love and respect each other? Well, if you were looking at them from the wrong side of the line of scrimmage, they could inspire not a little fear: fear that the Badasses would find a way to beat you, of course, usually in a come-from-behind fourth quarter, but also the fear that these men, my men, could just as easily separate your head from your body as they could erase a late-game deficit. When they hit, they hit with something to prove. Their *aura* hit.

"I swear, some teams didn't want to play against us; they'd

just try and lose," the delightfully crazed linebacker Phil Villapiano told me, the Raider of Raiders, the Jersey guy who lived for the rush of a brutal tackle. "We won a lot of games because people didn't want to fuck with us. They didn't want to rile us up. We won so many games when teams could have tried a little harder to beat us, but they didn't want to. It's like you don't want to fight Muhammad Ali. Ali drills you a couple of times, you fall down."

Football historians undervalue the Badasses. The record keepers rely on numbers. Numbers refer to quantifiable successes, and speak as if pro football teams were interchangeable machines. "Though the beginning of the '70s would be ruled by the Dolphins, and the end by the Steelers, the decade as a whole belonged to the Dallas Cowboys," wrote Michael MacCambridge in his definitive history of the league, *America's Game.* "They were the league's most visible, respected, resented and imitated team."

But those teams were not the most *feared*, and fear lies at the heart of a game in which a single blow can cripple you in a microsecond. Nor did the Cowboys have the most character—or characters. Nor did they inspire from the gut and the heart. Yes, the Cowboys would become America's Team, but didn't the very emergence of an America's Team—a national team—signal the beginning of the disappearance of football as it was meant to be played, the waning of the old, local game, when a football team represented a city's true work ethic? When its players weren't just individuals but a reflection of the identity of its city? In the '40s and '50s and '60s, American cities still turned out products that fueled the world economy, and football teams in cities such as Pittsburgh and Detroit and Chicago wore their football teams like proud insignia. In those years, professional football was still a worker's game. It didn't matter that some of those teams didn't win; they symbolized working-class eminence.

Besides, any team that was "America's Team" was, by definition, just as likely to sell jerseys in Des Moines as Dallas. Defined by Landry, a Christian war hero, and Roger Staubach, a Naval Academy clean-cut boy, playing quarterback in a city that epitomized New Wealth, the Cowboys' logo was nothing if not an early herald of modern America's instant-fame national ranking system for everything and everyone, wherein someone has to be the instantaneous best, the most recognizable, the champion, and can earn that perch and its attendant fame *American Idol*–style, without doing the work and climbing the ladder. Today anyone, out of nowhere, can be the Star: that supposedly hallowed emblem of the Cowboy team. And the star breeds stars, not brothers. It speaks of showmanship, not sport. Nor teamwork.

On the Raiders, a selfish drive to rise above the pack would have represented heretical behavior. "There was no superstar on the Raiders," the legendarily lovable, shaven-headed defensive end Otis Sistrunk, a veteran of football's minor leagues who reached Pro Bowl status wearing the black and silver, told me. "No retired jerseys. You had 45 players. You had a team"—a team perfectly designed for a town that occupied no place in the national pantheon of municipal privilege, or wealth, or respect, but went about doing the daily grunt work without reward, without national notoriety, in the shadow of the glittering, towered city across the bay.

If history reserves football of the '70s for the larger-than-life, star-emblazoned franchise, fine: for some of us the game itself will always belong to the anti-Cowboys, to the team with the dark, delightfully cackling soul.

"We used to say, 'You don't have to have a criminal record to play on this team,'" Duane Benson, an unheralded Raider line-backer of the early '70s, told me, "'but it really helps.'" The truth is, the Badass rosters included no actual criminals. Just men who delighted in living and playing somewhere outside and beyond the mainstream, and safely inside the Badass family, a team that found its bliss wearing black.

One other element distinguished my rebel squad, something obvious and infectious: the unmistakable delight with which they played their games, on the field or off. "They don't say you work football," the eccentric linebacker Ted Hendricks once said. "They say you play football." I was hardly surprised when Benson told me that he found the key to the Raider success in a place where others seldom look: in a team-wide vibe that stressed just how damned pleasurable it was to be playing a game with a bunch of teammates who exuded glee as much as they exuded menace.

"On the Raiders, there was a value placed on this notion of having fun," Benson told me. "It was such standard fare . . . to be a little bit crazy . . . to have fun. To have real *fun* and have real fun on an all-the-time basis. We always had more fun than whomever we played, during the week, and during the game. I've taken on other things in life [including four years in the Minnesota state senate] and still find it to be true: whoever has the most fun usually wins."

Or, as tight end Bob Moore, a Stanford guy, put it to me, summing up his Raider years, "Seven days a week, it was as much fun as a human being could have and still stay alive."

# PART I

# ROOTS, REBELS, AND RITES

## CHAPTER ONE

# The Immaculate Deception

ob Moore wasn't looking for a fight that night. The Raiders' tight end had planned to turn in early before the memorable opening game of the 1972 AFC playoffs. Like any proud member of the tribe, Moore was no stranger to the evening pub crawl, but public imbibing was not the wisest of ideas in a hostile city lathered in anticipation of its first postseason appearance in four decades, where celebrations were sprouting all over the city like Steeltown wildflowers. For all of their legendary revelry, these Raiders had generally known where to draw the line. The game always came first. Festivity, while an integral element of the Raider repertoire, had its own time and place.

So Moore and linebacker Greg Slough had decided to make it an innocent Friday night out and catch a movie—a gangster caper called *Across 110th Street*, starring Anthony Quinn and Yaphet Kotto. ("If you steal $300,000 from the mob," read the film's promo poster, "it's not robbery. It's suicide.") Then Moore and Slough hoofed it back to the team hotel—where they were greeted

by the sight of a well-fueled crowd gathered in front of the downtown Hilton, laying siege to the enemy's camp.

This contingent of fans, a splinter faction from an earlier downtown celebration thousands strong, had not gathered at the hotel on a
peacekeeping mission. They weren't willing to wait for the Saturday-
afternoon tilt at Three Rivers Stadium to vent their partisan emotions. They had assembled to deliver an advance decree to the visiting team: You're in enemy territory now. And they were armed.
Before the evening's end, one beer bottle would sail through a hotel
window, and another would clock a cop. Several arrests would be
made. Bob Moore had not figured to be among them.

The barbarians at the gate were polite enough to the two Raiders as they sidled forward through the mass, which was kidding
and jiving with the players but making way for them. Enemies
or not, they were larger than life. But when Moore met the wall
of blue that the city had enlisted to hold the frothing mob at bay
things grew ugly.

"We go up to the front, and there are these cops," Moore recalls now, lounging on the deck of his spacious home in the gentle
hills east of Oakland, its backyard shaded by tall redwoods, a home
bathed in peace. Beloved among his teammates then, and now a
Bay Area lawyer, Moore had joined the team in 1971 with a not-
atypical Raider pedigree. He had smarts (the degree from Stanford), he had workmanlike skills (averaging 25 catches from 1973
to 1976), he was the consummate team player, he loved a good
time, and he had an extra arrow often found in the Raider quiver:
defiance, especially in the face of a challenge. If you don't want us
to do it, that's reason enough to do it. This credo had always been
ingrained in the Raider DNA: Us against Them. Unfortunately
for Moore, on this night the opposition wore a different kind of
uniform—and it was armed with clubs. If Moore had been wearing
his own uniform, what followed might have been a fair gladiatorial
fight. As it is, this was no contest.

"We say we're with the Raiders and we want to go up to our rooms," Moore recalls. "This policeman kind of hits me and says, 'I don't care who the fuck you are. You're not getting to the front of this line.' I didn't think a cop with a nightstick was going to beat up an Oakland Raider in town for a playoff game. So I make a comment I regretted pretty quickly.

"I said, 'Look, motherfucker, I'm going to my room.'"

You called a riot-squad cop a motherfucker? Why? Moore thinks for a second, then answers: "It's sort of what people say at times when they're pissed off." Well, it's definitely sort of what a Badass would say, Stanford sheepskin or not.

"So then, *boom.* This guy comes down on the top of my head with a nightstick, which is like a baseball bat. Solid wood. The next thing, I'm on the ground. And I got a guy on my chest trying to beat the shit out of me, and another guy holding my legs. I'm trying to cover up, and I get my hands pulled away, and *bang,* I get it again. You get hit by one of these things while you're conscious, you think you're going to die."

"Motherfucker" was Moore's first Badass pronouncement. But he was just getting started. He lusted for Raider retaliation. Rationality had been replaced by Badass instinct. "They drag me away to a paddy wagon. I get in the back. The first guy comes in. I went after him. Just attacked him. Hit him with everything I had. He goes out and they slam the door. A couple minutes later the driver comes back and says, 'We're going to take you down and book you.' I said, 'Book me for what?'

"Then he sees I'm drenched in blood. He says, 'No, we're going to rush you to the hospital.' Turns out it wasn't bad. Seven stitches, cuts on both sides of my head. I was swollen like a son of a gun. I'm on the operating table and the young surgeon says, 'You're real lucky.' I said, 'You have to explain this to me. I don't feel very lucky.'"

Turned out the state of Pennsylvania had something called the doctrine of sovereign immunity. Which means you can't sue the city, only individual people. "So he said, 'Generally, guys who get this kind of treatment don't come here. We pick them up at the morgue after they dump them in the river.' I said, 'Thanks, that's comforting.'"

After they'd sewn him up, Moore was taken back to the police station to be booked. Madden was there. The mayor was there. The chief of police was there. But a deal was offered to Moore: If you don't sue the cop, you won't be arrested. His response would have done his teammates proud: "I said, 'Tell them to fuck themselves.'" Finally, Moore agreed to an alternative proposal: he wouldn't talk to the press while he was in town, and they'd let him go.

"The next morning in the locker room I can't get a helmet on. So [defensive lineman] Kelvin Korver had a big head, with, like, a size-eight helmet. They took his helmet, took all the insides out of it and made these Styrofoam donuts strapped to the inside. Everyone's crowded around me in the locker room before the game, right? So John walks up and says, 'Hey, Bob, with all due respect, we got a football game today. Tell them to go away.'" Moore's red badge of courage no longer counted on game day. Still, there was something reassuring about a Raider striking the first blows a full day in advance of the actual game.

"I don't remember a thing about the game," Moore says now. "I wandered like a mummy off the field, knowing we lost. But I had to figure out what the hell happened."

This, of course, makes Bob Moore unique among football fanatics. To the rest of the football world, what happened on December 23, 1972, remains indelible: what NFL Films would come to call "the greatest play in NFL history"—in a game that, arguably, despite its outcome, launched the Raiders' long, strange journey to the top. The catalyst for all to come.

For the Steelers, the game lives on forever, and the play remains a singular moment of glory. How else to interpret the statue of favorite son Franco Harris planted in a concourse of Pittsburgh International Airport? Does it show Harris slipping a tackler's grip? Sprinting or rumbling toward one of his 91 career touchdowns? Does it commemorate any of the hundreds of other great moments in the immortal Franco Harris's Hall of Fame career?

Of course not. It shows him reaching down to his shoelaces, gathering an errant football with his fingertips. For thousands of travelers, every day, there it stands: a very lifelike monument to a singular moment of (questionable) triumph.

"The Immaculate Reception? I call it the Immaculate *Deception*," Atkinson, the "Hit Man," says now, with only half a laugh. "We got fucked by a soft dick."

It made for a catchy sound bite, "the Immaculate Reception." But think, for just a second, about what this now-immortal phrase implies. Consider the phrase's original usage. To have an immaculate event, there had to be a miracle involved, right? And a god behind it? So isn't this the subtext of what the term "Immaculate Reception" suggests: that on the artificial turf of Three Rivers Stadium, with seconds left in a football game that the Oakland Raiders had more or less won, as Terry Bradshaw called the signals for a fourth-down desperation play, a beneficent god reached down and bestowed victory on a team that was otherwise unable to attain it on its own?

One narrator on a retro film clip subsequently called it "the greatest miracle in sports history." And miracles don't happen without divine intervention, do they? Any way you look at it, then, legend insists that it took Outside Help to defeat Oakland's Army of the Night on that December afternoon.

But why would a benevolent god intervene to help one football team beat another? Well, if one team was deemed good, worthy, anointed, and the other . . . demonic. If one team represented the staid old-world NFL's Rooney franchise, and the other represented the rebels of Al Davis, a man who bowed to no higher power.

In the end, what, really, does the phrase "Immaculate Reception" imply other than that the infidel band of marauders was poised to win the game and wreak havoc on the free world—until Someone decided to defy a defender known as "the Assassin" and drop the ball into the hands of one of the most loveable figures in the game? A man with his own legion of fans? "Franco's Italian Army" is what the T-shirts celebrating the Rookie of the Year read (which was cute enough at first glance, until you think about what Spain's Generalissimo Francisco Franco's regime stood for). But there was nothing not to love about Franco Harris. The Steelers' first-round pick, the biracial all-American boy, was as popular a player as the game would ever see.

No, on this day, the gods clearly had it in for the Badasses— "the Antichrist," says Atkinson, nodding, smiling, clearly proud of having been part of the dark side.

Of course, there was little question about whom the football establishment favored: that week, the guys in Pittsburgh had gotten a good-luck call from George Halas, officially giving the Old Humorless NFL certification to the Pittsburgh team. Halas had owned the Chicago Bears since its earlier incarnations, and was only five years removed from having coached the Bears for nearly half a century. Art Modell had wished the Steelers luck, too: the steward of the hallowed Cleveland Browns franchise. The Steelers had even gotten a best-of-luck message from Nixon: Mike Nixon, a former Steeler head coach. But a telephone call from the football fanatic president wouldn't have been too surprising.

No high-profile public endorsements of Al Davis's band of brutes were forthcoming. Nor was Moore's rumble the only pre-game omen that did not favor the West Coast challengers. The Raiders' plane had developed engine trouble at the start of their trip, and a replacement couldn't come in because of the fog. They'd had to bus to San Francisco for another flight east. Romantic fog might be a good omen for a team from the city across the bay, with its gentle, artistic aura of all things effete, but not for the guys from working-class Oakland, hometown of the Black Panthers as well as the black and silver. The week of this game, *The Black Panther*, the weekly "intercommunal news service" of the party, splashed "Season's Greetings from the Black Panther Party" on its cover—with a sprig of black holly adorning it: the hollowest of salutations, laden with dark irony. This was not the kind of town where Tony Bennett would leave his heart.

For the Raiders and their fans, this game would be the first step back to the long-awaited Super Bowl they'd been denied in January of 1968, a 33–14 drubbing in the second inter-league championship game against the Packers. This playoff game figured to launch them toward finally getting the rings they'd watched the hated Jets and Chiefs collect in the interim years. They'd be playing a team that hadn't made it to the playoffs in modern times, a team that had finished 6–8 the year before.

Steeler quarterback Terry Bradshaw had thrown as many interceptions as he'd thrown touchdowns in 1972. For 10–3–1 Oakland, 1972 offered a chance to return to supremacy after the aberrant 1971 season when, with much of the personnel from the team's previous incarnation slowed by age and injury, the team had missed out on the playoffs, and the Chiefs had won the division. (In 1970, the Raiders' eight victories had been good enough to take the division but, behind veteran quarterback George Blanda, they'd lost the championship game in Baltimore, to the Colt team that would win the Super Bowl.) In 1972, riding a powerful and unrelenting ground game led by the tanklike fullback Marv Hubbard (the man who once supposedly bet he could dive into a shot glass, and actually tried), the Raiders had pretty much put it away in week 11, when, with the division title on the line, they'd honed their game by routing the Chiefs, 26–3.

And Pittsburgh? No surprise that the town was in a bottle-throwing lather, with tickets being scalped for an unheard-of $50: playoff-wise, the Steelers were 0 for 39 years. In the first three years under Chuck Noll's stewardship, the Steelers hadn't had a winning season. But in 1972, in Bradshaw's second year, they'd won 9 of their last 10 and finished at 11–3. Individually, the "under the hill" gang averaged fewer than four years in the league, but with a defense anchored by Joe Greene, Dwight White, L. C. Greenwood, and Jack Ham, they'd given up a remarkable total of 15 points in their last four games and hadn't allowed a touchdown in their last three.

Now, the Raiders had returned to Pittsburgh to avenge the season-opening loss at Three Rivers, a 34–28 Steeler victory in which the Raiders had characteristically rallied from a 20-point deficit, but this time only to come up six points shy. The Raider-Steeler rivalry would, of course, soon become the game's most intense. "In a way, the teams mirrored each other," says Stabler. "You look at their tough blue-collar steel city, and our blue-collar city, both wearing black." But they were distinctly different shades of black. One signified industrial supremacy. The other stood for the dark side.

The game had featured a tense, wonderful battle of defenses, heavyweights gutting it out. Two-thirds of the way through the fourth quarter, the score was 6–0, Pittsburgh, on two Roy Gerela field goals. The Raider defense held Harris and the Steeler runners to 108 yards; Bradshaw completed all of 11 passes. "The best defense I faced all year," he would say afterward.

But veteran Raider quarterback Daryle Lamonica, ailing with the flu, had been ineffective, too: he'd completed just 6 of 18 passes for 45 yards. The "Mad Bomber" had been with the team since 1967, when he'd taken the Raiders to that second championship game between the NFL and AFL, not yet called the Super Bowl. But there was already some feeling on the team that Stabler should have been starting. Lamonica was not universally beloved, and the cool, high-living, high-profiled Snake was. But Lamonica had considerable physical gifts: he could throw the long pass as well as anyone, and certainly better than Stabler.

But now six minutes remained, and Madden figured that on this day the Bomber's time was up. In 1972, four years out of Alabama, the second-string Stabler had appeared in every game of the regular season, mostly in a backup-savior role, and he'd played effectively. He had completed 60 percent of his 74 passes during the year, including 10 of 11 in the second half of the season's final victory over Chicago, relieving Lamonica in a tied game to defeat the Bears.

So now Madden sent in the lefty, and a team that had lain dormant all day immediately responded to the laconic, eerily even-tempered Alabaman whose life philosophy, according to Stabler's own book, had been passed on from a hard-drinking dad: "Go for the good times when you can."

True Badass fans now had a glimmer of hope, if a slim one—and a glimpse of the future. Stabler engineered a drive that began at his own 20 and brought the Raiders to the Steeler 30. He called a pass, but in the face of an all-out blitz, he and his achy left knee took off and, with the defenders glued to their receivers, saw nothing but open field beckoning. He rambled an unlikely 30 yards down the left side for the go-ahead touchdown—holding the ball out like the proverbial loaf of bread, hair flopping from the back of his helmet, tucking the ball in and diving/falling across the goal line.

It was 7–6, Raiders, with 1:13 left. Three Rivers and the Steeler nation had fallen silent in disbelief. Score one for the Antichrist. Without the "Deception," this game would have gone down in history as Ken Stabler's Last-Minute Miracle Touchdown Drive—especially if the Raiders had then gone on to beat the Dolphins, which the Steelers didn't. (Then again, that year, no one beat the mighty white-clad Dolphins.)

"I guess it was kind of my coming out," Stabler told me, recalling the play as if it had happened yesterday but refusing to buy into the notion that he'd pulled off anything spectacular: "But that was kind of the personality of the whole team. It was, 'Find a way to win. No matter who does it, just get it done.'"

Now, with 22 seconds left on the clock, and stalled at their own 40, the Steelers lined up on fourth and ten. Or, as one commentator put it, "fourth and hopeless."

The play was called 66 Circle Option, with Bradshaw looking deep for the seldom-used receiver Barry Pearson, who hadn't caught a single pass all season. The ball was snapped, and Bradshaw faded back. But finding Pearson covered, Bradshaw was flushed out of the pocket, barely eluding the grasp of Raider lineman Horace Jones.

"Bradshaw avoided a lot of guys on that play," remembers Raider receiver Fred Biletnikoff. "We had the opportunity to sack him, and when he ran out, we still had the opportunity. He made a hell of a play just to get rid of the ball."

Bradshaw scrambled out to his right and, greeted by two lunging linemen in his face, threw desperately across the field, 37 yards diagonally downfield to his left, to "Frenchy" Fuqua, the running back who, to that point, had had a forgettable game, averaging just over one yard per run on 25 rushing attempts. On this play, Fuqua had run 25 yards down the left side, out of the backfield, and hooked in for the ball at the left hashmark. Safety Jack Tatum, that Assassin, patrolling the deep middle of the field, abandoned the tight end he was covering and took aim on Fuqua from behind.

Now, like the statue in the airport, time froze while the gods debated up on Olympus. "What are our options?" said Zeus. "Well," said Athena, "Tatum, the Badass of Badasses, is about to hit the Fuqua guy like a truck aiming for a squirrel. We can let him knock the ball out and give the game to Al Davis's guys. I kind of like that blond lefty quarterback, anyway. He has heroic qualities."

"No," says the Big Man. "Let's make that Italian guy the hero. Give the people what they want: good over evil. This one play will spur a Steeler dynasty. I love dynasties. Mine is eternal."

Well, it's as logical as what actually happened, isn't it? Harris wasn't even supposed to be near the ball. He was supposed to be blocking. He wasn't supposed to be anywhere near a miracle.

Today, there isn't a single Raider whose memory doesn't wince: NFL Films and YouTube be damned. The excruciating freeze-frames of the play remain as much of their everyday thought as the face they see in the mirror.

"I'm covering Franco," Villapiano recalled over a beer one day in an airport hotel in his home state of New Jersey. "When they snapped the ball, Franco set up to block. Now, in the NFL, when someone sets up to block, you run in and grab them, and it's pretty much over. I ran in and grabbed him, shoved him, and when Bradshaw rolls out to the other side, Franco just starts jogging down the field. I'm like, 'What the fuck is he doin'?' I'm just jogging right next to him. Then when I saw Terry throw the ball, I'm gone. I just shot over [downfield] to help. Then the ball bounced right . . . back . . . over my head."

Villapiano pulls on his beer. He wipes his lips. He shakes his head. "As I was sprinting toward it, it was going right over my head. See, I'm figuring Franco's running down the field, 'cause he's a rookie and he knows the coaches are looking at him. He's just trying to be a good boy. I always tell Franco when I see him: 'I was right on your inside. All I had to do was be as lazy as you. That ball would have come to me.' If I jog with him, it's over. Instead, I sprinted away from him. He kept running, and look what happened."

As one modern season bleeds into another, what happened at that moment only gains in historic momentum, if not in clarity. None of the recollections quite jibe on the details—where the ball hit, whom the ball hit—but all of them jibe on the weird geometry of what happened when Tatum, arguably the hardest hitter in the NFL, rushed from behind to level Fuqua.

There was no uncertainty in the Assassin's mind: "I hit Frenchy in the back," Tatum told me, "and the ball *had to* have hit him for the ball to have come back to Franco." Back then, the "two-touch" rule mandated that two offensive players couldn't touch the ball consecutively.

All three objects—the ball and the two players—came together as one. Out of the violent collision emerged the football, popping straight back downfield, like a leather spheroid shot from a cannon. Then the ball slowed, pulled by gravity. In all, it flew backward, where a football isn't supposed to go, for about seven yards, right into the path of Harris, jogging where he wasn't supposed to be.

Then Harris, trailing the play, as stunned as the rest of the world, reached down and plucked the ball from just a few inches off the Three Rivers turf, on the Oakland 42. Harris tucked the ball away and ran down the left sideline, stiff-arming defensive back Jimmy Warren at the 10, and took it into the end zone. Adrian Burk, the back judge trailing the play, signaled a touchdown.

The roar ballooned to fill the concrete cavern and echoed through Steeltown. Teammates and fans mobbed Harris in the end zone. But none of the Raiders were concerned; they figured it was an illegal play.

"I was on the right side," Raider cornerback and defensive captain Willie Brown recalls. "I saw Jack hit Fuqua in the back. The ball bounced off Fuqua, and I knew it was over right there. I said, 'Hey, great.' I knew it was dead. He hit the guy from the back. When you hit a guy from the back, it means you're knocking him forward. So how could Jack have touched the ball? I mean, come on, the laws of physics and the laws of common sense says there's no way Tatum could have hit it if he knocked Fuqua into the ball."

Brown smacks one hand into the other for emphasis. The passage of four decades has only heightened the image in Brown's mind. "He hit Fuqua, and Fuqua hit the ball. And I thought the game was over."

But referee Fred Swearingen had now gathered his crew for a consultation. In all the decades of the game, no one had seen a play as bizarre as this one. The officials huddled on the field as fans milled about on the perimeter of the field, eager to celebrate.

"'Oh, boy,' I'm thinking. 'Something's going on here,'" says Brown. "So the next thing I know, since I'm the captain, and so's Gene [Upshaw], we're running up to them and saying, 'The game's over.' They say, 'We don't know yet.' They kept saying, 'We don't know yet.' I'm saying, 'Bullshit. It's over.'

"Then I hear one of the referees say, 'Do we have security on the field? . . . If you do, I'm going to make this call in favor of the Raiders.' So someone says, 'Well, we'll get you out of here as fast as we can.'

"If they'd ruled in our favor, they would never have gotten out of there alive. That was the reason they changed the call."

Today, the Steelers' L. C. Greenwood agrees with Brown on one thing: it would have been ugly either way. Four decades of pent-up Pittsburgh frustration could have resulted in a near-riot if the call had gone against the Steelers. And if Swearingen ruled that the touchdown was legal, Greenwood figured, there would have been a riot anyway. Greenwood didn't want to stick around.

In fact, the defensive end who holds the Steeler sack record didn't think his team would get the first down, much less a touchdown. "I was actually headed for the locker room," Greenwood says now. "Then I heard the crowd cheering. I was actually running to the locker room to get off the field before people got carried away, as I expected them to anyway. They would have been upset if we had lost. Pittsburgh fans are pretty energetic fans. They don't like losing."

Greenwood wasn't the only player who was ready to call it a day. George Atkinson figured that the Raider celebration was just beginning. "I was on the other side of the field. I unsnapped my helmet. I'm headed to the locker room. It never hit me that it counted. When Jack hit Fuqua, and the ball ricocheted, I thought it hit the ground, from my angle. I also registered the two-offensive-players rule. So I thought, 'Even if Franco has it, it's dead.' The officials knew it was dead, too, [but] they couldn't reverse that call, man. In Pittsburgh?"

In the huddle, Swearingen canvassed his crew. Four of the officials said that they weren't sure what had happened. Two said that they thought that Tatum was the last to touch the ball. None of them had a conclusive answer. It had all happened way too fast. Swearingen then entered the Pittsburgh Pirate dugout and made a call upstairs to NFL Director of Officiating Art McNally.

"I ran out on the field," Madden remembers now, as irate today as he was that afternoon, "and they were all talking, and they said, 'Just get off the field; we don't know what happened.' I said, 'I *know* you don't know what happened.'

"Then I went off the field, and then they talked and talked and talked forever. Then the referee goes over and talks on the phone and comes out and says, 'TD.' I mean, that's not the way you call a touchdown! My thing, to this day, is if they knew it was a touchdown, why didn't they call it a touchdown? In the history of football, a touchdown is a touchdown! You don't have to go talk about it.

"And he calls it a touchdown. Well, what didn't you see before that, and what did you see after that? That was my argument. If you knew it was a touchdown, call it a touchdown."

Swearingen told McNally on the phone that he wanted to call it a touchdown, and McNally concurred. So Swearingen came out of the dugout and thrust his arms in the air: touchdown, 13–7, Steelers. Five seconds remained on the clock, time for a meaningless kickoff, followed by bedlam in Three Rivers, and devastation in every Badass soul. "We did enough to win," Biletnikoff says now. "To have something like that happen . . . It should have been an incompletion if it was that inconclusive. Shoulda went our way."

Linebacker Gerald Irons was the last Raider to leave the field, ignoring the scrum of Pittsburgh fans. He slogged over to the sideline, in a daze. "I think the officials saw the fans had been drinking a lot," says Irons, "so they pretty much wanted to get out of there. You can't blame them. It would have been nice if they'd sent security guards [so they could] make the right call."

On the other hand, maybe a true Raider fan would have a little sympathy in his heart for a call that might have hinged on the amount of libation the fans had consumed.

The phrase "cover-up" would become a more common term in the months following this game. But true Raider conspiracy theorists believe this cover-up was just as real as Richard Nixon's, and far more meaningful: that Swearingen, in the days before replay could officially be used to decide a play, wanted to know what the replay showed, in order to make his call.

"Joe Gordon [the Steelers' PR man] made the announcement over the press box PA system that they were looking at the replay," says Tom LaMarre, who was covering the game for *The Oakland Tribune*. "The NFL later denied it. Gordon would probably deny it now." (In fact, Gordon did deny it, in a *New York Times* article in 1997, in which he stated that McNally never did view a replay but was simply confirming for Swearingen the details of the two-touch rule. But why would a head official need a seminar on a simple rule?) "They couldn't admit McNally was watching it, because there was no replay rule back then."

The main network replay—as any viewing of it now confirms—was entirely inconclusive. There *was* another view of the play, though: a shot from the end zone behind Bradshaw, which NBC ran behind the credits at the end of the game. *San Francisco Examiner* writer Frank Cooney videotaped the telecast and later reviewed NBC's footage by freezing the frames. "It was really clear," Cooney says now of the end-zone shot. "Fuqua reached out for the ball, and it hit him in the arm as Tatum hit him from behind. I told Madden and Davis about it later. Davis, of course, was really pissed. He saw it as a conspiracy."

According to LaMarre, who saw Cooney's tape, the ball clearly flattens out on Fuqua's forearm. That tape has been lost to history.

"I saw McNally at the airport and he told me there was no doubt," Madden told a reporter for the *Tribune* a few days after the game. "But then I saw Jay Randolph of NBC Television, and he told me that there was no way to make a positive decision off the TV replays. Those are the same films McNally saw."

After viewing the game film on Christmas Eve, Madden told reporters he was certain that the two-touch rule should have been enforced: "What Jack did was give him a good shot from behind. Jack never touched the ball, which hit Fuqua on the shoulder pad . . . but there was no way they were going to call it the other way with all those people out on the field . . . I just think we were ****ed. . . ."

"They couldn't have any other decision with all those wild people on the field," Madden told the *Tribune*. "Something would have happened. Those people might have killed him."

Steeler owner Art Rooney Sr.—beloved Art Rooney, 71-year-old, cigar-smoking NFL patriarch Art Rooney—didn't even see the play. Before fourth down, he'd put out his cigar and left his private box early. It was Rooney's custom to visit after losses, but not after victories, lest he take away from attention that belonged to his team.

He was standing next to the elevator, listening to the roar of the crowd and wondering what had happened, when a guard ran up to tell him he'd won. When he got to the locker room, it was empty save a couple of trainers. He had no idea of the machinations taking place on the field. Finally, the door burst open, and punter Bobby Walden gave him the good news.

Then, after the team had joyously bounced into the locker room, Art Rooney watched coach Chuck Noll lead the team in the Lord's Prayer.

Divine Intervention indeed. Never was a post-game prayer more appropriate.

Asked about the play in his own locker room, Fuqua said, "I cannot tell a lie. No comment." Fuqua's comment to a Pittsburgh writer hinted at intrigue: "I'll tell you after the Super Bowl." But the Steelers lost to the Dolphins the following week, and the truth was forever buried. To this day, Fuqua won't admit what he knows, and according to Villapiano he dines out on his secret.

"I've seen him at the mic at various events many times," laughs Villapiano. "I've seen it at least five times: he has this whole act. Nobody plays it better than him. He pretends he's going to tell, that this is finally going to be the time he tells the world, then he starts fake crying and shaking and says, 'I just can't do it.'

"One time we had this big banquet, had everybody together—a bunch of Steelers, a bunch of Raiders—and he says, 'Tonight's the night. The world deserves to know. I've waited long enough.' Then he says, 'I can't do it. It's immaculate. Something that's immaculate—I don't have the right. If something's immaculate, that means God is the only one who can tell you.'

"It's beautiful, his act. He certainly knows. He knows the ball hit him."

But the truth is now revealed. According to Raymond Chester, Frenchy Fuqua *did* talk about it that day. Minutes after the play, on a visit to the Raider locker room, he spoke to his college teammate at Morgan State: Chester, who will never forget Fuqua's words.

"I can remember sitting in the locker room," Chester says now. "Frenchy came into our locker room after the game and leaned over my locker and said, 'It hit me.'

"'It hit me'—he absolutely told me that in the locker room."

Atkinson, then, has it right: deception had sent the Steelers onward and the Raiders stumbling home. The rogues had been unjustly denied.

The aftermath of the miraculous moment for Rooney and the Steelers provided some sweet reactions. The two most prominent telegrams of congratulations came from Frank Sinatra and composer Henry Mancini, a native of Aliquippa, Pennsylvania. Sinatra's read, "The following is an order: Attack. Attack. Attack. Attack." Mancini's read, "Congratulations on the Steelers' win. Where do I go to enlist in Franco's Army?"

For the Raiders, stunned disbelief and dismay provided the only post-game notices. Amid a sea of photographs in the next day's edition of *The Oakland Tribune*, one shot says it all: Stabler standing in dismay, his face buried in his left hand, his long hair draping over his hand. It's a classic pose. It is not commemorated by a statue in the Oakland airport.

"The photograph tells the story," Stabler says now. "It was the biggest game of my life at the time. You make a play, you do some things that give you the opportunity to get to the prize, you get that close, off a scrambling TD, and then you watch the things that happen in the next minute and four seconds? It'd put your face in your hands, too."

The play left a mark on every Raider, except, perhaps, Bob Moore, who was barely there to experience it. Moore played all of two downs that day, spending most of the day in a painkillered haze on the sidelines. The Raiders left town without getting the satisfaction they sought from the officials, of the game or of the city. The Pittsburgh police wouldn't identify the policeman who'd pummeled him. Moore's lawyer said he wouldn't sue if the police would just provide the name of the guy who'd beaten him.

Moore simply wanted to meet his assaulter face-to-face: "I said, 'Give me an hour in a room with this guy. No weapons. We'll either talk about it or beat the shit out of each other.'" Moore had no intention of actually revealing the guy's name. He just wanted a more primal, Raider-like resolution to the episode. But Moore got no satisfaction. The Pittsburgh police would not comply. His lawyer never heard back from the city of Pittsburgh after that distinctively Badass pregame ceremony. Moore didn't pursue the matter. Like the rest of the Raiders, he turned toward the future, secure in the knowledge that, from here on in, it was going to be Us Against Them.

"They were obsessed with the Immaculate Reception," says Betty Cuniberti, who would later cover the team for the *San Francisco Chronicle*. "It was such a wonderful fuel for their strange engine."

To the Raiders, that one play spelled it out in spades: they clearly had more to overcome than other teams. Their rebel image, their defiant owner, had stamped them as the enemy of civilized football. The stars, and the league, were aligned against them. From now on, if the gods had truly forsaken them, the team would have to reach the top banded as one, against all comers—including all conceivable powers who wanted to keep the rebels down.

"I actually always thought the NFL had a vendetta against the Oakland Raiders," Atkinson told me, and who can blame him? Considering the play by which the Badasses were so supremely fucked?

CHAPTER TWO

# The Early Years

Let's start with the distinctive, eternal symbol—virtually unchanged in half a century, an emblem with a visceral appeal. It didn't resemble the other benign, predictable, obvious logos of the early American Football League—Denver's bucking bronco; the Patriots' all-American tricorne-hatted soldier; Miami's leaping dolphin, with a tiny helmet crammed incongruously onto its head; or the Bills' slumping red buffalo, standing with its head bowed, as if awaiting the slaughterhouse.

No, the Raider crest displayed a singular attitude from the very start. "A guy with an eyepatch? Crossed swords?" says Stabler. "Black uniforms? Playing in the very, very tough blue-collar city of Oakland? It all fit like a hand in a glove."

Consider the nature of the pirate: a true outlaw, a man who defies societal strictures in order to loot, plunder, and seize whatever he desires by whatever means necessary. He is beholden to no one save his shipmates, vilified by conventional society but celebrated in fantasy. As far back as the numerous mentions in the lyrical lines of the *Odyssey*, the pirate who roamed the Mediterranean after the Trojan War was both scorned and begrudgingly admired. Not only did it take a lot of balls to raid a passing ship; it was a very tough and violent way to make a living. The pirate's turf was his own. He'd made the decision to sever himself from society's conventions, from order, but mingled with it when he had to, always on his violent terms.

Now let's think about how different history would have played out if the original choice for the team name had stuck: The Oakland Señors. Chet Soda, an original team general partner and a local businessman, was said to favor the greeting "Howdy, *señor!*" and envisioned cheerleaders with sombreros and serapes roaming the sidelines of Kezar Stadium, the team's first temporary home, up in Golden Gate Park. Never mind that the plural of *señor* is *señores*. Consider for a moment the bipolar effect on the team image had the original name stuck. The aura of Oakland's football squad, in a game of attack and mug and brawl, would have oozed a feeling of formal politeness: the Oakland Gentlemen? Would they have turned out to be a franchise without distinction? Would their style of play have conformed to the rest?

Instead, the team took the title Raiders, a fitting moniker for a team that would have to fight, from the start, for its share of the pie. The Raider franchise, playing just a few miles from an established NFL competitor, unsure that it could draw enough fans to survive, had been a last-second runt addition to the new American Football League in its first year, 1960; the charter AFL Minnesota franchise vanished when the National Football League, at the urging of Chicago Bears god figure Halas, put its own expansion team in the Twin Cities, the better to give Halas a local rival and cut down on travel costs. In part for similar considerations, Los Angeles Chargers owner Barron Hilton helped convince AFL commissioner Joe Foss, a legendary Marine flying ace in the Second World War and former governor of South Dakota, to grant an eighth league team upstate, in Oakland. This would give Hilton a

California rival—a rival that he would beat up on easily in the first three years of the league.

The delay in locating the team in Oakland had resulted in several of its first draft picks finding their way to other teams. The sorry squad that first played as the Raiders, in black-and-gold uniforms cadged from the University of the Pacific, won just six of fourteen games in its first year.

Chet Soda was soon gone from the ownership ranks. The team, now honchoed by principal owner Wayne Valley, a shrewd local construction multimillionaire, power broker, and former Oregon State lineman, was also poised to vanish from sight. Before the second season, which the team played at Candlestick Park (in a manner of speaking, anyway; they lost their first two games by a combined score of 99–0), Valley warned that the team would be gone after 1961 unless the city built him a stadium. San Jose was offering Spartan Stadium for 1962. God knows why. The Raiders weren't playing a brand of football you'd call professional.

Valley and his co-owners got their stadium. Sort of. Frank Youell Field was built for $400,000 and eventually held, when overflowing, close to 20,000. Named for a local sports enthusiast and city councilman who happened, appropriately, to be an undertaker by trade, the Raiders' home for the next four years was built on the site of former temporary housing for shipyard workers during the Second World War. The undertaker's park was likened by some to a giant erector set, although one critic compared it to a birdcage. Frank Youell Field's one concession to its crude design was the attachment of squares of colored plywood fastened to the steel girders that held the place up. "Reasons of economy dictated the omission of all frills," wrote one *San Francisco Examiner* scribe. "This Spartan design predominates the entire plant." (There's that Greek thing again.)

But a true football field needs no frills. All it needs is turf to be trampled.

The press-box food at Frank Youell featured pickles. In the stands, beer was sold by the can. But something about the bare-boned, intimate innocence of the place helped forge the first bond between team and fan, a frenzied, costumed symbiosis that, over the years, would prove to be among the strongest and most flamboyant and storied in professional sports.

"It was like a high school stadium, which made it kind of fun," Raider lineman Frank Youso recalls of that first year at Youell Field. Youso, a veteran of the Giants and the Vikings, and a man who tended to speak his mind to his superiors in the old league—including run-ins with Vince Lombardi on the Giants—was the archetypal Raider. "The fans were great fans. They'd not only fill the stadium; they'd stand about 10 deep around the sides, around the bleachers. They were always screaming and hollering. Swarming. I loved playing in that place. It was like playing back in high school again."

If both the team and its new home seemed jerry-rigged, this was all, somehow, the more fitting. From the very start, to be a Raider, landing in this fringe organization, was to immediately take pride in being slightly off-kilter. Lineman Dalva Allen had played on the first two Houston Oilers championship teams before being traded to the city on the wrong side of the Bay. "They said, to be a Raider," Allen told me, "you had to be half a bubble off." As in a carpenter's level. As in being a little bit off-center and unbalanced.

The most famous celebrity spectator at the undertaker's field? A film director, and not just any film director: a director of a world always slightly off-kilter. Alfred Hitchcock sat next to Allen's wife one day. "He invited us to come down and see where he'd just finished filming *The Birds*. And we took him up on it. Went down to Bodega Bay." The director of *Psycho* and the Oakland Raiders: a perfect match.

"To me, Frank Youell Field was bigger than life," said John

Herrera, now a Raider exec, then a teenaged ball boy. "It wasn't a little high school field to me. It was the Raiders' stadium, so it was impressive to me. The fans were always avid. Well, they became that way after Al turned it around. The first year there was kind of rough."

The team went 1–13. Most of the fans didn't care—among them Manny Fernandez, a teenager born in Oakland and raised in nearby San Leandro, and a huge Raider fan. Manny didn't care that the stadium was seemingly uninspired and the team's performance more so. "They hadn't gotten a reputation for being badasses yet," he told me. "All I knew was that we had a team of our own. It wasn't San Francisco we had to go watch anymore. We had our Raiders," albeit playing in a city that Fernandez the adolescent did his best to avoid. "Oakland in the '60s? Like any other war zone. Let's just say that as soon as we got our driver's license, we knew not to get off the freeway between San Leandro and the Bay Bridge unless you were willing to put your life at risk." Or wanted to mingle with the hardest of the hard-core fans.

Fernandez the defensive lineman would lose his love of the black and silver when the Raiders didn't pursue him out of the University of Utah. He signed on with the Dolphins, where he would pick up two Super Bowl rings and pit himself against the Badasses in some of the most memorable games the two teams would ever play.

"If I'd signed with the Raiders, it could have been my demise," laughs Fernandez now. "It was probably a good idea for me to get away from the Raider mystique. I could have been there giving Matuszak lessons on how not to behave.

"But by the '70s they were a bunch of winners who played hard, partied hard, and won a lot. I think most [players] of my era would have liked to play for the Raiders."

Today, other players around the league echo this last point virtually universally. In the '70s *everyone* wanted to be a member of John Madden's troupe. "They were a dynasty, man—everybody wanted to play for them," says Marvin Upshaw, a defensive lineman for the rival Chiefs in the '70s, and the younger brother of Raider immortal Gene. "They were respected throughout the whole league, because those guys were family, and everyone knew it."

"They had a coach who seemed like a great players' coach," says Fernandez now, "and they had an owner who took care of his players."

Well, they eventually would, anyway. First they needed a coach who knew what he was doing. The Raiders had lost 33 of 42 games in their first three years in existence. Then Valley looked to the south, to the staff of the San Diego Chargers, where he plucked the receivers' coach from Sid Gillman's staff and made what is arguably the most important hire in the history of American football.

"Al Davis," says Otis Sistrunk now, "is unique." Most of the time that's an overused and misapplied word. In this case, it's entirely apt.

He took over as coach in 1963. Thirteen years later, as Davis, by then the owner, led his team into the Super Bowl, the Raiders would be 133–46–11 under his reign: the best record in pro football since the day he first roamed the sideline. Between 1965 and 1986, none of Al Davis's teams had a losing record. For two decades, they would plunder the league, driven by the unrelenting will of the most curious, intriguing, and enigmatic figure the game has ever known.

## CHAPTER THREE

# "I Thought We Were *Better* Than the World"

The low-slung, gray, modern-sleek building tucked into an impeccably landscaped industrial park on Alameda, fronted by a man-made lake punctuated by two spouting fountains, could belong to any corporation's headquarters, save the undersize, round sign that adorns the black awning that fronts the place. It is not a corporate emblem announcing a high-tech company within, no modern graphic. The anachronistic Raider logo, the crossed swords and eye-patched pirate, suggests that, despite the slick façade of the place, the heart of the Oakland Raiders should not lie in a modern office park. It should reside a few miles away, on the other side of the estuary that serves as a moat between the island of Alameda and the heart of the city. Or back at the old, vanished Hotel Leamington, site of the team's early offices, or on the second floor above the Badasses' favorite old Oakland drinking haunt, Al's Cactus Room, also long vanished.

But here in Alameda, inside the thick glass doors and across a patch of carpeted silence, the receptionist perches at eye level behind a black, semicircular prow that halts your entrance immediately, so that the pleasantly smiling woman sitting behind her pulpit seems more like a sentinel issuing an existential challenge: You enter? It's all somehow evocative of what Willie Brown told me: "It was the Raiders against the world. That's where we took it." Us against everyone else—that's still what the old players remember, a sentiment they carry to this day. It was a slogan that fueled their fire. Not for nothing did the NFL Network cite the number one feud in the history of the league as "Oakland Raiders Versus the World."

Upstairs, in a huge windowless room free of decorative frill, in the innermost of black-decorated sanctums, the man sits at the end of a long table, wearing a Raider sweatshirt. Very quickly, the modern trappings of his large office seem to vaporize and vanish into another dimension; his presence is timeless. His features have aged, but their distinct angularity endures. This is a face carved onto an ancient coin, serious and imperial. To get a sense of being in the presence of the man, think in terms of a distant time, a distant place. Not ancient Greece, birthing its democracy. No, the context of the Raiders' ruler owes more to the warring Roman empire, which, for much of its time of glory, was dominated by one emperor, one ideology: to be the unquestioned, undeniable, dominant civilization on the planet.

"In order to run an efficient organization," Davis once said, "there has to be a dictator."

His hands beckon for me to take a seat. He does not rise or introduce himself. Of this there is no need. He instructs me to turn off the tape recorder. My time has been pronounced short, for his time is valuable.

So I ask him about that ideology: the Raiders against everyone else.

"I never felt it was us against the world; I thought we were *bet-ter* than the world," Al Davis tells me, his voice soft but his words hard. His eyes turn to meet mine and bore right through me; they are not eyes to be defied, or questioned.

He was born on the Fourth of July, 1929, raised in Brooklyn, the son of a well-off manufacturer of ladies' undergarments: a conservative, cerebral father who demanded intellectual rigor from his sons. Several things distinguished the young and ambitious Al-len Davis from the other kids playing basketball in the park in Crown Heights, football in the streets. Start with his gift of rheto-ric, his verbal dexterity. "Gold used to flow from his mouth," a col-lege friend once told sportswriter Gary Smith, in Smith's seminal profile of the man for *Inside Sports* magazine. His gifts of persua-sion would forever be one of his calling cards.

And he backed it up with toughness, despite, as a kid, his un-impressive physique. He played his sports tough, and he talked tough. "I came off the streets," Davis told me, but this is only truly accurate if you take it as a metaphor. "When your gang met my gang," he said in a 1969 interview, "and I got out in front to fight the other guy, I *had* to win." But this wasn't a dead-end, Sharks-vs.-Jets, survive-or-die kid. He lived in a stable, comfortable, secure middle-class home. He didn't burn to be the leader of a gang. He burned to win, period.

One thing was certain: he was always known for having the backs of his friends. From the beginning of his life, loyalty was everything; this is where the notion of Raider family was engen-dered. "People who knew him loved him," a childhood friend told his biographer Mark Ribowsky, "and he was a guy who'd absolutely go out of his way for his friends."

Davis's fascination with military history—specifically, the

Second World War, its battles, its strategies, its dramatic stakes—presaged his football success. His father's insistence that the boy pay attention to the fronts of battle nurtured a fascination with the war. He mapped army movements, learned to identify the generals and armies in the European theater. He learned of the blitzkrieg tactics of the Third Reich: its relentless attack, no matter what the front, what the terrain. No battle fascinated him as much as the German defeat of the vaunted French Maginot Line, in which the Germans had simply outflanked the supposedly impregnable barrier, outwitting their foes and then punishing them with a quick strike.

Davis's love of sports, distilled to its essence of winner-take-all, mirrored his fascination with war and larger-than-life world leaders. Weekly schedules handed out to Raider players would include the instruction that on Sunday, "we go to war." His passions for warfare and its tactics and his love of football strategy were parallel passions: football as surprise and speed, the latter being the one attribute his teams would always stress—not just down-the-field speed but speed at point of contact. Speed from side to side. Speed to the ball. Al Davis football was impatient football; quickness was all. Outrun and out-hustle and damn what anyone else thinks about conventional strategy. Al Davis was always looking for a way to get it done, and, as a rule, the more visionary, the better.

"The words 'cunning,' 'shrewd,' 'devious' don't have a bad connotation to me," he told Smith in 1981. "Look at the history of people in positions of leadership. They've said of every one of my time that he's devious—from Roosevelt and Churchill to Eisenhower, Kissinger, and Mao."

(It was in that interview that Davis was famously quoted as saying, "I didn't hate Hitler. He captivated me. I knew he had to be stopped. Jesus Christ, he tried to take on the whole world, the cocksucker." Years later, he would say, "I didn't tell [Smith] that.")

✕

"I believe in certain concepts, and I was going to follow them, as long as I wasn't going to hurt anyone else," he told me, choosing his words carefully. " . . . The idea is not to treat others the way you want to be treated but to treat others the way *they* want to be treated." It's a concept that helps to explain the success of the '70s Raiders: treating others the way they want to be treated. That particular compassion would be the glue that would bind the whole thing together, the trait for which his players recognized and rewarded him. He had amended the Golden Rule in a subtle but powerful way: for any relationship to function, you must consider the other guy's point of view. This is not a philosophy one immediately associates with Davis, but when it came to those who worked for him, it was his most memorable credo.

That belief, more than any on-field or draft-room tactic, sums up the most memorable of Al Davis's teams, where anyone, men of all shapes and stripes, many of them exiled from their previous teams, could find a welcoming nest. Davis wasn't trying to mold men into a football team; he was trying to recognize the shape of each of his football players and find a way to fit them all together.

"Al treated people like men," says Bob Moore. "Al didn't care what your color was, what your drinking habits were, probably didn't care about your sexuality. Didn't care about any of that shit. And that was the only team in the NFL like that, where someone wasn't passing judgment on your connections, who you talked to, whether you were gambling, all this kind of nonsense. All that mattered was what you did on Sunday. Remember, this was a football team where guys could show up Thursday at practice drunk and still play on Sunday. As long as you were sober on Sunday, that's all they cared about."

"We had the reputation of getting these castoffs, guys who couldn't make it on other teams," says Gerald Irons, "but who gelled with the Raiders, and ended up really blossoming, and doing terrific things. Other coaches and GMs would be saying, 'This is the same guy I got rid of?'"

For tradees, free agents, and the unofficial off-the-books taxi-squad roster Davis was rumored to have secreted around the Oakland area, there was always something about joining this band that elevated their game, no matter what their spotty heritage. "We had every reprobate in the league," says linebacker Monte Johnson.

Today, Davis refuses to go along with the notion that he had bred a legion of renegades. "Individuality?" Davis says. "Yes. But not rebellion. Not questioning authority." They never questioned *his* authority, anyway, unless they were negotiating a contract.

But lost amid the renegade image is another legacy of the Badasses: the level of the players' collective intelligence, a mirror of Davis's own. Whether it was advanced degrees, double majors, fascination with history or politics, physics or macroeconomics, the Badasses reflected their owner in this way: they seem to present an unusually high profile of thinkers, of men possessed of curiosity about things other than their beloved game, about things that rose above the battle on the turf. What other team featured a linebacking corps who discussed the Big Bang Theory in position meetings?

"You have to be smart to make real quick decisions," says Stabler, as football-savvy as they ever came. "A dummy, someone who lives in indecision, doesn't make a good football player. And Al was very aware of that. He liked the characters, he liked their passion, and he was aware that he could go and take players who had issues off the field and had struggled on the field and bring that player into this atmosphere among all these other guys who were the same way.

"It was like putting gasoline on a match. Boom! You got great, fun football."

Davis's passion for sports wasn't matched by great athletic talent. In high school, at the legendary Gothic palace of Erasmus Hall High School, in Brooklyn, his brand of tough street ball could never break him into the starting lineups. After stints at a small Ohio Lutheran college named Wittenberg, a transfer into Syracuse and another transfer to tiny Hartwick, in upstate New York, Davis settled back in at Syracuse, where he never really played varsity sports but somehow left the impression that he did by getting himself into team photos and wearing the university's athletic sweatshirts, and hanging with the athletes.

Unable to make the actual varsity football roster at Syracuse, he would sit in the stands, watching practice, observing Ben Schwartzwalder's strategies: his first exposure to big-time football tactics. Fascinated by the game, he soaked up the legendary coach's schemes just as he'd mapped the movements of the Allied armies.

At Syracuse another Al Davis trait emerged, at least publicly, that would be made manifest when he took over the Raiders: his insistence that race meant nothing. Black players felt comfortable around him. "I understood the blacks pretty well," said Davis to Gary Smith. This was a man, say those who know him, who held no prejudices. This wasn't just an enlightened attitude; Moore suggests today that the racial balance of the team, the prominence of Gene Upshaw and Willie Brown and Art Shell and George Atkinson as leaders, helped unite Oakland at an historic time, when American inner cities were roiling. Agents of racial and socioeconomic cohesion, Raider players were legendary for routinely mingling and drinking and hanging for hours with the legion of parking-lot fans after their games.

"In Oakland," Moore says, "a lot of lower- and middle-class families were great football fans. The tickets were four or five dollars apiece. After a game, the fans would stay, picnicking, partying, and we'd walk out there, from family to family, group to group: black, white, Asian. It was remarkable for its time. You'd look at the stands, and I'll bet you it was 50–50 black and white families watching a black-and-white football team down there—a team that was 50–50 black and white.

"And that was because of Al. He scouted small black colleges. And Al was the first guy to draft a black quarterback in the first round [Eldridge Dickey, in 1968, out of Tennessee State].

"And then, as a team, after a game, we're all drinking together. It didn't break down black and white. It wasn't blacks in one place and white players the other. We went to the same places, from Big Al's to the 19th Hole, from Clancy's to the Grotto. It's Upshaw, Shell, [Dave] Dalby, Hubbard, all drinking together after a game. That's the way things broke down on this team. I'll bet you didn't see that around the league back then."

Says fullback Pete Banaszak, "On our team, black or white didn't matter: you were part of the family. We all had respect for a guy's dignity, period. We didn't have groups of gangs or movements on the team. We liked each other. If anything ever bothered one of us we talked about it right away, any and all of us. The gyrations, the tension, never existed on our team."

"Your football team can go a long way in helping racial harmony, helping all sorts of harmonies," Stabler says. "A successful football team can take away a lot of frustrations in a city. You have to give credit to Davis for being able to see the type of players, the character, the personality that fit a tough town."

Al Davis had a habit of asking the question of people he'd meet, "What matters most to you: love, power, achievement, glory, or money?" For himself, he had no doubt about which attribute mattered most. "It's power," Davis told Gary Smith. "I don't mean

ruthless power. I mean control of my destiny. [Love] is the least
important of the five to me . . . I only want to be loved by certain
people: my players, the people I live with . . . not by humanity. I
push [love] away because I don't really need it."

But Al Davis didn't want political power, despite his fascination with world affairs. Davis never could have ventured into public
office. Politicians must pretend to embrace all sides. Al Davis saw
only one. "There were two kinds of politics for him," Raymond
Chester told me, "the politics of inclusion and the politics of ex-
clusion. You were the only team. You were part of the team. You
played at a level in terms of your effort that satisfied him, that satisfied all of us, and if that was the case, you were part of the politics
of inclusion."

And once you were included, you knew that the acceptance
went beyond a jersey and a paycheck. You were being judged worthy of joining the man's exclusive brotherhood. You weren't just an
NFL player. You were under the protection of Al Davis.

"I can't imagine ever playing for a different owner, quite
frankly," says Mark van Eeghen, Davis's Super Bowl fullback in
1976, an economics major from Colgate. "Al wanted to win football games. That's all he wanted to do. He was an owner you want
to play for. If you busted your butt and made full measure of effort
to win, he was loyal to you, and you could play for that. You can
play for anybody you can respect. That's how I viewed him."

As we speak, Davis is surveying a copy of his Hall of Fame induction speech for Madden, which lies in front of him on the table.
It is Davis's way of making a single point: any discussion of the
greatness of this team must center on the big man. The historian in
Davis wants to make it eminently clear that in this particular history, one man was responsible.

"This all took place with Madden as head coach," he says to
me, underlining the last four words. For Davis, the Madden numbers that testify to the coach's greatness aren't just the 103 regular-

season victories in ten years, the winning percentage of .763—both better than Lombardi's. They're his record against the other outsize coaching legends.

"John competed in the golden era of great coaches," says Davis. "In his 10 years he coached against many who are enshrined in the Hall of Fame: Shula, Noll, Brown, Tom Landry, George Allen, Weeb Ewbank, Bud Grant, Marv Levy.

"And remember now: this was John's first professional head-coaching job, and he did what we could call the impossible. He won more games than he lost against every Hall of Fame coach. His total record against them was 36–16 and two ties." I do not ask Davis whether he knew this by rote or had to look it up. I suspect the former. Just as impressive to Davis is Madden's Monday-night domination: an astounding 11–1–1.

"Now, no question," Davis concedes, "someone had to get those great players. But someone had to coach them. And you worked together."

And by all accounts, they did. Their shared love of strategy, of the game's nuances—of the power of the unconventional surprise in a game plan—led to a bond that went beyond any other owner-coach relationship.

"My office was right next door to Al's," recalls Al LoCasale, who served as the team's executive assistant from 1969 to 2004, and was hired within weeks of Madden's promotion to head coach. "That first spring, he and John would meet four days a week and spend a couple of hours talking technical stuff. I could hear these conversations through the wall, and it was just amazing, the level of football going back and forth."

When Al Davis makes it clear that my time in his presence has come to an end, it is an abrupt moment. He has very pressing work to do: rebuilding the image of a team that after a lifetime of supremacy has fallen on woeful times of late. Over the last seven years, they've lost nearly three-quarters of their games. *Forbes* magazine has ranked them the least valuable of all 32 teams in the league.

The current Raiders, after a series of uncharacteristically questionable top draft picks, are a far cry from the Badass era, which is forever commemorated in this office. A few feet away from where we sit, over Al Davis's shoulder, propped on a shelf, is a framed poster that features portraits of every member of the 1976 Oakland Raiders, a team that Davis himself places in the top five of all time.

"I've let it slip the last several years," he tells me. "That will tarnish a legacy that was tough to beat. But somehow or other I'll get it back before I'm gone."

So I ask him: Can he sum up those '70s Raiders? He does not hesitate in answering.

"There was no team that other teams feared more," Davis tells me. "No one wanted to play us. That's a sign of greatness . . . and dominance."

I am ushered out of the chamber by an assistant. Out in the parking lot, I take a last glance at the gray fortress. The face of the Raider symbol on the canopy seems to be smiling, a slight, ironic smile, like Al Davis himself, as we said our goodbyes. Somewhere back inside the citadel, he was plotting his next move against the grain.

## CHAPTER FOUR

# Al Davis Ascends

Davis landed his first assistant-coaching job within days of graduating from Syracuse in 1950. Having gotten an interview at Adelphi, on Long Island—after getting the interview, according to Ribowsky's biography, by possibly allowing the school's president to believe he was another Davis from Syracuse: the star running back George Davis—he was hired as a freshman coach. But whether he earned the job through guile or not, it was immediately clear that Davis knew his way around a football field: that first year, he caught the eye of legendary Lou Little, at Columbia. Little was so impressed with Davis's work that after a game between the two schools' freshman squads, he called Adelphi's head coach to ask Davis's name.

Davis's next coaching stint, after two years on Long Island, might not jump off a résumé, but anyone familiar with service football in the early '50s, when sterling squads stocked with college stars were so talented they'd scrimmage NFL teams, understands how serious military ball was, and how seriously the soldiers took their game: the ultimate in paramilitary competition. By combining his knowledge of military minutiae and college personnel—he'd been drafted into the army, assigned to Fort Drum, north of Syracuse—Davis wangled the head coaching job down at Fort Belvoir, in Virginia.

Recruiting from various college rosters across the nation—and wearing an officer's cap, even though he was a private, gifted with his own car and driver—the charismatic Davis commanded two barracks of football players and put together a team that beat national champion Maryland in a scrimmage. His Belvoir team went 8–2–1 and attracted the attention of coaches from the pros, including the Colts' Ewbank, who personally visited Belvoir to see Davis's team play. Just to the north, Ewbank was turning the Baltimore Colts from a doormat into a dominant NFL power. Davis's final act as an army coach was to appear before a House Armed Services subcommittee investigating reports of athletes on bases being given preferential treatment. Al faced the music and gave up none of his superiors. "You know how generals are," Davis told *Look* magazine some years later. "They want to win. This general gave me carte blanche. I also had very good contacts in the Pentagon that could move people. You follow me?"

After his discharge, Davis secured an unofficial scouting position with the Colts, who had signed two of his players. His next stop came at an appropriately named institution for a man who would later come to see himself under siege from the powers of the NFL: at the Citadel, in Charleston, South Carolina, after Ewbank recommended him to rookie coach John Sauer, a former pro.

Davis was hired as a coach and recruiter at the Citadel. His recruiting efforts weren't hindered by the Southern accent he'd picked up along the way: a pure affectation, he would later often admit. The Bulldogs hadn't won a game the year before. In Davis's first year, under Sauer, they went 5–4, their best record in 13 years.

At his next stop, in 1957, under Don Clark at USC, he served on the staff of a team that had been gutted by an NCAA scandal. In 1959, John McKay joined the Trojan staff and the team went 8–2. Al's name was linked to a minor recruiting scandal at USC. "I'm not going to say we were innocent," he would later say, "but everyone in America was doing it." The next year, McKay got the head job. Al was out.

In retrospect, it seems inevitable that the true Rebel with a Cause (right down to the pompadoured James Dean hairstyle) would get his first professional chance in the upstart American Football League. After all, the new league had a franchise right in town—right in USC's home, the storied Los Angeles Coliseum. The team was helmed by the legendary Sid Gillman, himself something of an oddity in football circles: a Jew, unable to gain a coaching foothold in the NFL, given to wearing bow ties and pants pulled up too high at the waist; as a coach, he looked like a geeky professor.

Gillman adored football strategy, preferring the film room to human company. He was a master at the x's and o's. Davis was more of a hands-on guy, already a savvy details coach who would draw the pattern in the dirt, get down on the ground with a receiver or a lineman or a defensive back to explain the minutiae as well as the basics. This Davis and Gillman shared: a love of the offense. Score, and score again.

"I had certain philosophies," Davis once said. "Number one is what I call the vertical game. We were going to stretch the field vertically. When we came out of the huddle we weren't looking for first downs. We didn't want to move the chains; we wanted touchdowns. We wanted the big play, the quick strike. They say to quarterbacks, 'Take what they give you.' That always sounds good to everybody, but I always went the other way: we're going to take what we want." In Al Davis's case, that credo could stand as a life philosophy.

In Los Angeles, Davis joined a staff that also featured Chuck Noll and, under Gillman, helped the Chargers get off the ground in style: relying, as most of the new AFL teams did, on passing for offense, on the air game as entertainment, they put together an eight-game winning streak in their inaugural season, losing in the title game to the Houston Oilers. "Three yards and a cloud of dust" was the other league's mantra. The AFL went to the air, and no team did so more than Gillman's Chargers, who averaged 46 points in the final four games of their first season and won the Western Division title their first two years.

By now, Gillman had struck up an alliance with his assistant. "Al thinks he's the smartest guy in football," Gillman once said. "He isn't. But he's going to be."

The 1962 season saw the fortunes of the Chargers plummet, despite Davis having lured Arkansas star receiver Lance Alworth into the upstart AFL fold after Alworth had been drafted in the first round by the 49ers, who were led by their celebrated quarterback John Brodie. Davis's powers of persuasion were too silken for Alworth to overcome. The 1962 Chargers, now in San Diego, won only four games—two against the woeful Raiders. But up the coast, things were going far worse. Wayne Valley, his club in debt, looked down to Gillman's club for a man who could save the Raiders' fortunes.

"We needed somebody who wanted to win so badly," Valley would later say, "he would do anything. Everywhere I went, people told me what a son of a bitch Al Davis was, so I figured he must be doing something right."

On January 1, 1963, Valley and Ed McGah, the Raiders' two general partners, met with the Charger assistant and allowed George Ross, the *Tribune*'s sports editor, and Scotty Stirling, the team's beat writer, to sit in on the meeting. According to Ross, the two men did not impress Davis. "I'm not running a school to teach owners football," he reportedly told them.

"In the interview, he looked more like a boy than an adult," Ross told me. "But he was very impressive. He was obviously interviewing from strength. He had learned an awful lot at San Diego. He knew enough to be an impressive interview. He was the only person interviewed for the job."

According to Ross, Davis would come to refer to Valley and McGah as "my two dummies." They were impressed by Davis's obvious all-encompassing knowledge of the game, as well as his overarching passion for it. Davis wasn't as impressed with his potential bosses. "At the end of the interview," says Ross, "Davis came over to talk to Scotty and me and observed that the two Raider owners didn't even know how to interview him." Ross stayed in touch with Davis over the next week. "He was questioning whether the Raiders were going to stay in Oakland, whether there'd be a stadium, whether or not the thing was worth taking on. I was eventually able to convince him that not only were the Raiders viable [but] that Valley alone was rich enough to take over the whole obligation if he had to."

Davis was legitimately concerned that this most ragged franchise might fold its tent, playing in a struggling league. So he asked Ross for assurances that both the owners and the local paper were committed to this team.

The brotherhood with the press did not last. As the years passed, the Raiders became a team that didn't ever seem to need the press—not because they were *against* the press but because the press wasn't relevant; they weren't *us*. "He built a fence around us," Tom Flores, his quarterback in the '60s, told me, "so we were all protected from the inside. He didn't let a lot in from the outside."

Wayne Valley wasn't overly fond of Al Davis from the start.

It was soon apparent that Davis wanted to exclude Valley and McGah from the football side of things. Davis's knowledge of the game, his emotional involvement with each contest, dwarfed his employers' engagement with their product. "His relationship with Valley was always a problem," says Ross. "When they hired Davis, Valley assumed that he would be called in to talk about football things, but Davis treated him as a football man would treat a rich owner. He would meet with Valley when he had to, but didn't enjoy it much."

Davis and Valley would never get along. "He's a winner," Valley later said, "but he's the most obnoxious person I've ever met." But Valley once also said, "If I said Al Davis is lovable, I'd be a liar. But you don't have to love Al Davis. You just have to turn him loose." There would never be any love lost between the two. They were cut from entirely different cloths. Over the years, Valley's resentment at Davis's perceived power-grabbing would come to an ugly head when Davis managed to pry the team away from its original owner.

But within days of their initial meeting, Davis had a three-year deal as head coach and general manager. "I have sole and complete control of the operations of this football team," Davis told the press, lest there be any doubt.

He was quick to start remolding the sorry bunch. Less than one month after taking over the team he brought in Art Powell, the New York Jets fleet receiver who had played out his option. He inherited the gifted running back Clem Daniels and began to use him as a downfield receiver out of the backfield. He turned to Flores, the first Hispanic quarterback to ever start a pro game in the United States, to alternate with "Cotton" Davidson. Flores would become his quarterback and receiver coach during the Badass years, then coach Davis's Super Bowl–winning teams in the '80s as the first Hispanic head coach in league history. (Years later, Davis would hire Art Shell as the first black head coach in league history.)

Davis took the rest of the ragtag assembly he'd inherited and effected one of the most remarkable turnarounds in football history. After going 1–13 the year before, the 1963 Raiders won 10 of 14 games. Powell was All-League. "He took some has-beens and made them into a football team," Dalva Allen says now. "What he did that first year was like that old story: a white guy rides a horse until it dies on him. Then an Indian rides it another 10 miles. That's what he did with us. He rode us another 10 miles."

He looked for every competitive edge, from the very start. There wasn't an opposing coach in the league who didn't think Davis was above subterfuge and spying to gain the beloved competitive edge. Madden would write about Chargers head coach Harland Svare talking to the lights in the visiting locker room at the Coliseum: "I know you're up there, Al Davis." Davis supposedly said afterward, "The thing wasn't in the light fixture, I'll tell you that."

The eternal suspicion that Davis watered the coliseum grass before every game? Probably apocryphal. The coliseum field was below sea level, set a few hundred yards from the estuary. It needed no help to stay wet. But it never hurt to have opposing coaches think he'd gone out of his way to tip the scales in his balance.

Davis's love of the downfield strike—"He once told me, 'If I get to the other guy's 40, he better look to his end zone,'" Ross remembers. "'Whether we score or not, we are not playing for 10 yards; we're playing for the ballgame'"—translated into a ridiculously prolific offense. The 1963 Raiders averaged 42 points in their last three games and beat Gillman's Chargers twice. And a formerly docile team grew so aggressive that they led the league in takeaways. The reporters named Davis the coach of the year in the American Football League.

But to many of the players on Davis's first team, the new

coach had already endeared himself in the preseason of that first year, when it was revealed that a 1964 exhibition game slated for Mobile, Alabama, would be played in a segregated stadium. Davis was outraged.

"He called a team meeting and said that the black players wouldn't have to play," Dalva Allen told me. "It came from his heart. I don't know if any other coach would have done it. After Al told the [black] players they didn't need to play, Freddy Williamson was kidding me and Jackie Simpson, saying, 'I'll be up there in the stands with a cold beer, probably have a white girl with me while you get your ass run over.' Jackie and I said, 'We'll do that, then after that game we'll be drinking a cold beer as we watch them hang your black ass.'"

The game was moved to Houston, a more enlightened town, if not team; the original Oilers had only two black players.

In 1964, the team slumped, record-wise, winning just five games. But as far as Clem Daniels was concerned, his coach had a very good year—not on the field but behind the scenes. According to Daniels, Davis was tasked with putting out still another fire involving black and white players—perhaps the last time the Oakland Raiders could be said to have black and white friction. "We nearly had a race riot," says Daniels. "Fred Williamson had told me to meet him at the Miramar club one night, because this Swedish woman he knew was bringing her sister. Al kept the offense late, so by the time I got there, they were gone. So there was this one player—I won't name him—when I got there he was half-drunk and he said something about Williamson and these girls. I was ready to jump him, but Jim Otto held me back."

The next day at practice the black players had gathered at one end of the field and the white players at the other. "Al calls practice over," Daniels recalls, "and calls me into his office. 'What's going on?' he wants to know. I tell him to ask this other guy.

"He says, 'You know I'm Jewish, right? We've been through a whole lot, too.'"

Davis called an immediate team meeting. "'I will not have this bullshit in this organization,'" is how Daniels recalls Davis's words. "'If you're doing shit like this, not only are you off the Raiders; I'll get your ass out of football.'

"And after that, there was never a problem. If any owner will ever protect you, Al Davis will."

Then, six months after the Civil Rights Act had been signed by Lyndon Johnson, Davis stood up for the black players in the league during one of the most remarkable moments of race history in sports. The boycott of the AFL All-Star game in January 1965 has been lost in the mists of not only football history but civil-rights history. At the time, though, the boycott represented a truly revolutionary act. Ask any of the men who participated in this physical manifesto. It was a John Carlos–Tommy Smith moment, years ahead of the Olympians' fist gesture. It was also a statement made by a new league that averaged 40 percent more black players per team than its rival league.

The game had been scheduled for January, 1965, in Tulane Stadium in New Orleans—one of the 13 cities that had approached the AFL about joining the league as an expansion team. But as soon as the 21 black All-Stars began to arrive in New Orleans, it was clear that the town was less than eager to see them.

Clem Daniels caught a flight from Oakland to Los Angeles, with black players from other teams. "We get out of the airport," Daniels told me, "and we see a line of cabs, 15 long. None of them move. Finally someone tells us, 'You'll have to catch one of the colored cabs in the back.' The colored cabs? That's when we figured out something wasn't kosher. So we finally get downtown and check into the hotel. In the elevator, the operator says, 'You're the first coloreds to stay in the hotel.'"

In the hotel restaurant, a woman moved her coat away from

a black player's. In the clubs to which they managed to gain entrance, they were mistreated. Later that night, the players gathered
in the hotel and discussed a boycott. The vote was 18–3 not to
play the game. Daniels, one of the majority, flew home, where he
fielded a call from Davis's secretary: the game had been moved to
Houston. AFL commissioner Foss had sided with the players—
after hearing from an outraged Al Davis. Word of Davis's stance
spread, and not only heightened the respect of his own black
players; it made the team all the more attractive to black players
around the league.

Five days later, the West won the game, 38–14. Cornerback
Willie Brown, of Denver, was named the game's defensive MVP. It
took Bronco head coach Lou Saban two more years to trade Brown
to Davis in Oakland. There, Brown would become, arguably, the
best cornerback in football.

In 1965, Davis's last year as head coach, the team won eight games,
finishing second to Gillman's airborne powerhouse down the coast
in San Diego. Davis's key draft acquisition had been All-American
receiver Fred Biletnikoff, out of Florida State. Pursued by the Lions in the NFL, Davis, ever mindful of theater, of a chance to rub
it into the face of the senior league, got the intense, talented kid's
name on a contract first—and ceremonially staged a mock signing
on national TV, with Biletnikoff performing the honors under the
goalposts after the Gator Bowl.

With Powell, Biletnikoff, and Daniels, Davis lost just five
games. "He built this team," says Tom Flores now, "starting in '63,
in his image. With his philosophy. His style of coaching. Drafting
for speed. He was involved in it all. And the tenor of what he put
in was continued."

But he would not coach again. He was destined for a more

powerful office. Both leagues were hemorrhaging money as they tried to outbid each other for draft picks. With its NBC television contract, and its ability to attract the likes of Joe Namath, the AFL was no longer just a pesky upstart league; it was proving a serious threat to the established NFL. Behind closed doors, a merger was already being discussed between executives from both leagues.

When Joe Foss resigned as AFL commissioner, in January of 1966, Valley decided to nominate his own coach for the AFL commissioner's job. Davis was approved, after some lobbying by his owner, at the league meeting in Houston, on April 28. The league needed a pit bull to take on the established league, and in Davis they had one. He promised that the league would fight for players in dramatic fashion. He envisioned a wholesale raid on the best quarterbacks in the NFL: a shot across the bow.

His brief coaching days were behind him. Had he continued? The late Bill Walsh, who served as the Raiders' running back coach in 1966 and whose 49ers would years later carve their way into football's annals, once said that "he was one of the greatest coaches I have ever observed," that Davis would have been "one of the greatest coaches of all time." His record? 23–16–3. Hardly Hall of Fame stuff. But perhaps men who knew him well for many years better represent the story of Davis as a coach. "If he'd kept coaching," Otis Sistrunk says now, "he'd be one of the top five in the NFL's history."

To a man who knew Al Davis better than anyone in the early years, he was "an exceptional coach—especially in the last two minutes." To Ron Wolf, his right-hand personnel man, it was Davis's relationship to the game he loved that drove him so relentlessly: the brashness, the rebellion, the careful cultivation of the image—all were secondary, says Wolf, to Davis's absolute, white-hot love for the game, and the people who were talented enough to don the uniforms.

"He liked that stuff about being a maverick and all that," Wolf told me, "but deep down it was always about the game and the people who played the game. I'll never forget what he told me once: 'You and I have to be careful. We're both very critical, and we can't be critical, because we weren't good enough to play the game.'"

If he couldn't be good enough to play the game, Davis *could* become the king of understanding it, of dissecting it, of dominating it.

But he'd moved beyond the routine title of coach. To be a head coach was to be part of a club—an elite one, granted, but merely one coach among many. Davis the loner had other mountains to climb. He was never meant to be a member of a boys' fraternity. He had his eyes on a larger stage. "I had made a vow to myself," he told writer Glenn Dickey, as recounted in Dickey's excellent *Just Win, Baby*, "that when I became commissioner I was through with coaching. I hadn't done all the things I wanted to do, like winning a championship, but I'd done enough. I don't care what others think, as long as I satisfy myself."

Ancient kings used to commission epics to celebrate their feats. Equally mindful of his public image, in the first press release issued to announce his appointment as commissioner, Davis asked the publicist composing the piece to include the words "dynamic" and "genius" in the copy. At his first press conference as commissioner, Davis told the assembled press, "I have dictatorial powers." He used those powers to declare an all-out recruiting war on those NFL quarterbacks, a full half dozen of them, including Roman Gabriel, of the Rams, who signed a three-year Oakland contract, to be effective when Gabriel's Rams contract expired. The Oilers soon announced they'd signed the 49ers' Brodie to a future contract. Neither ever played in the AFL, but the threats were real. Davis wanted to play for keeps. Whether Davis's aggressive tactics were the catalyst for the merger that had already been discussed for months is open to question. What isn't questionable is that, under Davis's aggressive watch, he was at the helm when history was made.

Had Valley kicked Davis up, sideways, or down when he convinced his co-owners to anoint his coach as league commissioner? Did he want Davis out of his hair? Or did he think the street-tough Davis would be the ideal man to stand up for the league at a time when its solvency was threatened? Probably both. Only the late Valley could have answered that question. The bottom line was that within a few months of Davis's appointment, the league had a merger agreement.

"We really did knock their ass off," Davis told me, with a small smile at the memory. "We forced the merger. We had won a war."

It was announced, on June 8, 1966, that the leagues would merge—in stages. They would not merge entirely until 1970 and pending Congress's subsequent approval. It was Pete Rozelle, the NFL's smooth-talking commissioner since 1960, who would serve as the combined leagues' commissioner. Davis would later say he didn't want the job. They were diametric opposites: the tanned, personable, PR-savvy Rozelle and the mysterious, driven, private Davis. "I didn't want to be commissioner," Davis told one writer. "No way. It's a desk job." The words ring true. Al Davis would never be happy unless he had at least one foot on the field.

"You don't understand Al Davis if you think he wanted that job, or that jealousy of Pete Rozelle . . . possessed him after that," Stirling, by then the Raiders' PR man, told Mark Ribowsky. "I know this for certain. Revenge and getting even is not in his nature. It doesn't make any fuckin' difference to him, 'cause he has other fish to fry."

In theory, with Rozelle's ascension, Al was now out of the

game. But Valley immediately brought his man back into the Oakland fold. He knew the game, he knew its players, he knew how to win, and he'd brought credibility to the team when it was still in its infancy. He had given Oakland an identity, and in a sport that was now capturing our collective imagination. Despite having no profound affection for the man, Valley convinced each of the Raider limited partners to give up pieces of their own ownership, which allowed Al to buy into the club. His title was managing general partner, and his contract was to last a decade. He would eventually leverage his stake into total ownership of the club.

"He wanted to be an owner," Valley said. "Davis is very image-conscious. He felt being an owner was a step up from being commissioner. Anything else would have been a step down."

The document that sealed the deal stated, "Allen Davis shall have the exclusive authority . . . to direct and manage the [Raiders] . . . and to do all things which he may consider necessary . . . in the best interests of the football team and the partnership."

"How Al ascended," Mark van Eeghen told me, "that's still a dark hole. I don't know how he did it. All I know is that we didn't have an owner who owned 7,000 hamburger shops or something. This man just wanted to win football games."

His new head coach—in the team's inaugural year in the coliseum—was John Rauch, the man Davis had hired as his first assistant coach back in 1963, out of the University of Georgia, where Rauch had been an All-American quarterback. But from the start, Rauch, not without ego, was worried about the shadow of the man over his shoulder, and even offered to step down once Davis's return was announced. Davis would not hear of it.

Off the field, Davis, Rauch, and Ron Wolf set about strengthening the foundation of the later years, In 1967, they brought in football-canny defensive coach Madden from San Diego State to coach the linebackers. Many of the players came from colleges that were far from top-tier, like Banaszak out of Miami in 1966, Gene Upshaw out of Texas A&I in 1967, and Art Shell out of Maryland State in 1968. And if they came from high-profile programs, it was often with an asterisk, like Stabler, who had been briefly suspended from Alabama, a left-hander in a sport whose poobahs believed that a lefty could never win. They were too flaky. They were too out of the box.

But through those three tumultuous and highly successful years, Rauch would never be able to countenance what he perceived as Davis's bigfooting of his operation. ("Dictator Davis does everything but take tickets," wrote Leonard Schechter in his insightful *Look* magazine profile in 1969, "and a coach is almost certain to resent the hot breath on his neck.") In 1968, Rauch's regular-season record was 33–8–0. He'd taken the team to that second AFL-NFL championship game. But Rauch and Davis were oil and water off the field.

On the other hand, in Rauch's first year, when the team didn't yet have its own practice field, the concept of the Raider family began to blossom. Davis's indifference to a player's outsize personality had resulted in a winning assemblage of loose, Badass precursors who bonded on the bus down to their practice field south of the city, in a high school that had been abandoned because it lay on the Hayward Fault. Well, of *course* the Raiders practiced on a fault. The Hayward Fault isn't as famous as the San Andreas, its neighbor. But the Raiders did everything they could to activate it.

"We had all the crazy guys rocking the bus on our way down there," linebacker Gus Otto told me. "We'd be going down the

Nimitz Freeway, and Ben Davidson and Dan Birdwell would be rocking the bus back and forth.

"But I'm telling you, those bus rides were a unifying factor. Taking the bus every day helped everyone get along. It was like the party we had after every game. It was family."

It was in Rauch's final year that the Raiders found themselves in the strangest of spotlights—well, technically outside of it. And, if you believe that the NFL gods had it in for the team and its fans back then, the Heidi Game simply confirmed the suspicion. On November 17, 1968, the Raiders won one of the sport's legendary contests—but virtually no one saw the ending. In retrospect, it's hard not to exploit the Heidi Game as the perfect metaphor for a team destined to make history by forever being involved in the epicenter of controversy, not to mention so many of the sport's most memorable games: a moment of Oakland Raiders triumph denied to those of us on the East Coast.

The rivalry with the Jets had been fierce for years, starting in 1967, when, before a game in New York, Joe Namath had insinuated that the Raiders' rough style of play went over the line, and that they were trying to hurt him. The Jets won that game. But during the rematch later in the year, the Raiders wreaked their revenge on football's prettiest boy. Lineman Ike Lassiter fractured Broadway Joe's cheekbone, but Namath stayed in the game. A few plays later, Namath scrambled out of the pocket and took a late hit from Davidson that tore off Namath's helmet with a sweeping forearm, a sequence immortalized in *Life* magazine on January 12, Namath's helmet flying off as he falls to the ground—a photograph that Davis later had blown up and mounted on a wall in the team offices.

The Heidi Game provided the Raiders' typical high entertainment and eight lead changes. Unfortunately, people watching anywhere but the West Coast saw seven. At exactly 7 p.m., with the Jets leading the Raiders, 32–29, and one minute left in the game, NBC switched over to its scheduled Sunday-night movie. NBC's thinking could hardly be faulted; Sunday night belonged to the nation's children; the time slot was the kids' last little moment of bliss before the school week began. On this night, NBC would be offering an uplifting made-for-TV movie about a Swiss orphan girl. Scored by John Williams, no less.

As *Heidi* time approached, people began to call the network to ask if it was going to drop the game. Network suits had already decided to delay the movie. But they couldn't get through to the man at the board in the studio. The flurry of calls, NBC executive Chet Simmons would later say, "literally blew out the switchboard." What the nation missed was the Raiders scoring twice in the final 42 seconds, and winning 43–32.

The protest that ensued from outraged fans carried a message: 10 years after an overtime game in Yankee Stadium had put the sport on the national map, in the Colts-Giants championship contest of 1958, the game had now sunk its hooks in so deeply that the *Heidi* fiasco made the front page of *The New York Times*, and the evening news on the network that had blown it issued a mea culpa. "Last night, somebody in the vast reaches of the NBC network didn't get the word, as in the Army," said David Brinkley, on *The Huntley-Brinkley Report*. "The result was that football fans, by the thousands, were roused to a cold fury. The fans who missed it could not be consoled."

The outrage confirmed a now-undeniable fact: football had worked its way into the nation's collective psyche. And the Heidi episode was the beginning of a Raider tradition: an instinct for being at the center of controversial and unorthodox games.

Far more heartbreaking to the team and the city was the final game of 1968, the final game of Rauch's career at Oakland, a season in which Rauch had taken the team to a 12–2 record, and yet another game against the Jets. But this time the AFC championship was at stake, contested in the windy bowels of Shea Stadium.

"Biggest game of my life," Jets receiver Don Maynard says now. "Just singing 'The Star-Spangled Banner' cranked me to the hilt. I was cranked up that whole game." This is the receiver whom Al Davis singled out to me as the one player who never got his "national due." When Al Davis, unbidden, decides to celebrate a non-Raider in a casual conversation, you'd best listen.

Halfway through the fourth quarter, an Atkinson interception and a Banaszak run of 4 yards had given the Raiders a 23–20 lead. That they were in the game at all was in large part due to Fred Bi-letnikoff; the sticky-fingered receiver had turned 7 passes into 190 yards. Now the Jets had the ball on their own 42. Maynard turned to Namath in the huddle. "I'd told Joseph earlier in the game, 'Joseph, I got a long one when you need it,'" Maynard recalls. "I could just tell from the way Atkinson was covering me that I could go long. We needed the score, and Joe said in the huddle, 'All right, linemen, y'all be real careful. We're gonna go for it. Nobody hold or nothin'.'"

Maynard beat Atkinson for a memorable 52-yard reception down the right sideline, but the pass was held up by the wind and Maynard's momentum took him out of bounds after his over-the-shoulder catch. But Namath hit Maynard again— his fourth receiver on the read—for a six-yard touchdown. On the ensuing march, as every disciple of Raider history will tell you, the Raiders were poised to go in for the winning score, but Lamonica's pass to the right flat floated over Charlie Smith's head—and, aided by the hometown winds, the ball sailed behind him. It was ruled a lateral. The Jets' Ralph Baker recovered, and the Jets won.

That night, at Namath's nightclub, Bachelors III, Maynard

recalls, "I got the coat check for my wife. One of my teammates looked at it and said, 'Hey: 43. You had his number all day.' 'I'll be,' I said. 'That's Atkinson's number.'" Maynard had Atkinson's number. Literally.

The Jets, of course, would go on to win the famed Super Bowl over the Colts, 16–7, which Namath had guaranteed. Another potential moment of Raider destiny denied by the fates.

According to Dickey's biography of Davis, during the Raiders' championship loss to the Jets, Davis was openly criticizing his coach in the press box, and it was common knowledge that Rauch was looking around for a new job, despite his stellar record with Oakland. That Davis's first coach would up and quit a championship-caliber team speaks worlds about the size and power of Al Davis's aura. It would clearly take a special kind of guy to coach for and coexist with the man. Rauch, not without ego himself, didn't have the psychological makeup to do so.

"Davis is a hard worker, and he'll do anything to win," Rauch said after he'd left the team. "I respect him for that. But here we were preparing for a championship game and a Super Bowl game, and he's got 15 reasons why I'm not a good coach. All he wanted was to run the show himself from behind his desk."

According to Madden, Rauch caught his entire coaching staff by surprise when he quit soon after the championship game loss to take the head job at Buffalo. (Rauch would flounder in upstate New York. His teams won seven games in two years, and then he vanished from the professional scene forever.)

In the next few days, linebacker coach Madden got a call from Chuck Noll, who had just been hired to coach the Steelers, offering Madden the defensive coach's position in Pittsburgh. Madden turned him down. He wanted to throw his hat into the Oakland ring. He'd been working for Davis for two years. He knew the system. More important, he knew the man. He had a sense of the particular kind of personality that was required of a man who was to work for a dictator.

The job John Madden had been aiming for his entire life was beckoning in his own backyard. And he would not be denied it.

**CHAPTER FIVE**

# John Madden: "One of the Guys"

Is it the greatest team ever? My Badass Raiders of the '70s?

"To me, it was," John Madden says, sitting in his office in Pleasanton, California. Madden's hands are jammed into a windbreaker, his legs khakied and askew, hair concealed beneath a baseball cap, feet clad comfortably in topsiders. A man at rest. He is not sitting at his large corporate desk, which is heavily rooted a few feet away. There'd be no room to *splay* behind that desk. Instead, we recline at a nearby table, two guys talking about a football team, no ceremony involved.

"When I went into the Hall of Fame," he tells me, "I had a party and showed old highlight films. I told the players that I'd started believing that thing about how players are bigger, better, faster, stronger now, and the game is better now, but when I look back at how we played it, and the guys who played, I realize that's not true.

"We *were* better," Madden says, his expression still buoyantly, roundly boyish at 73 when the subject at hand is the game he lives for. "Football is great now, but that doesn't means it wasn't great then. The stars then would be stars now. Freddy would be. Stabler would be. Bob Brown would be. Upshaw, Willie Brown, Shell, Otto, Ted Hendricks—they all would be." It's as emphatic as he'll be about his team. In an hour-long conversation, you won't find John Madden indulging in any "look at me," self-aggrandizing nostalgia.

All you need to know about Madden's down-home style is his ride. He'd arrived for the interview driving a white, frill-less Ford pickup, not a beetle-y, carapaced SUV, an Escalade or Porsche Cayenne, or a car with a driver. No custom plates. Just a pickup that speaks nothing of wealth, or distinction. It's a ride you'd never give a second glance to. The parking place he's pulled into doesn't display a sign reading, "Reserved for John Madden." It's just a parking place. He's parked the pickup in slightly askew fashion in the slot and ambled in with a cup of coffee in his hands. Just a guy on his way to work.

Technically, the tan building an hour southeast of Oakland houses the family's property-management company, and a production company with a soundstage that doubles as an amphitheater for Madden's Sunday football fests—nine monitors, including the main screen: 9 by 16 feet. The screens are ringed by dozens of chairs, for friends and family. It is here that Madden still lives football—and, ironically for a man who made a brief impression on the public landscape as an actor for a beer company, he does so without commercials. Madden takes his football watching seriously. It's his custom to rank all eight games he's watching, from best to worst, and to display the number one game at any particular time on the big screen. But if the Big Game goes to commercial, it's immediately replaced by the next-ranked game that's not in commercial. Madden still likes his football straight-up.

"Red Bear Inc.," reads the sign outside the building, the name signifying the alma maters (Harvard and Brown) of his two sons. Their offices flank the west side of the building. But the sign outside ought to read, simply, "The John Madden Building," because the first thing you encounter upon entering the place, through a nondescript door, before you see any people, are displays of ancient football equipment. Leather helmets. Leather shoulder pads. Old cleated shoes. And a couple of professional football's first face masks: metal devices that the players wore over their noses and mouths, with a distinctly medieval feel to them. The equipment that belonged to the first real Badasses.

In a sense, the hallway that leads to his office serves as a football museum. In another sense, it's just Ur-Madden, as if to let a visitor know immediately where the priorities of the major domo lie: an allegiance to a time back when men played the game unencumbered by modern techno-pads, or even regard for their own bodies. He says that the motif is meant to display the evolution of equipment. But there's little modern equipment to be seen, save a scuffed Raider helmet, from the Badass days. The most significant artifact, the one closest to his heart, is not on display. It's out back: the seven-man blocking sled he salvaged from the Raiders' revered old training camp up in the outback of Santa Rosa, the Badass playground.

Unlike Davis's sanctum, Madden's large office is bathed in light: two walls of glass let the sun flood the place. The walls are festooned with photographs—of Raider teams, yes. And of Lombardi. But other photographs hang on these walls, too: an historic nineteenth-century shot of the fabled Dakota building, in New York, where he still has an apartment, and a photo of the Golden Gate Bridge under construction. The one photo of Madden, hanging on the wall behind his desk, is small, with a fine-art sensibility; he's glancing away from the camera in this shot, and you can barely tell it's him. This is an office entirely without ego.

But here's the weirdest thing: the dominant piece of art in the office is not a football photograph or a football plaque. It's a large oil painting that hangs directly behind his desk, of a dark-blue, roiling sea, chaotic wave peaks reaching to the sky. It is a tableau devoid of anything but nature's unbridled might.

"I love the power of the ocean," he tells me. "It's never the same. You can sit in the same spot and watch it, and it'll keep changing."

The same can be said of the game, and his relationship to it. In his half century of coaching and watching football, John Madden has seen the game evolve, change with every season and era, but he himself never has relinquished the power and the glory that the Badass era bestowed upon him, whether on the sideline or in the broadcast booth. But Madden's power is a muted and unostentatious thing. There has always been to the man a self-assuredness—a command of his surroundings. It just happens to be wrapped in a guy who has never displayed signs of superiority: the only figure who ever could have guided and helmed this particular, peculiar, and singular ship.

He was hardly a household name, even in his team's hometown. The day after his hiring, the headline in *The Oakland Tribune* read:

RAIDERS NAME NEW COACH
PACKERS LOSE LOMBARDI

A few days later, the paper saw fit to finally identify him in a headline, but even then there was a suggestion of anonymity: "MADDEN: A Mystery Man."

This second headline had it so wrong and so right at the same time. The right part was that the press knew nothing about him, because no one had shown much interest in him, not with all the other bright lights surrounding the franchise. With an owner like Davis, reporters weren't spending a lot of time writing about a linebacker coach in polyester pants who'd never sought out a moment of publicity in his life.

But he was hardly a mystery. This was as unfiltered and uncomplicated and unmysterious a man as had ever roamed a sideline. This was your dad, your uncle, your brother. The guy you watch a game with, or talk to on the next stool over, after you've ordered the second beer, chomping a cheeseburger, without feeling as if you're intruding. This wasn't a domineering boss, arms folded, surveying the field like the principal in fourth grade. This guy talked with his hands, flailed his arms like an octopus's tentacles, the round face turning various shades of neon pink beneath the blond/red thatch a couple weeks past due for a haircut, by the standards of a real old-school coach. A guy talking to a player with Visigoth facial hair as if he was a comrade, not a legionnaire or a pawn. This was a large fellow with a disheveled feel to him who wore his average-guy-ness for all to see.

"John kind of looked like an oaf when he would dress," linebacker Monte Johnson says. "In practice he would wear the same polyester stretch pants, the shoes not tied, no whistle, a towel hung around the neck. He would chew on the towel, not as a pacifier but as a habit. Because it was there."

And now, in January of 1969, the team that largely belonged to a slight, mysterious Machiavelli was being coached by Al Davis's virtual physical opposite: a 260-pound teddy bear with no sense of "Us Against Them" about him. He was just one of us. When the eye of the camera focused on Madden, he would always seem refreshingly oblivious to our scrutiny, as if he could have been coaching a peewee team. In a profession teeming with men obsessed with their image, he didn't care a whit what we thought he looked like.

To a man—to a *man*—his players insist today that Madden was the perfect coach for this team of free spirits. Those are the exact words many of them use. Not one Raider I talked to spoke of him in any but those terms: that never has there been a better fit between a coach and a football team. Not just because he kept the rules and the strategy simple, and never tried to rein in their lives, but because he also never put himself above them.

"I was glad," says tight end Ted Kwalick now, "to play for a coach that treated you like a man, not like a kid."

To many, it went further than that. "You thought of him as one of the guys," says Willie Brown, echoing the oft-repeated mantra, "not necessarily as one of the coaches."

"I liked them," Madden tells me now, as if this wouldn't be self-evident, a given. "I liked all my players. I made a point of talking to every player every day. I'd walk up and down the locker room and talk to them as they'd come in, going into the training room, because I liked them. They were my friends. They're people. When you start thinking, 'How do you treat them?' you're thinking about it too much. You just do what's normal."

He was not without ego, of course; no one who strides the highwire of head coaching in the NFL can be wired selflessly. But he never let his ego get in the way. Not with his players, not to us fans.

"In the morning," says Pat Toomay, who came over from the Cowboys, "he'd be sitting in your locker with a cup of coffee and the paper: 'Hey, did you see this?' This is a coach interested in your opinion about something in the newspaper? Can you imagine that happening with Landry? In the Cowboy environment, you always felt like a freak or a piece of meat or some objectified kind of exotic hybrid. And here's a coach interested in what you think about something other than football? And what that creates is a bond: 'This is a guy I can play for. This is a guy where our interests are aligned. He cares about people who aren't replaceable parts.'

"There was a huge amount of respect. You could feel it. Madden wasn't going to bullshit us on any level. He'd stand there on the sideline, sort of helplessly, waving his arms, getting pink, but he gave over control, and it was great for the players."

John Madden reflected the team he coached: an obviously emotional fellow with character and compassion and substance and phobias and drive. He made you want to be one of them, didn't he? He made you desperately want *in*.

When Rauch left, Davis initially had his eye on men outside the organization, including Noll, with whom he'd worked on the Chargers. But when Noll took the Steelers job, Davis told his staff during a draft-preparation session that if anyone on the staff wanted to be considered, he'd be willing to listen. During the first break in that meeting, Madden, who was all of 32, walked into Davis's office and told him he was very interested.

A few days later, Madden made his pitch. "I went and told him, 'I know this team, I know these players. I know what they can do and I know how to get them to do it,'" Madden told me. "I said to him, 'Age is a number. If you're made to be a head coach, you'll be successful whether you're 32, 42, or 52. I don't have to wait 10 years. I know I can be a head coach.'

"I had a plan," he says now. "Because I had been thinking about this basically all my coaching life. Even as an assistant I'd thought as a head coach. Not second-guessing; first-guessing."

Davis was intrigued. There was more to his big linebacker coach than the guy who always seemed to be in a buoyant mood, who had a fondness for goofing around when he dropped by the Raider offices at training camp for some arm wrestling with the other coaches or players, or *actually* wrestling. Well, a fondness for any sort of contest at all.

"As the linebacker coach, he was one of the boys," John Herrera says. "He was just a guy. We'd have footraces out in the driveway up at training camp. Between the cars parked outside the rooms and the boundary of the motel, there wasn't any room to run. He'd put his big fat butt in front of me with the first step, and beat me in a 40. We'd mark it off. And he'd always win. He reminds me of it to this day."

At this, Madden laughs, the creases in his face turning upward as if every line and fold wanted only to return to the laughter that created them. "I beat his sorry ass. I stepped in front of him because I beat him."

"But I wasn't surprised when Al made him the head coach," said Herrera. "He had a certain presence about him that stood out from the other assistants. It's hard to describe it in tangible terms, but he had it."

Davis sensed that, somewhere beneath the big guy's jolly lineman persona lay a drive as intense as Davis's, if that was possible. "We were like kids," Davis told me. "We had our dreams. He had a big ego, I had a big ego, but we were smart enough to know we wanted the same thing."

Davis called for another meeting with Madden, and instructed him to tell no one. Madden was intrigued by the secrecy, and Davis sensed that this was the man for the new era. Davis wasn't looking for an authoritarian. He needed someone who understood people, who could relate to players in an age when they were becoming more individually empowered than ever before. The days of cowering before Halas and Paul Brown and Lombardi were gone. It was getting warmer and fuzzier out there, even in pro football.

"Those players needed someone who would lead them but not demean them," Davis told me. "Not drive them. They could win without that. He had a special talent at that. Football was going in a different direction. You couldn't dominate a player."

"And he knew both offensive and defensive football," Davis said. "He also had a feel for the passing game. He was on the staff. He was there." This wasn't just a matter of convenience; it meant that Madden knew the particular mind-set of the family. "And I also liked the idea that he was younger than me."

Davis was taking a huge chance. Madden would be the young-est head coach in professional football when he took over. Davis himself was only 40. The young, revolutionary Badass regime stood out like a neon blink in a game ruled by an older generation.

"I thought that he would be a great coach," Davis told me. "Anyone can see what a player is doing or not doing at the time; it was what you see in the future that matters: Can he coach? Can you develop him? I've seen it in a lot of young coaches. That doesn't mean they'll be successful with me. It's about the relation-ship. It's about keeping me informed. And vice versa. It's like a marriage. Believing in each other. Anyone can get married. But can you make it work?"

And, I ask, how deep was your involvement with making it work with your new prodigy?

"At the beginning, my role was one of direction," Davis says. "And then it became one of assistance."

Throughout the years, it has been suggested that Davis served as the second head coach of the team. But Madden's players never bought into that notion. Did Davis, the former coach, have spe-cific strategic ideas? Of course. Would he give advice to individual players after practice, which, under Madden, he virtually always attended? Obviously.

"I'm down the hall from the greatest football mind in the game," Madden once said. "I'd be a fool not to take advantage of that."

But the idea that Davis ran Madden? No one believes it.

"It was John's personality that drove that team," says Bob Moore. "That Al Davis was directing the team, calling the plays, doing all the stuff and John was just a hatchet man for him? That was absolutely not true."

"I think Al left John and his staff alone," Stabler told me. "I think he let John make the decisions. Davis had a lot to do with the draft, but as far as who plays? It was John."

Today, Madden insists that his players have it right. "Al's whole thing was finding personnel. But it was my team. That was never a question. Those things came up later. People had him calling plays and shit. But in those days players called the plays. I was never a headset coach anyway.

"I had a good situation. I always said that the fewer guys you have between you and the owner, the better. The best job would be Halas or Paul Brown, who coached and owned. The next best thing would be where you have an owner and you're the next guy. And that's what I had. It was a working partnership. . . . He was a team player."

And it was truly a front-office team. The main staff comprised all of nine people: Davis, Madden, Ron Wolf, LoCasale, and five coaches. And the offices they inhabited were intimate. There was no room for overlording, nor any inclination for it. "It wasn't like there was some big executive office—we were on the same floor," Madden says. "I mean, it was small. We were all there together. Al and I shared the same secretary. His office was right next door. There was his office, then a conference room, then my office, and in the office there was communication all the time.

"Hell, he was a friend. We used to have a box at the coliseum during A's games in the off-season, and we'd work during the day, and at night the coaches would leave and Al and I would go to the baseball game, watch three or four innings, talk, and go have dinner. We did a lot of talking at A's games. All football."

Madden smiles. "I don't know anyone like him. He is total football. If you cut him open, that's all that's there."

Pat Toomay puts their relationship in a slightly different perspective: the man in charge at the top, and the man who, ultimately, knew that his owner's expertise and ambition could help him achieve his own goals. "However he negotiated the space with

Al, whatever compromises Madden had to make, he made because it put him in the place he wanted to be. He was no dummy."

And there's no question about where he wanted to be. This Madden made abundantly clear, year in and year out. "At training camp," says Monte Johnson, "when we were all together for the first time, John would give his opening speech, and it was always the same: 'Our goal is to win the Super Bowl.' Not make the play-offs. Win it all."

CHAPTER SIX

# "Be on Time, Pay Attention, and Play Like Hell"

John Madden was raised in Daly City, a few miles south of San Francisco, the sports-loving son of a mechanic who had once given him some very sound advice, the kind of wisdom that most fathers are too dumb, or afraid, to impart: "Don't start working until you have to. Once you do, that's it. Put off working as long as you can."

In a way, he followed his father's advice. Football wasn't work. That doesn't mean he didn't have ambition. He just had the heart to follow his passion. When he came out of Jefferson Union High School, he was considering becoming a lawyer and pursued a pre-law curriculum for a while in college. "I changed that plan when I knew I didn't want to dress up and be in a suit," Madden says. "I knew I'd always be on the outside—and part of the game."

He attended four different colleges. He played on the line at the College of San Mateo, was recruited to and played for Oregon, moved on to a semester at Grays Harbor College, in Aberdeen,

Washington, where an off-the-field job was pure Madden: sweeping out a bar after the nightly poker game in the back. He moved back to California Polytechnic—Cal-Poly, down in San Luis Obispo—where he played both sides of the line; he would always see the game as a lineman, from the inside out.

So why in the world did he leave Oregon? He doesn't answer the question immediately. "I just didn't fit in there," he finally says. "First of all, I lived in a fraternity, and I'm just not a fraternity guy. I didn't like that thing where you're a pledge and some little guy is telling me what to do or he's going to paddle me? I didn't take to that too well." Fraternities take themselves illogically seriously. Madden's life has always been predicated on the opposite notion; declaring yourself to be elite speaks of pompous self-celebration. Madden belonged to the masses.

In 1959, the Eagles drafted Madden in the 21st round, but the rookie guard blew out a knee in a training-camp scrimmage. The subsequent operation on his ligaments put an end to his pro career before it ever began, but there was an upside to the injury. Arriving early each day for treatment on the knee, he was taken under the wing of legendary quarterback Norm Van Brocklin, with whom he'd watch film of upcoming opponents nearly every morning. The seeds of a coaching career had been sown.

He returned to Cal-Poly to earn a master's in education in 1961. Part of his master's program entailed coaching his first team: San Luis Obispo High's spring practices, which led to a coaching gig at Allan Hancock College, in Santa Maria, from 1960 to 1964. Madden began to seek out seminars taught by the best in the business. At one, he listened to Lombardi speak about the power sweep—for eight hours. Madden took notes as copious as you could take about a single play. He was insatiable. Somewhere inside resided a Davis-like drive.

At another seminar, Madden listened to John McKay pay tribute to the inventor of the I-formation, Don Coryell—the man who would come to revolutionize the game as the director of "Air

Coryell" with the Chargers in the '70s and '80s. Rather than seek out McKay after the seminar, Madden approached Coryell, who would hire him at San Diego State in 1964 as his defensive coordinator (and teacher of health education). During Madden's three years at San Diego State, the Aztecs went 26–4.

In retrospect, maybe Lombardi's lecture was the impetus for what would become Madden's most basic coaching axiom: if you keep it simple, and you drill the plays into your players' heads, so that even the least cerebral members of the team know what they're doing, then you're giving yourself a chance to win. The last thing you need, he always believed, is a guy worrying about his assignment, instead of acting on instinct.

"John has a great mind," punter Ray Guy says now, "but very few great minds make great head coaches. John's strength was that he had a way of making it simple. Whatever he was teaching us wasn't complex, something you couldn't understand. We wouldn't alter the game plan for this or that team. It would boil down to when the first ball is kicked, it's me against them. Line up and play."

"Teaching is repetition," Madden told me. "Coaching is the same way. Some of the players couldn't understand why I'd repeat everything. [Dave] Casper, for instance, got it the first time you said it. Hendricks? His IQ was off the charts. But in between there were others whom you had to show film of the play, then diagram it. And someone else who'd have to practice it and walk through it for two or three days."

Madden had three rules for his Raiders, and three rules only: "Be on time, pay attention, and play like hell when I tell you to." Nothing else mattered.

"I always knew that the more rules you have, the easier they are to break," he explained. "And once you break one, you may as well break them all. It's easier to have fewer rules but be a stickler on those rules. Things that aren't important, that have nothing to do with winning or losing, don't have to be a rule."

Like a dress code, for instance. Other teams made a point of spiffing up for the road trips—especially the arch-rival Chiefs. "They'd look like choir boys, all in their red jackets," remembers offensive tackle John Vella. John Matuszak, who would spend a few seasons in Kansas City before finding his home with the Raiders, in 1976, remembered the Kansas City lockstep conformity even more lyrically in his own autobiography: "Forty-nine large men wearing [red] sports coats offended my sensibility. . . . We looked ridiculous. We were the Killer Beets."

But under Madden, matters of sartorial decorum and conventional grooming pretty much flew out the window. Madden put no restrictions on his players' appearance; he considered them irrelevant. The Raider dress code was nonexistent. "I remember one time before a trip," recalls Vella, "Madden goes, 'Hey, guys, there's a few too many holes in the Levi's. Can we get the Levi's cleaned up a little bit? And, you know, I don't know about the sandals. Maybe you should wear some shoes. Can you wear some shoes?' That was the end of the speech about dress codes."

"I was coaching at a time when you had to wear white shirts and ties," Madden told me. "Well, you *don't* have to wear white shirts and ties. Facial hair? That has nothing to do with winning or losing. Those things weren't important to me. I didn't give a damn. Some teams were making their decisions based on stuff like that. 'I got to get rid of that guy because he has a mustache'? I always thought that was dumb."

How could you not love a coach who let his players express themselves as individuals? Who saw the idiocy in thinking that conformity could instill pride or encourage camaraderie? That very freedom off the field bound the Badasses.

"Any rule or regulation on the Raiders had to do with nothing but winning," says Mark van Eeghen. "Otherwise it was not a regulation."

Madden engendered an elemental way of thinking. He may have considered his players as men, and instructed them to treat their vocation as a job, but he taught the Raiders as he would have taught children. As highly intelligent as his Raiders were, we're still talking about a bunch of guys playing a kids' game. "As a coach," Madden once wrote, "the class that helped me most was child psychology"—which, of course, made him an ideal candidate for his future position. Of course, it wasn't just the Raiders who were more childlike than the pro football fraternity at large; they'd just act more playful than their peers on other teams, because Madden saw no reason to suppress their impulses to have a little fun.

Think about it: Ted Hendricks didn't ride a horse onto the practice field as a Colt or a Packer. Willie Brown didn't take his defensive backfield on a rock hunt during practice in the hills behind the training-camp fields as a Denver Bronco. Villapiano didn't hire any streakers to interrupt practice as a Buffalo Bill. Toomay didn't marry off a couple denizens of one of the Raiders' favorite training-camp bars as a Dallas Cowboy.

"On the field," says Stabler, "it was 'Go play.' Off the field, 'Go play.'"

The coach's acceptance of his merry pranksters is a subject that Madden is more than willing to address, even if he insists today that the lore of his team as a legion of outlaws has outstripped the reality. "The thing is," he told me, "you have a person, and he's made up of a total package. And you take all of the package. You don't just cherry-pick what you get. I remember one day I was walking off the field, and I was talking to our team doctor. I said, 'You know, we have doctors for everything now. Orthopedics, internal doctors, eye doctors, maybe we ought to get, like, a psychiatrist, a mind psychologist.'

"I'll never forget what he told me: 'You can do that, but you don't know what really makes a guy the person he is, and what trait it is that makes him a great player. You may remove that trait in bringing in psychology. And if you start messing with them, you may improve part of them, but the part that's improved might make them not play as well as they play.'

"I said, 'Oh, shit, forget I said that. There's no damned way I want to do it.'"

He pauses for a split second and then all of a sudden the crinkly, oval face animates. As if he's channeling himself, in some kind of personal séance. Now I have him back in the day.

"Did this guy do this or that?" Madden shrugs. "He was mine. That was the whole package. It was all acceptable. . . . You're not going to change them. You have to accept the whole person and whatever they're going to do. If I give Marv Hubbard a card that says, 'If you ever get in a fight again, I'm gonna cut you,' what's that going to do? Or if I tell someone, 'If you ever take another drink in a bar . . . ,' what am I gonna do?"

He answers his own question: "I'm not gonna do anything."

The old saying about giving someone enough rope to hang themselves? Madden gave them enough rope to *be* themselves. Lineman Mike McCoy recalls his first pregame meeting with the team, when he was stunned to see four or five players get up and walk out of the room to get a cab to the stadium—in the middle of a Madden chalkboard talk. "He doesn't even mind," McCoy says. "He knows they know what they need to know. And I don't think that's something you can teach or coach; I think it was just something he sensed. Basically, he was a laid-back coach, which was just right for this team. If he'd pushed and pushed and pushed, I don't think the Raiders would have won."

Of course, to be a good teacher you have to be intelligent, and none of his players doubted the breadth of his brainpower. He may have projected a goofy, everyman aura, but there was no question that the man possessed a knowledge of every aspect—technical, emotional—of the game. "Our nickname for him was 'Fox,' because he was so smart," says Stabler—when they weren't calling him by the other, more affectionate nickname: "Pinky." Madden wasn't particularly fond of "Pinky," as George Buehler, the right guard, discovered one day in 1972. Madden knew that Buehler, despite his Stanford pedigree, had trouble with names. One day Madden was goofing with the big man.

"He asks me, 'Do you know who Cliff Branch plays for?'" Buehler recalls. "This was Branch's first year. I say, 'He's with us. Is he a fullback?' Madden chuckles, and he says, 'How long did it take you to learn my name?' And I blurted out, 'You mean "Pinky"?'

"Madden's face fell. The smile vanishes. I can't believe it came out of my mouth. John being Irish, a redhead—obviously, when he got excited his face would flush and he'd turn pink. After about two seconds of twisting his face around, he said, 'Well, that'll end that conversation.' Then I said something about the weather and we went on from there."

The Badasses may have played like badasses, and partied like badasses, but none of them ever showed up on a police blotter (Moore was never booked). For all of the carousing, for all of the attitude, for all of their lives well lived, you never heard of a Badass on the evening news. The players chalk this up to Madden's appreciation of them as men who had the ability to draw their own boundaries, and didn't need a man with a metaphoric whip—or a phony Gipper speech—driving them on. They knew he had their backs. And they knew he hated phoniness, especially in his pregame speeches.

"It wasn't a lot of 'Rah, rah,'" Stabler says. "It was 'This is what we have to do,' as opposed to 'Go kick their ass.'"

This is not to suggest that the Madden practice or game-day demeanor was laid-back. This man could lose it. This was a dad with a temper. But even the eruptions were often practiced; a motivation drove the madness. Says Stabler, "I saw him come into dozens of meetings where he'd turn over a chair, raise hell, walk out, come back in, and wink. Like it was no big deal. That was his style."

Often Madden's eruptions were just a mind game, especially during practice. He even admitted this to Buehler one day, to the big guard's astonishment. On a special-teams day, Buehler was sitting on the sidelines, watching kickoffs, when Madden walked over to him and said, "I'll bet you that within five minutes I'll blow my top." "I said, 'You plan that stuff?' He said, 'Oh, yeah. I don't do anything haphazardly or emotionally. I take a critical look, and I see whether the team needs praising or being yelled at.' He says if he knows they need to be yelled at, 'I watch all the bad stuff. And I ignore all the good, until I naturally blow up.'

"Less than five minutes later, sure enough, Madden was screaming: 'Goddamnit! Get your asses . . .' And everybody straightens up. That's the way he coached."

The explosions came frequently, and democratically. "It didn't matter if you were heralded or you were an unknown," says van Eeghen. "He was a master of that. He knew everyone's hot spot. Knowing that everybody has to be treated equally, but maybe not all the time."

Van Eeghen vividly recalls learning his own lesson. Two days after he had tripped and missed a crucial block in a game against the Broncos, and watched from the ground as Randy Gradishar tackled Clarence Davis behind the line, the film review session was brutal. "Madden clicks [the play] over and over and over and over. Fucking 30 times. Then he gets up, rips the reel off the projector, throws it in the trash can, and says, 'Get out on the field.'"

Van Eeghen followed his teammates out of the room, tail between his legs—only to have Madden catch up with him on his way to practice. "Mark, I got to let you know—that was one of the better games you had for me, and I thank you for your effort," Madden said. "I took advantage of you because I wanted to make a point to the team and I knew you wouldn't take it personally."

Today, Madden will concede that some of his outbursts were less than spontaneous. "But whether it was premeditated or not, it would go away quickly," he told me. "Sometimes you'd raise your voice, and then it would just go away, and I'd just say, 'I had to do that.' Sometimes you felt you had to yell and scream. I tried not to do it to a player. I tried to do it collectively. There were some guys it didn't affect—they'd say, 'That's just Madden being Madden.'"

He knew when to loosen things up, too. Nose tackle Dave Rowe recalls the day a fight broke out in practice on a goal-line play, and Madden ran down to break it up. "They're having this punch-up, and he's going in between them and he slips. Everyone sees him fall, and the fight stops, and they all help him up. Then he says, 'We ain't having fighting.'"

Rowe figured that Madden would call practice over then and there. Instead, he lightened the mood. "That was a damn sissy fight!" he said. "I'll show you how to fight!" Madden started swinging his fists, comically. "And that defuses the whole situation. And we go back to practice."

Despite the well-measured eruptions, Madden practices were not known for their intensity. Players who arrived fresh from other teams couldn't believe the mellow tempo of Raider workouts. (Bill Walsh wouldn't allow anyone on a practice field to even sit down, under any circumstances; Madden let his players perch on their helmets whenever they wanted to. And they often did. Their helmets were the Badass bench.)

McCoy, who came over from Bart Starr's Packers, recalls his

incredulity at the relaxed atmosphere of practice. "I thought to myself, 'This is incredible. This is the way it should be.' He didn't want you to leave it on the field, so practices weren't what I was used to."

What McCoy was used to was hitting as hard as you could, every practice. What he was delighted to discover was that Raider practices had their own measured pace. One day, McCoy laid a hard hit on Pete Banaszak and was stunned to hear the running back say, "Cool it down a little. This is offense day. Today the offense wins. Tomorrow the defense wins." Meanwhile, McCoy feels Jack Tatum's hand on his back, signaling the same sentiment: Cool out, guy. Save it for the game.

To McCoy, the laid-back workouts directly contributed to the Raiders' legendary ability to come back and win in the latter stages of a game. "They always had the fourth quarter. And that's because they were rested."

Perhaps it's fitting to leave it to George Atkinson, of whom Madden was particularly fond, to sum up the man: "You had to take your hat off to Madden as far as keeping everything from going haywire bonkers, you know? He kept us aware of what our mission was. In order to keep all of us organized and running smoothly, it took a hell of a guy."

## CHAPTER SEVEN

# Summer Camp

The El Rancho Tropicana Hotel. It sounds like the fall-back plan on a family vacation, the resort of last resort, or a likely place to find a talking corpse in a David Lynch film. It most definitely doesn't sound like a professional football team's training quarters. But there it was—the Raiders' long-vanished shrine to summer madness, 60 miles north of Oakland. The team's arrival in 1963 represented a typical Raider out-of-the-box move. Everyone else trained on college campuses. Davis chose to inhabit a grade-C tourist motel. El Rancho exists today only in lovingly tended Badass memories.

The site of the old motel now hosts a line of Costco gas pumps. Across a hundred yards of parking spaces, where the practice fields once lay, now sprawls the Santa Rosa Marketplace mall: Office Depot, Best Buy, Target, Old Navy, Trader Joe's. The only archaeological vestige of a prior civilization is the Villa Trailer Park, directly across from the mall, announcing itself with distinctly '50s lettering on the sign.

You'd think there'd be an historic marker somewhere in the vicinity or, at the very least, a plaque. "There's definitely some ghosts around there," Fred Biletnikoff observes. "The grounds seeped beer."

"Of *course* we stayed at the El Rancho," says Dave Rowe. "Nobody stays at something like that. Football teams stay in dormitories. We stayed at the El Rancho."

The El Rancho complex actually consisted of several buildings: a normal motel, where visitors to the town stayed; an office building with a restaurant; and a square one-story motel annex that stood alone, out in the back, with a courtyard in the middle: "the Zoo," which housed the Raiders and the Raider offices. "They wouldn't let the other people near us," Pete Banaszak recalls with a certain amount of pride.

The tourist building boasted a pool. The motel owners discouraged the Raiders from using that pool, but with little success; you never knew what scantily clad women you might meet there. "One of the reporters stayed over there," remembers one player, who requested anonymity in exchange for the recollection. "I remember him leaving his room, and he didn't shut his door. That was a convenient room to use one time, after I met a lady at the pool."

Today the vineyards have made Santa Rosa and Sonoma County into a destination. The highways into town are flanked by perfect, undulating rows of grapevines, the leaves twittering in the breeze dotted by billboards advertising casinos (and, with half a shout-out to the old days, a number to call to obtain medical marijuana). Santa Rosa has become a town of sushi and Supercuts, bars with names like the Russian River Brewing Company, a place where you can get good Ethiopian food, a town so perfectly nouveau Californian that the prevalent downtown sound is the endless, high-pitched ping of the pedestrian crosswalk lights, counting down the seconds until you're allowed to cross the street.

No one disobeys the crossing signs. There's not a trace of anarchy to be found anywhere. Not a note of country or rock blaring from a Raider car radio. But back then there was hardly any traffic, and no need to monitor pedestrians, only to warn them to look both ways on nights when the Raiders were speeding through town to make the 11 o'clock curfew, or leaving El Rancho again after a cursory bed check. Or returning quietly, sufficiently lubricated in the much later way-after-curfew hours.

Back then, Santa Rosa was a country town, and for several dozen men enduring a full two-month training camp through July and August, pinot noir was not the beverage of choice.

"You were in the middle of frickin' nowhere," says the *Chronicle*'s Betty Cuniberti, who spent time in El Rancho. "You would no more go to Santa Rosa back then for a leisurely weekend than the corn country of Kansas. This was a redneck town. There was nothing going on."

But it was the perfect frontier town for the perfect outlaw team. "When we started going up there the people of Santa Rosa just embraced having a pro team," says Herrera, who helped find the sanctuary for Davis, miles from any scrutiny, behind which he could build his practice fields. "It wasn't just any team, of course. It was the Raiders—a character-driven team whose characters on the team got out into the community on a regular basis. These guys couldn't wait to get out. Every single night. What town is not going to embrace that?"

And what cluster of taverns, bars, and restaurants isn't going to embrace the summer circus that gave Santa Rosa an identity? For eight weeks every year, the little country town took on a whole new vibe. And a little extra income.

"There was no recession in Santa Rosa during Raider training camp," says Banaszak, the veteran fullback who enjoyed much of the after-hours revelry for a dozen years. "The owners of the establishments were overjoyed when the Raiders were in town. We were single-handedly boosting their economy. The hookers rejoiced.

"We'd show up two days *early*," Banaszak says. "We *loved* training camp."

Today, training camp tediously taxes players in the NFL, the low point of their year, an exercise in monotony. So what band of loons would want to leave home *early* for two-a-days in a sleepy, inland country town where the temperatures could reach 115 degrees at noon? Grown men who'd never grown up, who were eager to get back to summer camp—with its many annual rituals, from the tavern tournaments to the remote-controlled toys, from the annual late-August parade of cars and pickups on Rookie Night to Pass the Pitcher Night. Eager for a two-month vacation with the family, playing a game they loved by day, playing games by night. That's who.

"It was just kids having fun and life being good," says Stabler. "We couldn't wait to get to training camp, to get away from wives and girlfriends, play some football, have a few drinks at night. And do that for eight weeks."

Yes, the daily schedule involved football. The two-a-days in Santa Rosa were the hardest practices they'd endure during the season. The players are convinced that many of their fourth-quarter comebacks were due not only to relaxed regular-season workouts but to the two-a-days in the Santa Rosa heat, which shed the offseason poundage and prepared their legs for the season to come. "Madden worked the piss out of us in training camp," Banaszak says. "These guys today go out in their underwear and baseball caps and sunglasses and don't put pads on. We practiced twice a day in pads."

Speaking of underwear, some of the storied libidinal craziness at the El Rancho, according to Stabler's own book, took place in the quarters that he shared with Biletnikoff, Banaszak, defensive end

Tony Cline, and linebacker Dan Conners: suite 147, with Stabler and Cline in one room, the other three in a second. "The collecting of female undergarments," Stabler wrote, "became an annual rite of training camp for many of the Raiders . . . I liked to tack my collection up on the walls."

Today Stabler refuses to reaffirm the tale. Players avoid questions about panties. A few players do recall collections pinned to the wall of suite 147, but Stabler deflects queries about his own tale of collecting such artifacts, a thrice-divorced bachelor no longer eager to surf the craziness of the past.

"Hey," says Banaszak, by way of explaining his teammates' unwillingness to fork over the details. "Some of these guys got grandkids now." But "Rooster" can't forget a particular pair, draped on a lampshade: "Mesh."

But even the two-a-days were not often without some sort of diversion. Like the day Ted Hendricks set up the Cinzano umbrella on the Santa Rosa practice field, so that the post-workout refreshment could be served up in high style. "I borrowed it from one of the Italian restaurants in Santa Rosa," Hendricks recalls now. "I put it out there for the afternoon practice, right in the middle of the field. With a table and two chairs." He enlisted another player to serve as waiter, with a towel draped over his arm.

But that one paled compared to Hendricks's most storied stunt. For a break in routine, the team was practicing a few miles to the south at Sonoma State's modest football field—an idyllic, secluded natural bowl, flavored by the soft northern Californian summer air, bordered on one side by a low, grassy hill and on the other by a stand of tall, fragrant eucalyptus trees, which on this morning looked down upon a cluster of men in football uniforms, stretching at the start of the afternoon session.

Madden gathered the players together to begin the practice. "Where's Hendricks?" he asked.

He was answered by a man in a Raider uniform and pads emerging from behind one of the end zones perched astride a large roan horse and wearing a black German army helmet embellished with the Raider logo on each temple. Expertly, Hendricks galloped the horse onto the field, dismounted at the 50, and announced himself ready for practice. "Instead of having a long spear," Monte Johnson remembers, "he had an orange traffic cone on his hand."

Madden was entirely nonplussed. "On another team," says van Eeghen, "you start a practice like that, and someone's gonna be fined, demoted, or sent home. But it had nothing to do with lack of respect. He was on time, he practiced hard. He didn't violate anything. John loved that. You can't script stuff like that. That's what our team was about."

"It really just happened by chance," Hendricks says now, playing it all down, unsuccessfully. "A friend's daughter was taking her horse out to ride nearby. So I asked if I could borrow the horse for about 15 minutes. Madden had everyone gathered together. That's when I rode out onto the field. I galloped him up to the 50, jumped off, and said I was ready. It didn't faze the team. Or Madden."

"That's nice, Ted," Madden said. "Now get rid of the horse."

As far as his teammates were concerned, Hendricks was not to be outdone. He soon had his copycats. Team legend has long held that Hendricks enlisted the streaker who enlivened another particular practice, but this was a Villapiano production. "I thought I'd send a treat in for the boys," Villapiano recalls. "I got a girl from one of the clubs and gave her fifty bucks. She put on white sneakers and white socks. And nothing else." To earn her fee, Villapiano had instructed her to run around the two practice fields.

"They always kept the fence around us closed because they didn't want people watching," Monte Johnson remembers. "All of a sudden the gate opens just a crack. And here she comes. And she is buck naked. She was a pretty girl. She was a very appropriately built young woman. And she starts running the entire length of the field. She then turns around and starts to run on the other field, and she gets winded . . . she can't run. She has to start walking, she's lost her breath.

"Madden doesn't know if he should be mad or he should laugh."

Was she really pretty? Says John Vella, "I don't know if I was looking at her face."

Football notwithstanding, the days' revelry didn't start until much of the team—and always the offensive linemen—hit the Bamboo Room within a few minutes of the end of afternoon practice. They would shed shoulder pads, helmets, and jerseys and file into the otherwise inconspicuous little tavern, with its typical red roadside-bar sign spelling out its name in white neon. And order up their pitchers.

About a fifteen-yard slant from the team's tiny locker room, the Bamboo has now been replaced by a veterinary hospital, which somehow seems fitting: animals are still being serviced on the spot. The Bamboo was nothing less than a shrine, a temple beckoning brightly. "One pitcher and you'd be shit-faced," says Banaszak. "At five we shower, five-thirty we're in the Room slompin' 'em down. Then we walk over to the Rancho for dinner. One night Pops [Jim Otto] is stumbling, bouncing off the wall. 'Rooster,' he says, 'it was too much, too soon.'"

When Davis asked Herrera to find the team their secluded camp back in 1963, he hadn't instructed Herrera to make sure there was a bar next door, but it turned out to be a brilliantly Badass move. The college dormitories where other teams trained that didn't feature taverns within a stone's throw of the locker room lacked a distinctly intimate rec room where a player could further bond with his teammates. Only a Raider training complex could feature a Bamboo Room.

"We'd have those two-a-day practices," Duane Benson recalls, "and after those, in the heat, after a beer and a half you were so shit-faced you couldn't make English a language. You'd suck them down, because it was a pretty cheap high. Pitchers of beer was the stable offering. Everyone was into volume. I don't remember anyone drinking out of a bottle."

Vella's earliest memory of the Bamboo was also one of his sweetest, back in 1972. "I gotta take you guys for a beer," Otto told Vella and Dave Dalby, rookies who had no idea if they'd crack the roster. "You're way too tight out on the practice field. Lighten up." It was in the Bamboo Room where Otto let Vella and Dalby know they'd made the team. Well, of *course* Badass personnel decisions were confirmed in a bar.

It didn't take the big-hearted Dalby long to make the Bamboo his second home, with his confreres. Dalby, the unofficial director of a summer-evening social schedule that included tavern tournaments of all shape and stripe, took his role pretty seriously. "Double-D had one of those hats that Fred Flintstone used to wear at the lodge, furry with horns on it, like a buffalo head," remembers quarterback David Humm. "He'd always wear that hat in the Bamboo Room.

"The rest of us just had orange baseball hats with 'Bamboo Room' on them. We were over there so much, we finally got a hammer and nails and we hung the Bamboo hats on the inside of the wall that surrounded the practice field. So after practice, we'd pick up our hat on the way out." Thus did the orange Bamboo hat become their second helmet.

They called their Bamboo bartender "our Queen." When the

Queen announced that she was going to marry one of the Room's denizens, the Raiders held a wedding at the bar. Toomay performed the ceremony for a fee of a hundred dollars: "The Reverend Tombstone," says Banaszak, "from the Church of the Holy C-note."

Villapiano was the ringbearer. "She comes in a white dress. The guy she married was in a cowboy hat and boots. She thought it was legit. It wasn't, of course. We all chipped in and got them a week in Lake Tahoe, and a police escort on the way out of town."

And why, pray tell, was she the Queen? "Anyone who served us pitchers," Foo says, "and was nice to us—she was a queen."

According to Benson, it was at the Bamboo that Villapiano got the nickname "Foo." (Foo's other nickname was "Ginzo," a vague reference to his Italian origins.) Benson was trying to say "Phil" but, due to copious amounts of liquid refreshment, the syllable came out slightly askew: "Foo."

They all had nicknames. King Arthur. Foo. Snake. Rooster. Boomer. Piggy. The Governor. The Hit Man. Fog. Scrap Iron. Matzoh Ball. Assassin. Tooz. Zhivago. Stump. Dr. Death. Ghost. Kick 'Em. Chicken Skin. Buckethead. Jethro. Augie Joe. And, of course, Pinky.

Pitchers at the Bamboo, though, served as only the opening act for the Badasses' evenings out, which took place in two unofficial acts: pre- and post-curfew forays. The two hours between the end of evening meetings and curfew didn't furnish enough time to sample the myriad delights of the country town, with all of its various attractions, its tonics promising to loosen up the dings and bruises.

The first (tolerated, if not necessarily sanctioned) chapter of a routine evening would begin with the rumbling of the engines in the U-shaped back driveway of El Rancho as soon as the evening meetings let out. "Getting out after the meetings was kind of Le-Mans style," says Humm.

The Raider game plans were notoriously simple, anyway. The sonorous drudgery of the endless summer evening meetings (especially following a lengthy post-practice refueling at the Bamboo Room) only served to whet the Badass appetite for the second act of the nighttime escapades. And as soon as the meetings ended, the players were invariably eager to make the most of their freedom.

"We'd hit five bars in two hours," says Banaszak of his brethren in suite 147. "The Bamboo Room, the Music Box, Melendy's, the Hilltopper, and the Hofbrau. The Music Box was a strip-mall tavern. Melendy's featured a long bar with a jukebox and booths. We'd roll dice. Whoever lost the dice game bought the first round."

"Melendy's was out on the highway," Benson says. "It didn't have much local color. Local people didn't go there. You'd get the riffraff coming through." Exactly. "We'd accuse Snake," says Banaszak, "of studying his playbook by the light of the jukebox at the Music Box"—although Stabler by his own admission seldom, if ever, studied a playbook.

"We couldn't wait to get out of meetings, do the circuit. There was always a game plan to the madness," Stabler says of their night crawls. "We had all the stops worked out, the same music stations on the radio. We ran in cliques like a pack of dogs, like a pack of wolves."

The first chapter of the evening revelry would end with the traditional sound of cars screeching back into the El Rancho parking lot to beat the 11 o'clock curfew. None of the coaches needed clocks. The traffic jam told them all they needed to know.

"I'd come in there every night, and there was a long, long driveway to the back," says Banaszak. "I'd peel off down that driveway, squealing the tires, at about 50 miles an hour, at five 'til 11. That was my way of letting the coaches know I was there. They'd hear the tires and say, 'OK, Banaszak's in, we don't have to check his room.'"

One evening, Banaszak was a little overzealous upon his return and scraped Stabler's Corvette in his haste to beat the clock. "I go in the room and I see Snake sleeping. I bang him on the shoulder: 'Hey, I kind of hit your car coming in. It didn't look too bad. Rub it out with Turtle Wax.' He got up real early and I'd torn the fender off. Next morning he's banging on my door raising all kinds of hell."

That's when there *was* a Stabler car. One morning the Snake discovered that his wheels were missing. He accused Banaszak of hiding his ride. "'No,' I said, 'I didn't fuck with your car.' They'd repossessed it." (Despite being one of the highest-paid players on the team, Ken was always a little nonchalant about his money.) "He gets on the phone. He says, 'You motherfuckers, you cocksuckers, you come up here and take my goddamn car? People are out there robbing people and you're repo-ing cars?'" Other teams' quarterbacks might be out polishing their cars. Only on the Raiders would the team leader have to buy back his own car.

Of course, not every stop on the circuit suited every personality. "I didn't hang at Melendy's," receiver Cliff Branch protests. "I didn't go to the Bamboo Room, because I wasn't much of a beer drinker. I'd be at the Music Box, where the girly-girls were. We're talking '70s, remember. Good dancing music and girly-girls."

When Stabler and Banaszak were on the town, simply being Raiders out on the circuit wasn't Badass enough. The two old buddies had to take their recreation a step further. When they hit the circuit, they liked to leave their old identities behind and adopt alter egos. "We wanted to be something different than a football player," says Banaszak. "I always liked to tell people in the bars, 'I'm a doctor. I went to Harvard.' 'Really?' they'd say. 'Well,' I'd say, 'Miami is the Harvard of the South.' Kenny was always a crop-duster from Alabama. If we woke up with a hangover, it'd be 'I've got a low ceiling.'"

They'd play their roles right to the hilt. "They'd never crack a smile," says Benson. "They could keep that deadpan look, and in the places we'd hang out, by and large they could pull it off. The deal, the unwritten rule, was that you couldn't break up their act."

Being a fullback on a dominant professional team wasn't glory enough? "I have no idea why," Rooster told me. "Maybe it was a frustrated dream of mine. So I'd just say, 'I'm here on a doctor's convention.'"

Stabler had a particular fondness for cropdusters because one of his dad's best friends flew one of the little planes. Stabler's alter ego involved piloting a biplane. "Kind of like driving a race car. You're wearing the little leather helmet. I admired those guys. They were characters, diving down through the pecan trees and under the power lines." Or, in Stabler's case, fantasizing on a barroom stool, bathed in the light of the jukebox. Getting off the ground—only just in his head.

Getting back on time, before 11 o'clock curfew, was considered semi-imperative: a fine of several hundred dollars on a $20,000 salary represented a gouge of considerable scratch. The night Stabler, Biletnikoff, Banaszak, and Cline blew a tire two miles from camp resulted in fines all around. They were a half hour late. As Stabler later told it, Banaszak was too drunk to change the flat. "I think I walked home that night," Rooster recalls now, a little vaguely.

Round two of the evening's festivity began as soon as a coach tasked with bed check verified that the players were back in their rooms—at which point the more adventurous, risk-taking members of the pack of wolves would venture back out again.

"The rooms at the El Rancho opened onto a courtyard, but they also had a door on the backside, right on the parking lot." Coach Bob Zeman would pull back the sliding glass door on the inside, say, "Are you here?" then leave. "The moment that happened," says Banaszak, "as soon as they would turn the corner, guys were bailing out the back door into their cars. It was like the Daytona 500 leaving the parking lot. Everyone knew it. But that was part of Madden's philosophy: 'I don't care what you do Monday through Saturday. As long as you show up Sunday and play your heart out. And don't let anything happen that will have an impact on Sunday.'"

But Madden wasn't always so understanding or sympathetic. One evening, Bob Moore stepped out the door and was heading for his car when he found himself face-to-face with his coach. Madden chased Moore back to his room. "He's knocking, shouting, 'Lemme in! Lemme in!' The phone starts ringing, and we assume it's John to chew us out. We don't answer.

"We get up the next morning, thinking, 'Holy shit, this is gonna be really bad.' But we pass him at practice, he's going the other way, and he just says, 'How ya doin?' I don't know if he had his boots full that night or what. But it did scare the hell out of us."

Obviously, the Badass power structure wasn't completely tolerant of the excessive escapades. Lines had to be drawn somewhere, and at least some of the time. At the very least, there had to be the *appearance* of some sort of discipline. And no one knows if it was Madden or Davis's idea to plant one of the team's gofers in the bushes next to the driveway one night to take down license-plate numbers. But everyone remembers that it was Upshaw who called the police after noticing a shadowy form lurking in the foliage. Uppy told the cops that there was a Peeping Tom in the bushes.

"The cops come and take him away," says Moore. "And the exodus starts again."

✕

But on what other team would the coaching staff virtually sanction the breaking of curfew? When I ask Madden, it is clear that he is a little less than pleased to be discussing the cowboyish aspects of his football team, when we could be talking about more relevant issues—like the games themselves. His coaching did, after all, make the annual championship games into a virtual Raider ritual. But he warms up to the subject of the nightly escapades quickly, because, in its way, the sanctioned revelry cuts to the core of his coaching philosophy: the fewer the rules, the better. The closer a team grows. And the more enamored it becomes of its coach.

"Maybe that goes back to the way I felt about fraternities," Madden told me. "People aren't made to live together and stay together that long. We'd go for two months in training camp, and to believe that men are going to go stay in their rooms and practice football for two months, you're nuts. They had to have fun."

Did you know that other teams didn't do all that stuff?

"No," he admits. "I know it now. I didn't know it at the time. I thought that was all normal, that other teams did it. Because it was normal to me. I would have done the same thing, the things they did."

"Oh, yeah, we knew what they were doing, going out after curfew," Bob Zeman told me. "You could hear the cars start up in the parking lot while we were in meetings. We knew what was going on, but the guys always got back OK and were ready to go the next day. We didn't go around and double-check. We were up there in Santa Rosa for so long in those days that it actually helped. I think it got them all together."

But what about the fines? A few hundred bucks is a lot to pay for a couple of extra beers. "Well, if there were fines," Zeman says, "John might have given them back to them, if they complained." Besides, some of the coaches could sympathize. Once in a while after a late meeting, they'd go out for a beer, too. "Sometimes we saw them out after curfew. We just didn't go out with them."

To one Raider, offensive tackle Bob "Boomer" Brown, a literally larger-than-life legend among the black and silver for his exploits both on the field and off, fines were not a deterrent. One morning after Brown had shattered a curfew, presumably to take a trip down to the city, Moore asked him if he'd been caught. "I don't sneak out. I leave at 10 at night," Brown answered, "and just leave a blank check signed on my bed, and if they come in and fine me, they can just fill out the check."

Moore told him that if he wanted to pay a little less money, "you can follow us out of the parking lot at 11:05."

Not Boomer. He had his own way of doing things. There are few Badass sagas as vivid as those involving the legendary Hall of Fame offensive tackle Robert Stanford Brown.

By the time Bob Brown arrived in 1971—the Raiders were his third team—his reputation was well established: a very smart, standout football player, unafraid to speak his mind, and able to back it up with action. "Any time I got a good [hit] in there," Brown once said, "it'd take a quarter out of the guy." He meant a quarter of a game.

Asked for comment for this book, Brown politely declined. He asked that I include two things: "John Madden was the best coach I ever played for" and "It was by far my best experience with other players." When I asked him whether he wanted to help me modify or embellish or retract some of the Boomer stories, Brown laughed and said, "Let's let it all be a mystery."

So we'll let his teammates do the honors.

"He shows up in '71, the first day, in a Cadillac, wearing a basketball shirt, with this huge upper body. And he's got a driver," says Duane Benson. "Shit, the rest of us were driving junkers, and he shows up with a driver, and a suitcase full of pistols. It was like I told [linebacker] Gus [Otto]: 'I don't the think the son of a bitch needs a pistol. He's got arms as big as your legs.' He fit right in."

But the ostentatious ride was just Brown's first act. The second one attracted even more attention. After he'd changed into his uniform on his first day in camp, exposing incongruously skinny legs to counter the enormous upper body and wide shoulders, he didn't wait for practice to start. He needed something to attack—and immediately. So he walked straight across the field, lowered into a three-point stance in front of the goalpost, and, well, bulldozed it.

"I swear, those goalposts were four-by-fours," says Banaszak. "He snapped it right in half. My eyes fell out of my head. You got to remember that every weird guy who ever played football those days came through the Raiders."

The Eagles had traded Brown to the Rams in 1969 when he vocally protested the firing of general manager Joe Kuharich. In those days, the NFL wasn't big on guys who spoke out. On the Rams, he made his presence known in a duel with one of that team's leaders. In Ram practice, he would line up against "Deacon" Jones, not only the best pass rusher the game has ever known but an early proponent of the head slap, wherein the defensive lineman would try and disconcert his opponent with a blow to the helmet. Boomer didn't like the head slap. One day he asked Jones to refrain from the tactic. At a subsequent practice, as Madden told the story, Jones reapplied his massive hand to Boomer's helmet, and withdrew a bloody mitt. Brown had replaced a small screw that held a helmet pad in place with a longer screw.

In Oakland, without drawing blood, he managed to make an impression on Foo that might as well have been an upturned nail, when he asked the linebacker to stick around after practice one day to help him on his pass blocking. "He tells me, 'I'm going to get back off the ball and you're going to try and get to the quarterback,'" recalls Villapiano, a man who tends to pepper his vocabulary with a specific profanity whenever he's telling a tale. "I fucking come upfield, hard, come in, make a move—the fucking guy blasts me in the stomach, nearly fucking kills me. I go, 'Bob, what the *fuck*?!' I mean, we didn't even have helmets on.

"I called him 'El Boomo.' We'd go to Golden Gate and Bay Meadows and play the horses. You should have seen his outfits. You'd get on the airplane with him, he'd have these tight spandex pants, 300 pounds, with a silk guinea T-shirt showing off these huge muscles, gold chain, a fucking hat, fucking boots. You'd go, 'What the fuck is this?'"

On the plane, Boomer was always up for a card game. Receiver Mike Siani recalls one flight when Boomer was backing a losing card player as the plane approached the airport. Boomer would bankroll anything, flashing his wad of cash. "He refused to sit down. The flight attendant asked him, like, eight times. 'We're not stopping this game,' he said. 'I gotta get my money back.'"

Boomer lived life loud. Well, with a little help from his ordnance. Ask any teammate about the Boomer and they'll tell you about three things: his massive upper body, his aggressiveness as a blocker, and the pistols. According to Dickey's book, Marv Hubbard told the tale of the day when Brown had been beaten consistently on the line in an exhibition game. Afterward, in the locker room, he slipped a gun into each of his two under-arm holsters. "You can't block him," Foo said to Boomer, "so you're going to shoot him?"

Another night, the team awoke to a shot ringing through the hall. "We're all ducking and running down the hallway like the black plague's here," Benson says. As the story goes, Brown had shot out his television and, while his teammates hid from sight, Boomer simply found one of the team's gofers and handed over a twenty to get the set replaced.

"He was something of a nighthawk," Banaszak says. "He'd walk around at two in the morning, and one night he was out taking a piss and shot a gun into the air. Madden got pissed off. He didn't want any firearms around."

But there's no Boomer gun tale that can rival the night he shot Willie Brown's mattress. Willie and Upshaw were roommates, down from Boomer's room, who would pay frequent visits to raid their refrigerator. "Gene and I would be watching TV," Willie says, "and I'd be telling Bob to do this, do that: 'Bob, cut the light out.' Then I'd say, 'Get me some cheese.' Then I'd call him back and say, 'Bob, get me a soda.' Then 'Bob, turn off the TV.'

"So the next time, he comes back and *'Bam! Bam! Bam!'* Right into the bed. Not near me. He wasn't trying to hit me or anything like that. I backpedaled in that bed so fast. Hell, I was scared to death. He says, 'That'll teach you to make me your [servant].'"

"I do understand that he once chased Al [Davis] with a gun," guard George Buehler says. Gus Otto heard it a little differently: "The story had it that he was negotiating his contract with Al, and that Al didn't want to give him a raise, so he pulled out a gun and set it on the desk. I don't know if he got the raise."

For Madden, the old offensive lineman, Brown brought veteran leadership—after all, he did make the Hall of Fame at right tackle, and was voted into six Pro Bowls—and an infectious style of aggressive play. The big man's determination to assault the goalpost was just a hint of the style he brought to the football field, and for Madden, all memories of the Boomer begin and end with his technique—specifically, as a pass blocker. It was Madden's belief that just because a lineman is backing up when he's blocking for the pass, that doesn't mean he has to be passive. You can do some damage from the pass-blocking stance if you're attacking even as you retreat.

"That's what Bob Brown did, and that's what he taught our guys. They were tough anyway, but from Bob they learned that even in relatively passive situations they could be aggressive. You feed off Boomer Brown's aggression on your offensive line, and pretty soon everyone's playing that way."

And the guns? "I think I got rid of those," Madden says with a vague frown. End of the firearms discussion.

This much we know, this much is dead certain: there was a motel-room lamp concealed under the covers in Santa Rosa, where a player was supposed to be. Where it gets all fuzzy is exactly who the player was, or which coach busted his ruse. But in the end, does it matter whether it was Fred Biletnikoff or someone else who was actually out at the Music Box or Melendy's or the Hilltopper? Whether an assistant coach or Madden himself made the discovery? That several of the Raiders are now prone to play down their prior exploits is understandable, if a little baffling. It's as if age has shed their youthful skins. Perhaps they believe their frivolity diminishes their statures as football players when, in fact, it only embellishes them.

So in the meantime, let's let Banaszak's version stand, if only because his details are the best, and Rooster, once a great fullback, is now a great storyteller. "One night I didn't feel like going out. Fred wanted to go out after bed check. I was tired. I said, 'Fuck it, Fred, I'm staying in.' So Fred puts two tennis shoes under the covers, took the pillows and rolled them like legs, then he grabbed the lamp off the table, and put it in there, and tucks his hat in there. It looked pretty real."

Madden was doing the bed check that night, as Banaszak re-calls it. "I knew it was Madden because he never wore shoestrings in his sneakers and you could hear his feet dragging on the side-walk outside the window."

Madden slipped the key in the door, reached in, and flicked the light switch—whereupon the empty bed lit up. Madden walked over and switched off the lamp. "The next day at morning practice," says the Rooster, "he calls the team up. 'By the way, Biletnikoff, I came in last night and your head lit up. Gonna cost you.'"

One thing Banaszak vividly recalls is the night Biletnikoff drove linebacker Dan Conners's car back from a good night on the circuit, driving through some bushes, and doing wheelies in front of the Raider offices. Madden was up, of course. He was legendary for his late-night film viewing.

"We were all shit-faced that night," says Rooster. "It's amazing when you're in real good physical shape how you can do that. Anyway, Madden ran out yelling, 'What the fuck is going on?' Fred was smart enough not to get caught. To this day, Madden probably thinks it was Conners."

Just another chapter in the chaotic, joyous carnival that furnished the legends of a Badass summer camp. Their nightly antidotes to the daily grind remain as vivid in their memories as the games themselves. "But what we did off the field," Biletnikoff tells me, a little reluctant to relive the storied nights, "was never a reflection of what we did on the field. I guess we can all put it that way. What we did off the field was a whole other different thing. Certainly what we did off the field . . . well, we had fun."

## CHAPTER EIGHT

# Fun and Games

Not all of the evening sojourns were devoted to suds, women, and song. Santa Rosa wouldn't have been a summer camp without the intramural tournaments, like the Gus Otto Memorial Bowling Tournament. This wasn't actual bowling. This was an electronic machine at a tavern, of course. That tourney began innocently enough, when the quartet of Benson, Villapiano, Moore, and Otto decided to make the place a regular evening stop, lured by the lights and jangle of the bowling machine.

After Otto, already a bar-shuffleboard champion, left the team in 1972, the action ramped up in his honor. No one who left the Raiders ever stopped being a Raider, symbolically. Your name forever lived on. And that year featured the first Gus Otto Memorial Bowling Tournament. The place generally held about 30; the night of the tournament, capacity would double. Villapiano and Moore sat in chairs set up on the bar, the better to serve as chairmen, overseeing the action and making rulings on the game.

But no Raider tradition was more hallowed than the training-camp air-hockey tournament, which grew from routine diversion to beloved ritual. This one grew out of a charity basketball game between the Raiders and the Rams in the 1973 off-season. The halftime festivities included man-on-man tricycle races. When Foo beat Rams linebacker Isiah Robertson and got his pick of prizes, he chose the air-hockey table. That summer, Foo brought the table to camp and then transported it to Melendy's for the inaugural version of a tradition that would endure for several years. The players paired off into two-man alternating teams. Villapiano, once again, presided as the chairman.

"The number one rule for the air-hockey tournament was 'Cheating is encouraged,'" recalls Monte "Matzoh Ball" Johnson. "Number two was 'It's only cheating if you get caught.' What the air-hockey tournament revealed was how we played football. There were rules, but there weren't rules."

The summer after the inaugural tournament, the profound seriousness of the ritual became apparent. The team had lost its first few exhibition games, Foo recalls, and spirits were low. "We were playing terribly," says Villapiano. "It seemed like no one gave a fuck." And while the Raiders were always nonchalant about playing exhibition games that didn't matter, this time the clouds were ominous in Santa Rosa. Somehow, the team needed a spark. "So Madden catches up with me one day," Villapiano remembers, "and says to me, 'What the fuck kind of commissioner are you?'

"I say, 'What are you talking about?' He says, 'You know what I'm talking about. We can't win until you start this fuckin' craziness.'" And so Villapiano set the wheels in motion for another tourney.

"It's like any other business," Villapiano says. "When you look back you say, Maybe it would have been better if you cut back on some of the craziness—the bowling tournament, the air-hockey tournament, Rookie Night. But Madden loved it. And as soon as he told me that, we mobilized quick."

"That was one of the great things about John," Biletnikoff says.

"With the tournaments, they'd always try and give him the date in advance, so we could have extra time off that night. Of course, we still had to break curfew."

Drinking at the tournament, of course, was mandatory. "When we got Dave Rowe in 1975," defensive tackle Art "King Arthur" Thoms says, "he didn't drink, so they tried to disqualify him because his alcohol blood level wasn't high enough. I think he had a sip of beer to qualify himself."

Can it be coincidence that it was the summer of 1976—when the team would finally win its ring—that the tournament reached its pinnacle? That air hockey became the Raiders' second sport of choice?

In search of a tournament queen with a higher profile than the local talent, telephone calls had already been made to Elizabeth Ray; it had been two months since the Washington, D.C., call girl had been implicated as the central figure in the sex scandal that had brought down Representative Wayne Hays. Apparently, her social schedule was already filled.

Nonetheless, this was going to be a tournament for all time. Johnny Vella (J.V., "the Italian") was in charge of writing the program, replete with odds for, and commentary about, the various teams' chances. Villapiano posted the rules—on the fence surrounding the practice field. The actual regulations for this particular event have been lost to history, but a rules listing from the tourney a few seasons later gives us an accurate idea of the tone of the event. Among them:

Cheating is encouraged.

Motherfuckages and verbal abuse of opponents is encouraged.

No physical abuse to table, players, or judge (penalty: one

unmolested free shot; guilty party must cruise with the
Tooz).

Long-sleeve shirts are illegal (Tooz will remove all sleeves
personally).

All hosebags must be registered with Rooster.

Drunkenness is mandatory—urine must be clear.

Rookies cannot win.

Phil Villapiano Most Disgusting Player Award will be presented to the most outrageous display of buffoonism or
illicit behavior.

Ray Guy Poor Sportsmanship Award to the biggest shitsport.

The air-hockey tournament was to be held two days before the
final exhibition game against Los Angeles, and Cuniberti wrote a
feature story on the tournament, a tale that ran on the front page
of the paper's sports section the morning of the event. Her story
led with a Foo quote: "If I was the coach, I'd say, the hell with the
Rams. Let's just practice for the tournament."

The rest of the story featured detailed commentary on the various two-man teams, including odds and handicapping: Foo and
receiver Mike Siani were favored: "No human can beat me," Villapiano said. Zeman made the boldest prediction: "We will not
only repeat as Most Valuable Cheaters," he boasted of himself and
partner Biletnikoff, "but we will be the most spectacular team. We
have perfected a mind-boggling technique which will upset the
tournament."

It wasn't just mind-boggling. It was prestidigitatious: finger-
boggling. Cheating was refined to a fine art. "Everybody was always trying to find their way of getting the advantage," recalls
Zeman. "So one day when the players were at practice, I went into
the room where they kept the air-hockey table. Then I measured
the goals. Then I went out and got some hard, transparent plastic.
You could hold it in your hand and slide it on across the goal, which

was an inch high, four or five long. In the tournament, we slipped the plastic in the goal when someone took a shot."

Let's not even ask how Zeman was able to slide unnoticed out of practice. A six-year veteran of the AFL, he'd been hired by Madden to mold a defensive backfield. By 1976 he was the de facto defensive coordinator. But on this day, his priorities clearly lay elsewhere. Let's chalk it up to a coach whose competitive edge fed off the demeanor of his men. Of course, another thought immediately comes to mind: the family of the Badasses was not only willing to welcome coach Zeman into its weird fraternity, they considered the popular coach as one of the family—so much so that he was known among the players simply as Z.

"Oh, they'd always invite me to come along," Zeman says. "No one thought anything of it. The players accepted us. They all knew what we expected from them. We also knew on the days we were going to relax [that] we were going to be ordinary people with everybody else."

As the tournament began with more than a dozen teams, Z's ploy was working well. "Since it was a dark bar," says Banaszak, "you couldn't tell. The puck would look for sure like it was going in, and it wouldn't, and you'd go, 'Wow. What a great save!'"

But when they got to the final round that night, fate intervened. According to the very bendable rules, sometimes two players would be playing at once, and sometimes just one, depending on whether or not your partner was attending to other priorities at the bar. When he got busted, Zeman was a one-man team. And despite the supposedly inviolable insistence on cheating, this strategy went a little too far for the judges.

"Z screwed it all up," Biletnikoff says now. "We were doing good. We had gotten into the finals." Then Zeman took a clear shot at the goal and missed it. The puck ricocheted clear down to the other end, bouncing off Zeman's plastic shield. "And that's how

we got caught. We had done a great job of it to the final. We had
to forfeit the game."

Others would argue that the Biletnikoff and Zeman bust did
not provide the highlight of the air-hockey tournament's history, that the Plastic episode paled next to another tournament
that very well might have involved some plastic itself: the tournament where Carol Doda, the most famous topless dancer of
all time, *did* actually visit, as honorary queen, and used her own
somewhat natural endowments to stop shots, invited by Biletnikoff.

"She put her tits on the table and blocked shots with her tits,"
says Foo. "She was a hit."

Pressed today on the veracity of that incident, Biletnikoff falls
silent for a moment and then answers in tones and language you
might use in a witness box, before 'fessing up: "At that period of
time . . . yes. I did get her."

How did you approach her?

"We had mutual friends," he says, preferring to leave it at that.

No one recalls who actually won the tournament in 1976. But Villapiano recalls the reaction to the *Chronicle* article vividly: "I walk
into breakfast, and fucking Madden, the great psychiatrist, kicks
open the fucking door, almost rips it off and breaks the glass. He
says, 'You don't worry about the Rams? Why don't you get the fuck
out of here?'"

His troops' revelry didn't bother Madden; he was all for the
tournament. It was that the revelry had been revealed. And Madden subsequently did his best to kill the messenger. He invited

Cuniberti into his office—and lit into her. "He was furious," she recalls. "'I can't believe you wrote this story.' He was so mad that his face was red and there was this vein standing out in his forehead." She failed to see the problem.

"'It has nothing to do with football!' Madden ranted. 'Women shouldn't cover football. This has nothing to do with football.'"

Cuniberti vehemently disagreed. "'I think how people on a team get along with each other has a lot to do with how a team performs on the field,'" she told him. "Yes, I said it was a bar, but it wasn't the night before a game.

"Then I get the word that he wants to see me again. Now what? I go into his office, and he goes, 'You know what I really hated about that story?' I said, 'No, what did you really hate about it?' He says, 'My wife really loved it.'"

The air-hockey tournament found its way down to Oakland—with predictably mayhemic results. The publicity had reached the ears of the executives at Coleco, the manufacturer of the table, who offered to hold a banquet tournament at a restaurant in Oakland. Two dozen Raiders were accompanied by cameras from the local TV stations. The Coleco people were seated on one side of the room, the Raiders on the other, and, of course, this being the Raiders, a food fight ensued.

Villapiano remembers the president of Coleco throwing dinner rolls. Foo won't elaborate on how he retaliated, but we can assume he was not a passive bystander.

✕

Training-camp pub rituals culminated with the final ceremony, just before the team broke camp: a parade through town on Rookie Night, when the newbies were officially welcomed at a bar that regularly featured local strippers. The winners of the various tournaments were honored, after riding through town in the back of various pick-ups—including, according to one player, Dan Con-ners's El Camino, with a bra draped on the trailer hitch—and on at least one occasion, with a police escort, the winners of the tourna-ments pitching candies to the roadside kids.

"It was a huge event," Banaszak recalls. "Like a ticker-tape pa-rade. Usually we had to kick in some money to clean the place up afterwards. We'd always end up throwing food at each other."

Today, tight end Ted Kwalick doesn't remember the procession. "The parade?" This most proper and gentlemanly businessman shakes his head. "A lot of that stuff that happened, man, you gotta realize, we weren't sober."

The Santa Rosa fun and games weren't all fueled by liquor, of course. This was the '70s, after all. "We used to have a smoking room at the El Rancho," says Art Thoms. "We changed the closet into the marijuana room. We didn't put any clothes in there."

The Badass non-drinkers—well, the relatively temperate ones—reverted to adolescence in another way. But they were no less seri-ous about their off-field distractions. You have to wonder what the dog happily swimming in the middle of the slow-running, peaceful Russian River thought when it spied a remote-controlled, two-foot-long model speedboat, painted black and silver, screaming through the water right at its head. Did it have time to notice the Raider decal on the craft's meticulously painted hull? It certainly must have heard the high-pitched whine of the oversized motor that its creators, little kids in bodies the size of refrigerators, had mounted on its fiberglassed balsa-wood body. To Dave Rowe and George Buehler, who had assembled it at El Rancho, it was the sound of a finely tuned watercraft giving off an ecstatic scream, freed as it was from the El Rancho pool. To the canine, it must have been the sound of a predator alien.

"It ran right across the dog," Rowe recalls. "It may have hit its nose, or it may have just scared the poop out of it. That dog took off. I had that thing wide open, going 30, maybe 35 miles per hour."

That a small boat could attain such speeds testified to the diligence that these kids brought to their craft. "Football was secondary when we were in training camp," Rowe says of the remote-control crowd. "We only did three things in training camp. Practicing, eating, or working on those stupid cars and boats and planes."

Which is to say: not every player fled the final meeting, tore off in their cars double-time, and prowled the circuit. Instead, several of them hightailed it over to the Coddingtown hobby shop, in a shopping center north of town, domain of "the RC guy"—the remote-control guy—who presided over a showroom of high-end model kits. "We spent every night in that shop," Rowe says. "It's amazing how much money you could spend on that stuff."

"We all made remote-controlled models," says Monte Johnson. If Johnson's name has tapered into obscurity, it's not because he wasn't a very good linebacker; he was calling the defensive signals during every huddle in the Badass glory years. Chalk up Johnson's anonymity to his wisdom in those days, spending his time not shattering curfew but, armed with glue, using a watchmaker's precision, assembling his vehicles. "I made a sailboat that I sailed in the motel pool. I actually kept that sailboat for 20 years until it finally made it into the trash can."

Buehler, the Stanford guy, captained this crowd. George's boat was a thing to behold: a more conventional craft, a replica of the kind of '50s-style steering-wheel speedboat you'd see on some private Adirondack lake. Only a little bit smaller. But as far as the boats went, nothing was as glitzy as Rowe's canine-hunting speedboat. "I had to help him build that one," says Buehler, the eccentric technician. George would rather talk remote control than football, as we sit over iced tea at a Denny's in a small town outside of Pasadena. George is wearing red-white-and-blue suspenders and a straw hat that makes him look like a very large Amish farmer. "We laminated the balsa wood of Dave's boat so it painted up real nice. Yeah, that one would really move along pretty good."

"You gotta understand that we were all competitive," says Rowe. "So this was all about who has the biggest, the fastest, the baddest, and the best."

After the miniature boats came Buehler's miniature tank, which has taken on mythic proportions in the storied retellings of its journeys across the courtyard of the Zoo, not in the least because the man behind it was the right guard they called "Fog," because he seemed so often to be in one. The nickname is one that George could do without these days, but his teammates, with fond recollections, insist that it was entirely apt. "George gave you the impression," Johnson says, "that he lived life in a fog bank." That he was a hell of a guard is something no one disputes; that his name is lost in the annals, despite a distinguished 10-year career with the team, might have something to do with his misfortune of playing across the center from Gene Upshaw, who never met a camera he didn't like. Which is not to imply that George was mute. Just . . . different.

"He'd say the strangest things," says Banaszak. "One time in the heat of battle against the Steelers, I was wearing new shoes. We're in the huddle, and his eyes look up at me, and he says, 'Rooster, why are you wearing those nice football shoes out in the rain?' I say, 'George, we're down on the 20, we're playing the Steelers, and you're worried about my shoes?' With all us heathens and jaloobies, here's this prim and proper guy. He never swore. And he never held."

"Pete liked to mess with my head," George admits now. "He'd ask me stuff like 'The thermonuclear separation of the atom is a quotient of what?' The truth is, I never did graduate. I flunked chemistry. But I told the guys that just getting into Stanford was like getting a doctorate at one of their schools."

This is a man who used to fashion explosives out of matchbooks, which he would place under teammates' toilet seats. One time, when the team had to spend a week in a hotel in East Orange, New Jersey—and the clerks had to ask him to cut down on pilfering the matches at the front desk—George added homemade cannons to his arsenal. "I made those out of ankle tape and tubing," he told me, not without some pride, "and I decided to put one of my bombs in the barrel, with a time-delayed fuse in the bomb. We were on the third or fourth floor. The thing is I didn't realize how short the fuse was going to be. It blew up 10 feet out of the barrel. Then I dropped one down on the street and it went off as a car was going by."

Buehler's tank resides to this day in his home. Some football players display their trophies. George cherishes his tank. "The original idea was that I'd be able to send it over to the office, and Ken Bishop, our secretary, could stick my mail on it and I could bring it back. But every once in a while it would go crazy. It would get caught in the carpet of the office. It never actually succeeded in getting my mail.

"It was the wrong tank for the job."

✕

At some point, the boats and the tanks gave way to the cars. Some of their teammates favored speed in real cars, of course, but for Buehler, Rowe, and Ray Guy, the model cars were the only cars that counted. For these guys, competitive beer drinking wasn't nearly as fun as racing cars in El Rancho's driveway. What Ray Guy sacrificed in speed he made up for in remote-control maneuverability. Befitting the best punter the game of football has ever known, Guy had to have the most impressive vehicle in the toy-car fleet.

"I had my Wild Willy," Guy recalls, his deep Georgia drawl slathered over his words like syrup. "It was a Jeep. When kids came out—kids were always coming out to the El Rancho to see the players—what I'd do is get up on the breezeway of the motel, out of sight, and have the Jeep hidden between a couple of cars.

"Then just as soon as a kid would come out, I'd run the Jeep out, have it do a wheelie, run it back between the real cars, then ease it back out there into the middle of the driveway and turn it toward the kid. I'd run it at him, stop it, and run it. Inch by inch. They didn't know where it was coming from."

Rowe's car was a miniature Indy machine, with oversized tires, painted black and silver, of course. "We'd jack those suckers up, put the big tires on them, and, man, they'd go." A veteran of four other teams, Rowe is quick to point out that he never dabbled in toys in any of his other training camps. Only on the Raiders would you find a defensive lineman spending his downtime building intricate toys with such diligence. "We never did anything remotely close to that with any other team," he says. "Are you kidding? The coaches would have had a heart attack."

"Only on the Raiders," says Guy.

Eventually, the ground represented too tame a frontier for the toy crowd. The wide-open Sonoma Valley skies beckoned. And so the RC collective took to the air. As a rule, their intricate flying machines spent more time on the ground, whether whole or in pieces, than they did in the warm currents above the peaceful Santa Rosa hills, which rose behind the training fields. Like the day when a Buehler machine met an untimely end at the hands of tight end

Dave Casper, who swatted it out of the air when it ventured too close to the big guy. Banaszak swears it was a Casper helmet that brought the beauty down. (Casper, unfortunately, chose not to comment for this book.)

On another day, one of the Buehler creations ventured too close to another species of mammal. One of the hillsides out beyond the fenced-in practice fields was a horse corral. "So he's worked really hard assembling this big plane," Rowe tells me, "and he's flying the plane out beyond the field. He has the control in his hand. All of a sudden you hear this 'wwwhhhaaaaaaaaw,' this high-pitched screeching. I look through the glasses. It's going down. I'm shouting, 'Pull back! Pull back!'" The plane plummeted smack into he middle of the corral. The horses were freaked. "The plane was busted to smithereens."

Keep in mind that this was not an out-of-the-box airplane. It cost Buehler, king of the remote controllers, $500 to buy, build, and customize. Its skin had been molded to its frame by his meticulous use of a hair dryer. It had taken him a month to build. The wingspan reached a good four feet, which must have made it look like something akin to a condor to the horses beneath it. "I forget about the horses," says Buehler. "I jump the fence and run 50 yards to the middle of the corral, to my where my plane was, and I'm assessing the damage. Then I look up and there are these two horses side by side stomping the ground. Ready to charge."

This was a man who made a living facing snorting defensive linemen. But he wasn't quite certain how to block a four-legged adversary. "All of a sudden, I'm going, 'Aw, shit.' Rowe comes up and grabs a big blue wing while he's yelling, 'Whoa, boy, *whoa*, boy . . .' I took the rest of the plane and flew over the fence and left Rowe back there to deal with the horses."

If the summation of all of the RC endeavors adds up in the negative column in terms of actual mechanical success, Buehler shrugs this off. To George, all things considered, it was time and money well spent, considering the alternative. "All of the guys on the team thought it was very childish to be building model airplanes and boats. I would be in at night rather than being out on the town and so forth. But, of course, after Stabler wrote his tell-all book, everyone claimed they were out buying airplanes."

All of the extracurriculars had this in common: for a team that lived and breathed to beat the opponent, the games furnished nothing but another form of competition. And the competitions were never-ending. Like the one to see who could put the weirdest or largest object into the Gatorade bucket: jockstrap, socks, helmets, and other unnamed artifacts. For the summertime Badasses, all of life was a contest.

"I think it was all a natural extension of what we did for a living, whether it was conscious or unconscious," Duane Benson says. "Obviously these are grown men playing little boys' games. If you suggested any sort of game, this family mind-set we had every day led to other players getting into any kind of game pretty quickly"— like the competition to see who could sweat less. On a football team. During practice.

"What kind of team competes to see who could sweat the least?" asks Rowe. "We would. Everybody would throw in twenty bucks to see who would sweat the least in practice. Guys would be standing around, and [linebacker coach] Don Shinnick would say, 'Monte, get in there.' Monte'd say, 'I can't play. I haven't been sweating yet.'"

There was even a contest that related to football. As Stabler recalls it, it was a team-wide thing: "We used to put aluminum garbage cans against the fence, and everybody's trying to get the ball in the can." Wagers, of course, were placed. "Guys would be down, like, $35,000," Rowe remembers. "Unbelievable. Obviously, I never saw anyone pay off."

The winner would invariably be the ultra-accurate Stabler, whose usual opponent would be suitemate Biletnikoff. "They'd have these challenges," says Kwalick, "but Stabler was so precise. He'd never miss. Freddy would say, 'You're too close. Move back.' Snake would still drop it in. Then 'You're too far left. Move right.' Kenny'd still put it in. 'OK, you gotta bank it.' And he'd still make it. Then Freddy would hit the rim. It'd bounce out."

The very first unofficial competition in Raider camp remains one of the stranger duels in football history: an ongoing battle of the intellects, between linebackers Benson and Otto.

"I'm going to ask you about the breed of beef cattle called Herefords," Benson, the animal-genetics expert and future state senator, would say to his friend as they sat on their helmets on the sideline. Or huddled up. Or lined up for another endless practice drill. Or afterward, in the shower. "I am not going to ask you the color, or where they originated. That would be too easy. I'm going to ask you another question: what's the color if you cross it with an Angus?"

"I'm not going to ask you the height of Everest," Otto would counter. "That's too easy. What's the height of Pike's Peak?" Or the second-tallest waterfall. Or the third-longest river. Otto was the trivia master of mountains and waterways. "Well," Otto says now, "when you go to the office, you want to have fun, don't you?"

"Gus would just deflate you," remembers Benson. "I'd study all off-season. But Gus was a very cerebral guy. For years he wrestled with whether we'd put a man on the moon or whether the whole thing was staged in a studio in Los Angeles."

"Yeah, it was always rivers, mountains, and streams; I have no idea why that was my topic," Otto ("Augie Joe") says now, as if it's weird that I'm even asking, as if having a running quiz show between two linebackers was the most normal thing in the world. "Sometimes we weren't all that exact. I do know that Pike's Peak is 14,110 feet. And that Everest has somehow gotten seven feet taller, according to the almanac."

"Heaven forbid if we played 20 years together what the game would have been," says Benson. "Self-surgery or something: 'Take out your appendix.'"

Roadhouses and juke joints. Streakers and suds by the pitcherful. Barroom queens, galloping horses, and squealing tires. Mind games and miniaturized, motorized mayhem. Tavern tournaments and a pirates' parade—with a little football thrown in.

The reach of the annual Badass training-camp festival went far beyond the summer. If you're looking for reasons to explain the annual Raider dominance of the 1970s, start with this ultimate family reunion. The bonding power of the El Rancho escapades sowed the seeds for each superior season to come.

## CHAPTER NINE

# The Oakland Circuit

**W**hen the team broke camp and headed back to Oakland, all the requisite Badass skills finely honed by months of grueling afterhours workouts, the taste for nightlife hardly abated. New contests awaited, like the shuffleboard tournament at a place called The 19th Hole in Alameda. Whereas in Santa Rosa drinking circuits were varied and compelled mostly by different factions (the vets on the circuit, the linemen ensconced in the Bamboo), back in Oakland tavern life was pretty much team-wide, more of a family affair, kind of like an army unit that had done its training at a far-flung domestic base then flown into the real war zone.

Down in Oakland, the mantra was one for all and all for one. On Sundays, the revelry always started with the weekly post-game party, hosted by Davis, win or lose—in the earliest years, at a place called the Edgewater West Motel.

"That was one seedy place," Villapiano says now. "I mean, this was a dive." In a time when salaries were closer to minimum-wage than white-collar, a free, all-you-could-eat-and-drink meal was like manna from the gods. The party was as highly anticipated as the games, not just because of the generosity of Davis, but because of the chance for 40-odd families to hang and get to know each other: the neighborhood cocktail party writ large.

"But, remember, the NFL was just getting started, and these teams didn't have a lot of money to spend," Villapiano recalls. "The Raiders were the only team that threw a full-fledged party for all the players and their friends. And if you didn't go, someone would be down your fucking throat. We all went, we all had a good time . . . and shit happened."

"The great thing about the Edgewater parties was you'd get to know everyone, and that had a lot to do with the team's camaraderie," says Benson. The bond that the fete symbolized was emphasized in a conversation Benson had with Davis a year after the owner moved the team to Los Angeles, in 1982. "'How's it going?' I said. He said, 'It sucks. When we would go to the Edgewater, if one or two people weren't there, everyone would wonder where they were. In L.A., one or two people showed up.'"

"Everything was always family with the team," says Madden. "I used to let my players and coaches bring their kids to Saturday practice for home games. I had my two kids, too. Then when we all went in, to take off the pads and shower, the kids would play a game on the field—on the game field, the day before a game. Those were great practices. They were fun. You could still do that back then, still have fun."

Madden says that his biggest shock when he went into broadcasting was the silence that enveloped other teams' practices. No one seemed to be having any fun at all. "The funny thing is I thought we were normal. Then I went out there and it turns out we weren't. It was normal to me. But what we did, I guess it wasn't normal to NFL teams."

✕

On Tuesdays, the Raider chalkboard featured a roster for an entirely different kind of game: the weekly afternoon golf tournament. Madden didn't participate, but he took delight in seeing the matchups scrawled on the board. "We had a two-man scramble match," says lineman Steve Sylvester. "Dalby and Upshaw were always partners, they both cheated, and everyone fell in line after that." The ten teams would sprint right from practice to the golf course, and Madden would let them out early if they'd played a particularly good game. "He always loved to stand there with a towel over his shoulder, bottle of Maalox in his hands, looking at the matchups."

The weekly Camaraderie Night, though, held on Thursdays, once the game plan was in place, stands as the most sacred tradition of all. Attendance was mandatory. "Everybody had to be there; we didn't accept excuses," says Foo. "We'd tell the new guys, 'Tell your wife anything, but you gotta be there.' No wives. No friends. No girlfriends."

On the Oakland circuit, the first stop was always, without exception, Al's Cactus Room, located in the center of downtown, just off Webster Avenue on 19th Street. Al's was nothing to look at from the outside, just like the Bamboo Room, but it was a shrine for the football team within. "It was in the middle of nowhere," says Villapiano. "During the day downtown, there'd be life down there—the corporations, the workers. At night? Nothing. Nobody. Except for the Raiders. The place would be packed, with Raiders and with fans."

The enormous jukebox favored Al Green, Marvin Gaye, and Otis Redding, but the true Cactus Room soundtrack was the banter between player and fan.

"The Cactus Room was kind of like a Cheers bar," Stabler recalls. And, of course, everyone knew their names. To this day, no one knows why it was called the Cactus Room, but everyone remembers its proprietor: the biggest Raider fan of all; wearing his black-and-silver T-shirt emblazoned with the number 1, Al Punzak stood somewhere between 5'2" and 5'6", depending on who's remembering their favorite saloonkeeper. How sacred was Big Al to the mystique? He was Villapiano's daughter's godfather. Only the Badasses would bring a barkeep into the family.

"He'd make these delicious beef ribs for us," Mike Siani remembers, "and every player who walked in had a drink named after them. Mine was a 'Mike Special.' It had something to do with Bailey's Irish Cream. We paid nothing, for anything. Of course, part of why he did it was because it brought hundreds of people into his restaurant every week."

"He was the sweetest man of all of them," says Foo. "Al Punzak: our Hungarian guy. It was the perfect hangout. Big long bar, and down at the end he had this bell. As soon as you'd step in, he'd ring the bell, and it was 'Villapiano in the house! Ken Stabler in the house!' Big Al would feed us booze and food. We had no money. I couldn't pay. Who could?"

Few of the Raiders ever went upstairs at Al's. That privilege was reserved for the old Raider Frank Youso, who returned to town on business in the '70s. "Big Al said, 'You can stay in my apartment upstairs,'" Youso recalls. "'Keep the door locked. If you hear anyone banging on the windows, there's a .45 under my pillow.'"

The next stop on the regular-season circuit took the team out of the deserted reaches of downtown to Jack London Square, down on the waterfront. Well, what better neighborhood for the renegades to inhabit than a few square blocks named for an avowed socialist (he twice ran for Oakland mayor), member of the Bohemian Club, and author of *The Call of the Wild*? The square wasn't the tourist mecca it's become now, just a cluster of bars planted on the fringe of an industrial district, and its most frequent visitors in the '70s wore black and silver.

"After the Cactus Room, we'd head to the Grotto to eat, then to Clancy's, Uppy's," Banaszak says. "Christ, we were drunker than skunks. But we had a way of policing each other. If a guy was too drunk, we'd always find a way to get him home."

Gene and his brother Marvin owned Uppy's on the Square. One wall of the restaurant featured a mural of a cotton field, a reminder of the Upshaws' impoverished south Texas youth. "Hello, Snake," Stabler heard one night at Uppy's, and turned to see Huey Newton, cofounder of the Black Panthers, standing at his side. Well, of course Newton knew the Snake. One Badass to another.

"Bobby Seale would come to practice sometimes," says Willie Brown. "The Panthers loved the Raiders. They were part of us. All the different organizations and groups that were disengaged, we took them in and brought them in and accepted them. That was our style. The Angels? That's part of us. The Panthers? That's part of us. We didn't think of it then as what it means today." According to Gene Upshaw, as quoted in a 2007 magazine piece, Seale and Newton were Raider fans "because they admired the team's fierce sense of loyalty."

They were all part of a gritty city, just a few bridges distant from San Francisco but light-years removed from that glittering burg across the bay. Oakland was the nation's largest port: a transit town for freight, not a destination for tourists seeking High Culture.

San Francisco fomented the flowery voice of the psychedelic and weeded-out and birthed the music that was the backbone of the Woodstock generation. Oakland was known for fomenting the distinctly unmelodic sounds of an entirely different kind of revolution: the rhetoric of the Panthers, founded in 1966 (the year Al

Davis joined the Raiders' front office), with their mantra of violence. "We greet you with the revolutionary fervor of the people," announced one Panther official at a rally at the time. "We greet you with the gun."

Oakland had been Hells Angels country for a long, long time. In October of 1928, in the middle of filming his epic World War I film *Hell's Angels*, Howard Hughes moved the shooting up to the Oakland airfield. Three pilots were killed during the shoot. The title was adopted by a bomber squadron during World War II, and in 1948 the outlaw motorcycle gang, founded down in Fontana, adopted it as its name—along with the symbol of a skull with wings. Kind of like crossed swords behind a helmeted pirate, when you think about it.

The Angels didn't hang at Uppy's, though. It was at a faceless downtown bar near a fight gym that Biletnikoff used to frequent, where Snake had his first drink with Sonny Barger, the legendary Angel leader. "I was always a huge fight fan," Stabler says, "ever since I was a kid and I'd watch the Friday-night fights with my dad. Freddy and I used to go to this gym in Oakland, right downtown. Freddy would live in there and watch the fighters work out."

One day Stabler met Biletnikoff at the place for a drink and a game of nine-ball. "There was a guy at the bar with a sleeveless jean jacket that says 'Hells Angels' on the back of it. Everybody knew who we were. So he introduced himself, wanted to know if we wanted to shoot a game of pool with Sonny Barger. And we did."

"There was one story," Art Thoms recalls, "that Stabler was out drinking with the Angels 'til 6 a.m. He went to the game; they'd go home and watch him on TV and pass out."

It was the beginning of a beautiful friendship between Barger and the Raiders. "I used to lift weights with Sonny over in a gym in Hayward, on East 14th Street," says Villapiano. "Sonny and his bodyguard were serious lifters. Matuszak and I would meet them there a lot in the off-season. If you met them at a bar, you'd have beers together. They'd be on the sideline during the game—you'd see Sonny a lot. Just like the Panthers were there."

"Oh, yeah, we had Black Panthers and Hells Angels both identifying with us," George Atkinson says. "We were real, man. There was no pretentiousness."

It was a few years later, before his final Raider season in 1979, that Foo and a minor chapter of Raider/Angel history managed to blemish the friendship—an ugly episode that nonetheless emblemized the solidarity of the team.

Curfew had long passed up in Santa Rosa, and Villapiano was absent. The bed-check coach didn't want Foo to get in trouble, so he was asking various players if they knew where he was. Foo had been spotted at various locales during the evening, but no one had seen him for a while. By now a group of players had gathered in the courtyard, because it was unusual for Foo to be out by himself. Finally, recalls Buehler, "all of a sudden, around the corner here comes Phil, a bloody mess. Shirt torn. Sort of stumbling. Didn't look good. They got him over to the training room."

Today, Villapiano is reluctant to recount the incident, even after the passage of more than three decades: "It's a very touchy thing. These guys play for keeps." It had actually happened in the parking lot of the Bamboo Room. Villapiano was in a foul mood: he was being shifted to inside linebacker. He'd severely pulled a muscle in practice and knew he wouldn't be practicing the next day. So he hung around for a few extra beers, came out, and saw a couple of guys leaning on his car.

"I said, 'Get the fuck off my car.' The next thing, I got a hammer to the side of my head. If I don't know Sonny, I'm probably dead. As soon as I mentioned his name, those guys stopped." It wasn't as bad as it looked, he says. "Head wounds just tend to bleed a lot."

The team's response? To a man they wanted revenge. Jack Tatum urged Foo to rally the troops. "I say, 'No, we don't want to go there, someone's going to get hurt, it's going to ruin our season.' But I've never seen the Raiders mobilize like that."

"Guys are yelling, 'Let's go! Let's go!'" says Buehler. "Coaches are literally pushing us back in our rooms because guys want to go get the Hells Angels. Madden was out there: 'No one's leaving!' Even in those days, that would have been crazy. But we were young and nuts and ready to go."

The tale has a happy ending. A week later, at afternoon practice, some unexpected visitors appeared on the sideline: a dozen Angels on their Harleys. "'Rooster, I made up with them. I had to invite them to practice,'" Foo told Banaszak. "'I forgot to tell Madden.' Madden says, 'What the fuck?' He's ranting and raving. Finally Ginzo has the balls to tell John how he'd made up with them. After that, they were our best buddies."

The normal mode of transportation in Oakland, from Al's to the Square, or anywhere in between, would have naturally been a cab, or a player's car. Not for the Junior Board. The Junior Board was not to be confused with the Senior Board, comprising the vets like Stabler, Banaszak, and Biletnikoff. The Junior Board was a fluid half-dozen-plus guys—Thoms, Vella, Moore, Villapiano, Sistrunk, Siani, Dalby. The Juniors tended to stick together all season long. Hence the need for the limo. "We were doing so much together during the week," Vella says, "we thought, 'Why don't we get a limo so we can go places as a group?'"

So King Arthur took the reins. "We had a lot of Board functions, so we had to have the Board Limo," says Thoms now. "We all kicked in, like, $500 apiece." It was a huge, used limousine. It was black, of course. "Couldn't have cost more than $2,500, tops."

("King Arthur was kind of fucking strange," Banaszak notes. "He would travel with a Snoopy lunch pail under his arm. I have no idea what he kept in it.")

Typical of the Badass' woolly aesthetic, the Junior Board's ride did not dazzle with chrome. It was frayed at the edges, designed to simply get the job done. A pure Raider ride.

"It was a big, black, piece-of-crap, run-down limo," Moore says. "Hell, it must have been 10 years old." But contrary to legend it was not a hearse, as Banaszak recalls—even if it makes for a good story. No, the occupants of the Board's ride were very much alive.

The limo's prime function was twofold: to serve as transportation to the games and to usher the Board in style to postgame affairs. Its faux-impressive stature empowered Thoms to just pull it up in front of a tavern of choice and leave the vehicle unattended as the Board piled in for a drink. Or several.

"After the 49er games, we went down to a bar on Union Street in San Francisco," Thoms told me. "One time we parked right in front, and we put all our girls on our shoulders and walked into the place. The bouncers weren't real happy. They tried to keep us out, but we weren't leaving. The 49ers weren't very good at that time. That might have been the night Villapiano got up on one of those tables. He was singing along, and he fell off the table. He cut himself pretty bad. I think he pulled a groin, too."

It would have made for an interesting injury report that week. Villapiano: lacerations, pulled groin due to excess vocalization and liquid consumption. No matter what the episode, you could always count on Foo being in the middle of it.

"Another time we used it to go to a Boz Scaggs concert," Thoms recalls. "He was a Raider fan. Used to say I was his favorite player, actually. So I pulled the limo up to the very front of the place, and there was this line of people waiting to get in. There was this little area, this red zone. I backed in and I hit the curb and the tire blew. It was like a shotgun going off. Everyone turned and looked and we just walked in. I left the limo there.

"It's a miracle," Thoms says now, "that I didn't get sued." Or that they could all fit into the limo.

Thoms kept their ride on call at all times. He would hire a kid who worked at his laundromat to pick him and Sistrunk up at the Hilton on Sunday mornings and take them to the coliseum. And so early-arriving fans at Raider games would be treated to the sight of the limo pulling up to the stadium and disgorging a very strange-looking pair of men: the long-haired Thoms and his partner, the shaven-headed Sistrunk.

"Otis and I were 'Salt and Pepper,'" Thoms says. "Everyone had a gimmick. You had to have a gimmick." This gimmick owed something to one of Hollywood's most forgettable movies ever: *Salt and Pepper*, with Sammy Davis Jr. and Peter Lawford. Well, Sistrunk *had* signed with the Rams originally because he wanted to be in Hollywood. (He would eventually even make it into film, with a cameo in *Car Wash*.)

"He was black and bald and I was white with long hair," says Thoms, "so I'd wear a black hat, he'd wear a white one. He brought the cigars. We'd smoke the cigars on the way to the stadium."

Well, it was fitting that they arrived at their home field in style. Because the stadium, of course, was their ultimate hangout. If the Raiders owned all corners of the city, as well as every haunt and heart in Santa Rosa, the true capital of Badass camaraderie was the coliseum. For all of their after-hours revelry, at the end of the day—and night—the one place where they truly came together for fun and games was on the field, where the Badass brand of football was played by men who plied their trade the way they lived their off-the-field lives: with abandon, on the edge, as one, and taking no prisoners along the way. At the coliseum the Oakland Raiders were most at home, hosting a municipal party for 52,000 friends, and for those of us in the nationwide gallery who liked their football to be played as it was meant to be played: by brothers.

# PART II

## BADASS FOOTBALL

## CHAPTER TEN

# Guy, Foo, and Freddy: Building the Foundation

**M**emories of the Immaculate Deception had lingered all winter. In a very short time the play had taken on a fabled luster, savored by the football nation at large, a slam-bang, dramatically physical spectacle that instantly and forever carved its way into our sporting subconscious—which made it all the more of a stab in the heart to the Raider nation.

"We saw the play in our minds," Gerald Irons remembers. "We had nightmares. Several times I would wake up in the middle of the night seeing that play. When we came back in '73, it was still the talk. But in a way it added incentive."

Davis, Wolf, and Madden had already built a strong foundation on defense, thanks in large part to the first two rounds of the memorable '71 draft. Because "we needed to get tougher," Davis told me, they'd first taken Tatum out of Ohio State and then Villapiano from the much-lower-profile Bowling Green—two men who would forever symbolize the black-and-silver's bloodlust on the field. The two had little in common personality-wise: Tatum, sinister of appearance, largely kept to himself, while Villapiano, everyone's instant friend, was as gregarious a man as ever walked the earth. But both possessed the two essential defensive Raider tools: they were the two most white-hot-intense men on the field—and they lived to hit. Both savored the sensation of a bell well rung.

The Tatum pick was a no-brainer. A versatile defender who'd won every award you could think of at Ohio State, including national collegiate defensive player of the year in 1970, he played "monster back": safety, cornerback, and linebacker. As for Villapiano, he'd been fantasizing about wearing the Raider uniform ever since Thanksgiving of 1970, back in Jersey, when he and his family had been watching the Raiders play the Lions in the traditional Turkey Day game. Oakland lost that one, but it wasn't the score of the game that had intrigued Villapiano; the Badass attitude on the visitors' sideline reached right out through the screen and hooked the kid.

"They were trying an experiment on the broadcast," Foo recalls, "and they were mic-ing the sideline. And you hear the players saying stuff like 'Get that motherfucker' and 'You fucking asshole.' They had to turn the mic off.

"The profanity was so bad my mother was saying, 'Who are these hoodlums?' Meanwhile, I'm saying to myself, 'Man, I'd like to be a Raider.'"

The game flowed in his blood. His dad, the athletic director for the Asbury Park (New Jersey) High Bishops, stored the school's football uniforms and equipment in the garage, whetting the kid's appetite for his future vocation. The Bishops' colors? Black and blue. Villapiano was the only sophomore starting on the team, doing what he'd always done best. "I just loved to fucking *tackle*, from the beginning," he says. "I thought it was the coolest thing in the world to tackle somebody."

Oddly enough, the young Villapiano's most memorable tackling day occurred at a baseball game. During his freshman year in high school the Jersey kid proved his physical mettle, with a battle he savors in memory. "There was this fucking kid," Foo recounts. "He was the bully of the neighborhood. Thought he was a hot-shit running back. And I knew it was going to come down one day when we'd have to fight. It was just gonna have to happen.

"So one day we're at a Babe Ruth game, and I said to him, 'Look, instead of fighting, why don't you try and run through me?' There were like twenty-five guys standing around, and so we clear out a lane. No pads. So he tries to get by me, and I fuckin' smash this fuckin' guy three fuckin' times. I just killed him. I rammed him so fuckin' hard, I knew I could do it. I just knew I could tackle him, and I did. It made me feel so fuckin' *happy*."

When his dad took a new job at a neighboring high school, Villapiano had to transfer schools. Ocean Township wasn't like Asbury Park, which had won the state championship in Foo's sophomore year. At the new school, they had to borrow helmets from one school, jerseys from another. But he attracted enough attention to get an athletic scholarship from Bowling Green.

"I was getting zero attention [in college], except for the Browns and the Giants—Alex Webster was their coach, and he was a Jersey guy," he recalls. "Then I played well in the Blue-Gray game, and another five or ten teams get interested, and I get invited to the Senior Bowl." Al Davis was, as always, in attendance, and while Jack Youngblood, of Florida, was named the defensive star of that game, Davis took the time to congratulate Villapiano afterward. Foo had made a slew of tackles, and he took Davis's post-game compliment of "Nice game, son" as an encouraging sign.

He may have been from a small school, but Bowling Green had sent a handful of players to the NFL—including All-Pro receiver Bernie Casey in the '60s—"and Al didn't give a fuck where you were from as long as you could tackle." After that game, Villapiano began to hear from scouts that he might go in one of the top rounds.

It was the last he'd hear anything from the Raiders until draft day, in January. Phil decided to hold a party for all of his friends and stocked up on multiple cases of beer. The draft wasn't televised, but that didn't hamper the festivities.

"So people start drinking at, like, ten. I wouldn't let anyone get near the phone. My mother calls, like, a hundred times. Now it was about noon, and nobody's called, I say, 'Fuck this, let's drink.' I figured I wasn't getting drafted. Everyone was getting *so* fucked up."

It was at 5:30 that the phone finally rang. Foo's girlfriend answered it and said the Oakland Raiders were on the other end. "I say, 'Get the map! Where's Oakland?'" He grabbed the phone and, through the beer buzz, heard Ron Wolf's greeting.

"I was pretty fucked up, but at twenty-two, you can get sober pretty quick. Wolf didn't care anyway. I say, 'What round was it?' He says, 'Second.' He says, 'We've been following you, and we really like the way you play. You could be a great Raider.'

"I think, 'Holy fuck! That's great!' Wolf says, 'Tomorrow we expect you to be in Oakland.' And that was the end of my education. I was in Oakland the rest of the school season. When I get out there, the first thing Madden says, he tells me, 'You're not gonna understand what you're doing out there. Don't worry about it. We just drafted you to make tackles.' I thought, 'Holy shit! How easy is that?'"

Not as easy as he'd hoped. Injuries to the linebacking corps in training camp and preseason thrust him into the starting lineup on opening day against the Patriots, and for Villapiano the transition was semi-traumatic. Bowling Green, Ohio, was one thing. The angry mammoths in black and silver were another. "You'd come off the field, everyone wanted to 'motherfuck' you. Jim Otto, Blanda, Madden—I had, like, fifteen coaches. I mean, *everyone* would motherfuck you. 'Cause you're playing, and you're a rookie.

"I'd have rather covered kickoffs and called it a day. I was so nervous at the start I can remember not being able to eat. The only thing I could get down my throat was lobster because of the melted butter. I was too afraid of fucking up. I was a fourth-team linebacker, and everybody gets hurt and now I'm first-team linebacker on opening day."

He would be the NFL's defensive rookie of the year, starting all 14 games. He didn't excel because of size (an inch over six feet, a dozen pounds over 200). "Why do you pick Villapiano?" asks his buddy Bob Moore, rhetorically. "Because he tackles everyone within fifty feet of him." Foo played with wild abandon, entirely unrestrained. On any given play, he was likely to either make a tackle on any part of the field or run himself out of the play because of blind, balls-out adrenaline.

"Phil was just a great tackler—a *great* tackler," Madden told me. "We'd had a bad year at tackling in 1970 [despite winning the division at 8–4–2]. I said to Al and Wolf, 'We want to take our first two picks and draft the best tacklers in college football. I'm tired of missing tackles.' You can teach it and coach it, but you can't practice live tackling. So if you can't practice it, you better go get it. We drafted Tatum one and Villapiano two, and we never had a tackling problem after that. All you need is a couple of them, and everyone else feeds off them. He was a hell of a linebacker."

And a great storyteller, right? At this observation, something like a frown clouds Madden's face: "Some of his stories are a little far-fetched." John Madden is not enamored of this ongoing characterization of his team as a posse of Badasses, of fringe personalities.

Madden would prefer to be known as the coach of an immortal football team. "The further you get away from the '70s," he told me, "the more of the lore you hear. But the truth of the matter is that we had a great core of very strong individuals. And if we had some guys who were a little off, they were the periphery."

But Villapiano, like Hendricks, like Casper, like many of the characters, was hardly on the periphery. He was always around the ball, taking his craft very seriously. "I always tried to figure out where a guy didn't like to get hit, you know?" Foo says. "Some don't like to get tackled around the neck, and I was really good at that. Knees. Ankles. Chest. I'd always try and hit them where they didn't want to get hit.

"And I was always trying to make the perfect tackle. You know how in the rodeo the cowboy lassos the bull around the back of his feet and pulls, and the bull goes down real quick? That's the perfect fucking tackle to me. Some tackles were just so perfect and effortless that you *and* the running back enjoyed it."

Maybe all you need to know about Phil Villapiano's mind-set on the field can be summed up by a recollection from defensive lineman Kelvin Korver. "I remember Foo coming back to a huddle one time. He got beat on a play, he was all dingy, he was hit so hard, and he's all wide-eyed. He says, 'Did you see that hit? Did you see that SOB? He cleaned my clock! This is the most fantastic game in the world! I can't wait to get back and do it again!'"

Villapiano didn't limit his lust for hitting to regular-season games, either. Consider his running duel with Kwalick, the All-Pro 49er tight end who would become his teammate in Oakland in 1975. Banaszak relishes the memory of Villapiano's exhibition-game duels with Kwalick as a 49er almost as much as Villapiano does.

"The week before one game against San Francisco," Banaszak told me, "Madden is telling him, warning him, 'Keep your jock on. This son of a bitch is *all-world*. He'll knock your dick off.' Now,

Phil was a very emotional and excitable guy. When you got Phil riled up he was bouncing off walls. And that week I had him ready to play. I said, 'Ginzo, I want you to knock that fucker's dick off. He's not as big and bad as Pinky says. Pinky will shit in his pants when you knock his dick off.

"Ginzo says, 'Rooster, I'm going to get that cocksucker right on the first play, right from the get-go.' The first play, they get the ball, they come out. Kwalick lines up to the strong side. He's next to our bench side, right? I'm hollering at Ginzo, 'Knock his cock off!' Ginzo gets up in his face, like one foot away. The ball is snapped—and all you see is blood flying out. Five flags come running into Phil's back. He's knocked the piss out of Kwalick. I think he knocked a tooth out. Blood shooting out everywhere. Phil was like a razor blade. When he hit you, he cut you up. This was a forearm right to the face. The ref says, '41, you're outta here!'

"I'm going, 'Ginzo, way to go!' I'm jumping up and down. Phil's going, 'Did I get him, Rooster? Did I get him good or what?' 'Yeah,' I says, 'you got him good.' Then Madden grabs me: 'What the fuck? You got him thrown out. Jesus Christ. Now he's no good to us.'"

That was actually the third bout with Kwalick, says Villapiano, wanting to set the record straight, and eager to elaborate on the rivalry, for it was always when the stars were standing opposite him—Russ Francis, Kwalick—that the gleeful demon emerged in Foo. The first time, they were both thrown out. The second year, Kwalick suckered him on a reverse. "I'm bleeding everywhere," Villapiano says. "The ref stops the game because I'm bleeding so much. I went to the wrong bench, and I was still yelling at him.

"It was the third year we never got past the first play. Madden was nuts. But it was always Banaszak's fault."

✕

The 1971 draft also brought in Clarence Davis, the running back out of USC, who would figure in the team's two biggest victories of the era with his slicing running and undersung blocking, and tight end Moore, who would be a reliable, sure-handed receiver and blocker until Casper replaced him in 1976. Moore fit in with the Raiders nicely from the start. He studied law at Stanford, where he earned the degree, but put law school on the back burner when he began to attract attention on the Cardinals' playing fields—not always for the right reasons. As a starting pitcher on the baseball team, playing down in Santa Clara against Stanford's rival, he managed to hit both of the All-American Strain brothers with pitches, causing a riot behind the stands between members of each school's football teams. Anyone who can prompt a fist-throwing melee without laying a punch of his own clearly had the Oakland Raiders in his future.

The '71 draft paled next to the 1972 crop, in which Davis and Wolf found not only two-fifths of the offensive line that would take them to the Super Bowl—right tackle Vella and center Dalby, originally selected for his long-snapping skills—but two receivers who, along with Biletnikoff, would make up one of football's consummate receiving corps. Mike Siani, chosen from Villanova in the first round, would start every game that year, and the Raiders took Cliff Branch in the fourth round out of Colorado, to serve initially as a punt returner.

Siani, a Staten Island kid with a Badass soul, was a possession man. Branch, from Houston, was nothing but pure speed. That the Raiders' top choice came from a small school better known for its basketball and track-and-field teams may seem weird on the surface, but the move was entirely in keeping with the team's draft-day philosophy, according to Wolf: "We didn't have any restrictions on what program they'd come from. We were trying to find football players. It didn't matter where they were or what their level of competition was. It was how good they were."

For Siani, like Villapiano, the transition from Villanova provided something of a shock, but in a slightly different way. Siani didn't know exactly what to expect, but it was nothing like what he encountered on his first day as a Raider: "I walk into the locker room at Santa Rosa, and my locker is with Biletnikoff, Stabler—all the wide receivers and running backs and quarterbacks are together. And I thought I was walking into a jail cell, instead of a football locker room: 'Who's got the cigarettes? Who's got the cigars?' The language . . . I thought, 'What in the hell is going on here?' . . . The hair, the mustaches, the sideburns . . . if you looked at those guys—Snake, Freddy—they looked like Hells Angels." Funny thing about that.

Siani adapted quickly. "Mike was right in there with the rest of us," says Villapiano. "He was a fucking wacko."

If Davis had the last say in the drafts, a close second belonged to personnel man Wolf. Yes, he's the same Ron Wolf who rightfully earned considerable fame as the GM of the Super Bowl Packers—just a younger version, and an integral, if then anonymous, piece to this puzzle. More than one player cites Wolf as the unsung hero of this tale.

"I heard about Wolf long before I saw him," Tom Flores recalls. "In camp, I'd walk by this one room where he hung out. It was always dark. All I could hear was the sound of this old Bell & Howell projector. I'd think, 'Who's that guy?' No one knew what he looked like. You just heard about him. But you never saw him."

"Ron Wolf was a one-man full-time personnel staff," Madden says, in near reverence. "And he was the one man who could *be* a one-man staff. I mean, Ron Wolf knew *every* player everywhere. Ron Wolf's mind was amazing. You could ask him, 'Ron, there's this junior wide receiver someone told me about at Alcorn,' and he would know him. He didn't have to go through notes and read stuff. He'd say, 'This is who he is, and this is what he does.' He truly had a photographic mind."

"I was just one of those guys lucky enough to be along for the ride," Wolf says now, and you are welcome to believe him if you want. But the consistent excellence of those Raider drafts, from the mid-'60s until he left in the late '70s, suggests otherwise.

Wolf never had his eyes set on the front office, but he'd had his brain wrapped around football from the start, working in 1963 for a publication called *Pro Football Weekly*, a small bible for the true fans in those days, which Al Davis read religiously. When the editor of the magazine met Davis, then the Raiders' head coach, at a wedding, Davis mentioned that he was looking for someone who knew players from the inside out. Davis knew the game, had always been thorough in his knowledge of the college landscape, but he needed someone to help him blanket that landscape with an extra radar.

"Al had this desire to always find a sleeper," Wolf told me. "Someone no one really knew about. We hit with a couple of them," he says, with no discernible trace of irony (they hit with a lot of them). "We always tried to pick the best player for the Raiders. There wasn't anything like need for position or that type of thing. To be perfectly honest, what Al Davis did was design that team, in his mold. Those of us who were there can take some credit, but really and truly, with the exception of Lamonica (John Rauch pulled the trigger on that one), those were all his trades. From Willie Brown to Ted Hendricks . . . I look back at the moves he made, and they were remarkable moves."

And if the corps that Wolf and Davis assembled takes the award for eccentricity, outrageousness, and, well, *lore*, Wolf insists that it would be a mistake to overlook the true character of these characters. "That myth of rogues was kind of perpetuated, but by and large they were pretty good people. And even better football players." Then, Wolf wasn't hanging at the Bamboo, or cheating at the air-hockey tournament, or riding in the parade. Or doing bed-checking.

Wolf *would* know about finding gems. As the general manager of the Packers, he would bring in an unknown named Brett Favre from the Atlanta Falcons.

The surprising clouds of cigarette smoke that Mike Siani had inhaled back in '71 were billowing out of the best receiver the Raiders have ever known, one of the men who made this team so easy to identify with. On the field, every time Fred Biletnikoff caught the ball and cut upfield, his hair would flap out of the back of his helmet like the mane of a blond horse. His eyeblack glistened like vampiric mascara, his skinny physique seemed no more muscular or toned than the average fan's. His uniform, instead of being contoured and skin-tight, seemed to flap in the wind. And he caught virtually every ball thrown his way.

"I've seen players today drop more passes in one game than I ever saw Fred Biletnikoff drop in his career," Siani says.

By the end of Freddy Biletnikoff's 14-year career, he'd gathered five miles worth of passes, including 70 postseason receptions, a Super Bowl MVP trophy, and a berth in the Hall of Fame—testament to a work ethic the likes of which none of his teammates had ever witnessed. Biletnikoff would hold his own post-practice practices, accompanied by his own bag of balls, snagging extra passes from Stabler—25 corner routes, 25 curl-ins. When Stabler had had enough, Biletnikoff would find someone else to throw him the ball, mentally preparing himself for any and all situations he might face in a game. Biletnikoff's workouts furnished the stuff of legends.

At just 6'1" and 180 pounds, he was determined to do whatever he could to give himself an edge.

"My rookie year," says David Humm, "I decide I'm going to stay out as late as the latest guy, and it was always Fred. I would work out with Freddy and his bag of balls, jump rope, hit the speed bag, do all this stuff in cycles." The speed bag, Madden says now, was Biletnikoff's way of keeping both hands in sync; one of the keys to being a good receiver, Biletnikoff believed, was having both hands always in place to catch the ball, both hands always working together. And his footwork was as precise as a ballet dancer's.

"I'd say to him, 'You done?'" Humm recalls. "He'd say, 'No, no, no.' I mean, we'd be out in the dark working out by the light of the back door."

"Freddy represents everything the team was," says Stabler, who counts among one of his own career highlights the day he threw the pass that made Biletnikoff the Raiders' all-time reception leader. "He wasn't the biggest, and, hell, *I* can outrun him. But he had a tremendous heart. He'd always find a way to come up with the ball—those rawboned hands always snatching a ball out of the air when you needed it most."

Biletnikoff, a modest man as a player and a modest man now, plays down the notion that he was doing anything exceptional with his post-practice routines. Like Villapiano, he was possessed with refining his craft. "I just loved going out there and staying after practice," he says now. "It was fun to be able to think about your routes, your footwork. I mean, the ball's not always going to be perfect. I liked being able to think about how high it might be, how low, covering my ass and catching all of those balls, too. You got to practice like you're going to play."

Born and raised in Erie, Pennsylvania, Biletnikoff was the son of a welder who'd been a boxer in clubs when Fred was a little kid. "I came from a tough background. I came from a neighborhood where it was very full of ethnic groups—Russians, Polish, blacks, Italians, some Jewish, some German—and you were brought up playing sports, because that's all you had. Nobody had a lot of money. You played within the neighborhood. You played against guys older than you, and those older guys kicked your ass."

Among his teammates, the Biletnikoff rituals resonate in memory nearly as vividly as the receptions. Let's start with the carefully shredded uniform. Biletnikoff would alter his garb like a meticulous tailor from the other side of the looking glass. If you're looking for a single symbol to represent the Raiders' innate disregard for outside authority, Fred's uniform is as good as any: an emblem for the whole team's disdain of petty rules and meaningless structure. The NFL had uniform dress codes, and the man they sometimes called Zhivago didn't. Freddy looked like a mailman in a shredded football uniform.

"Well, you can't go out on the field unless you feel good," he says now. "The more comfortable you make yourself, the better you feel. So to make the uniform more roomy, I would cut underneath the jersey, underneath my arms, so you'd feel like you didn't have a jersey on.

"Then I'd slit the back of my pants, because they were real tight pants. It looked ragged, but it was comfortable. And right where the jersey comes around the front I'd slice that down, so it wasn't so tight around my neck." Not to mention spatting his shoes with tape up to the ankle and wrapping his forearms with tape. It all made for a unique look—and brought Al Davis no end of consternation, as Pat Toomay recalls.

"One time we won a game in Cleveland, late in the year. There are three buses for the players afterwards. I always got on the last one, and this time there was just Fred, Snake, and I in the back.

Snake has a pint of whiskey in his bag. They have a drink. We're about ready to go. Then Davis gets on, the last guy. He sits behind the driver. And he turns and looks at the back, and stands up, and holds up a letter from the league, and points to it, and says to Fred, 'You cost me another $2,500 with the way you mess with your uniform.'

"Biletnikoff says, 'Fuck you. You told me, "Whatever it takes."'" Davis looked at him, and he laughed, and sat back down, and just shook his head.

"Fred says to me, 'I guess I told him, Tombstone,' and off we go."

The Biletnikoff ritual that stands universally enshrined in the team's collective memory, though, is the vomiting. It was Fred's habit, as he waited out the endless hours before the game, and the tension built, to visit the bathroom and disgorge whatever might be lying in his stomach. No one had any idea what Biletnikoff was disgorging, since no one saw him eat before a game, just chain-smoke his cigarettes.

"Madden made the comment one time," says Monte Johnson, "depending on how many times he threw up, you knew what kind of game he'd have. I think it was superstition, but whatever it was, Freddy would disappear into the bathroom, calling dinosaurs. That's what we called it, because he would make these odd, groveling, groaning noises. Like a dinosaur might make."

"I was just real nervous and intense," Biletnikoff explains now. "It was the waiting, waiting for hours. Every game to me wasn't just a game. It was a big game. Every game meant something to our team, and to me. The thought that you were never prepared enough when you went on the field, putting that on yourself is going to make anyone sick—until everything starts. And then you're fine. Then everything falls into place."

The Biletnikoff catalogue of eccentricities must include the Stickum, a gooey adhesive paste, which helped him hold on to the ball. Biletnikoff would apply the adhesive to various parts of his body: on his forearms, his socks. Biletnikoff wasn't the ochre-colored adhesive's first user, only its most famous; punt returner and receiver "Speedy" Duncan was using Stickum down in San Diego, and equipment manager Dick Romanski procured some of the glue for Fred to try. On a team where the rules were always malleable—where you did whatever it took to win—the stuff was clearly within bounds. Besides, Stickum was legal back then, if frowned upon by purists.

"It looked like a huge gloop," says Stabler. "From afar, it looked like it might be a four-inch bloody gash seeping through his socks. After he catches that first pass you have to go right to the official and get a new ball, because that one was all sticky. He was that way the whole game. Madden swears he once caught a pass that stuck to his forearm." Stabler laughs. "Freddy was just a mess."

"You needed paint turpentine to get it off," says Banaszak. "Fred would have it everywhere. His uniform. His head. His nose. His mouth." (Then again, Banaszak would know. He was not averse to using it himself in later years, along with fellow fullback van Eeghen.)

"It took me a day to wash off Biletnikoff's helmet," says Romanski now. "But he didn't really need it. He just used it to remind himself to hold on to the ball. Not that he needed to. Best pass catcher I ever saw."

"It was more psychological than anything else," Biletnikoff insists. "I never used it in practice or training camp. Only games. The biggest thing was you were able to hold on to the ball when you were fighting with the defensive back, and you have to have any opportunity you can to get a grip on it.

"But, yeah," he admits, "you're going to pull some balls out of your ass with it on . . . Sometimes it helped a great deal."

But it was so sticky it attracted the turf and the dirt like a magnet. "Whenever he fell he'd try and protect himself and turn to where he didn't get his hands in the dirt and the grass," John Vella recalls. "I'd be across from him in the huddle, and there were times when his fingers would be stuck together, and he had a bunch of grass stuck to them. Stabler would be calling the play, and Freddy would be saying, 'JV, help me out.' I'm reaching over to separate his fingers because they're all stuck together."

Biletnikoff's hands were covered with so much Stickum that he couldn't peel the paper off the sticks of gum he chewed during the game. The task of putting them into Biletnikoff's mouth fell to Romanski: "Every time he came out of the game, he had to have new gum. He was superstitious. He'd want spearmint sometimes, Juicy Fruit another. It was always three sticks. I'd mix 'em all up and he wouldn't know the difference."

"At halftime," Siani says, "Fred couldn't hold the cigarette. He'd have Romanski actually hold the cigarette for him so he could smoke it."

One other piece of the puzzle had come together in 1972, but not from the draft. Otis Sistrunk never went to college. He sprang like some ageless, mythical figure from the soil of the minor leagues.

In the summer of '72, the Rams had a surfeit of defensive linemen, and Davis was reportedly interested in Jack Youngblood. But he returned from a trip to the Ram camp, at coach Tommy Prothro's invitation, with unexpected news: they have a completely unknown guy, name of Sistrunk. And therein was born another legend. A few years later, when *Monday Night Football* commentator Alex Karras would note the steam rising off Sistrunk's bald head during a game and remark that Otis, with no college experience, had come from "the University of Mars," he wasn't far off: Otis Sistrunk's professional career theretofore had consisted of playing for the Norfolk Neptunes.

Wolf didn't think the Rams would trade Trunk, but they did, for a mid-level draft choice. "It was an unbelievable acquisition," he says. "This guy was exceptionally quick. He could play the run and he had a burst of speed and a surge to the quarterback. You'd think the guy was a number one pick. The fact that he was a minor-league player? Incredible. It's all a tribute to Otis's stick-to-it-iveness. Refused to give up on his dream."

He was raised in Columbus, Georgia, in a family of 10 kids, son of factory workers; during high school he moonlighted at a cotton mill for $1.05 an hour. After high school, Sistrunk moved to Wisconsin, where he got by on odd jobs and played semipro ball for $75 a game. A friend turned him on to the Continental League, where he played three years for the Neptunes before a Ram scout invited him to camp. Consider it a stellar college career, only without the college part.

"When I got to Oakland," says Sistrunk now, "John told me later, they knew nothing about me. 'Did he just get out of jail, or what?' They were taking a chance. 'Who's this guy Treetrunk?' So you come in with your big cigar and your dashiki, and you start doing your thing."

Madden's first question of the big man was what position he played. "I said, 'All four.' He said, 'Which one do you want?' I said, 'I play all four. Just say the magic word. Whatever makes the Raiders win, that's what I'll play.' When you make a boast like that, you better back it up. So I played in the first exhibition against Baltimore, and afterwards he said, 'You proved it.'"

"We had no background on him," Madden says. "We had no idea how old he was. And I never did know. I saw him at the Gene Upshaw memorial and he looked the same then as he did when he played for us. He looked old then. When he played for us he could have been anywhere between 30 and 60." And starting at defensive end by opening day? "He was that good. He was just a natural defensive lineman," says Madden.

Sistrunk would be named runner-up for rookie of the year, whatever his actual age. Two years later, he'd play in the Pro Bowl. Two years after that, he'd be wearing the championship ring. But he'll forever be known for the Mars line, and he is more than happy to live with it. Fame comes in myriad forms.

"People really want to put a tag on your back, I guess," he told me. "Doesn't matter to me. 'University of Mars' worked fine for me. It's not like it was cognac coming off my head. It was steam."

Befitting their contrarian ways, the Raiders bolstered their roster in most unorthodox fashion in the '73 draft. Oakland's previous resident punter had been a guy named Jerry DePoyster, who'd spent two years with the Raiders. He'd been an albatross around their neck. He had three punts blocked in '72. So for the first and only time in the history of the NFL, a punter became a first-round pick. According to Madden, it was the only time that the entire staff, from Davis and Wolf on down, had completely agreed on a first-round pick. (Then, according to Bob Zeman, no matter how many coaches and personnel people were in on the draft preparations, only one man's opinion ultimately carried weight: "Of course, Al would make the final pick. It might be 10 to one against him, but he'd make the pick.")

"There was no argument from any guy in the room when we decided on Ray Guy," Madden says now. "[DePoyster] had to catch the ball against his body, and you wondered if he was ever going to get it off. Every time you go to punt, you wonder, 'Is it going to be blocked, or dropped?' I said, 'I don't want to go through this again.'"

Why had an NFL team never used a top pick on a punter? Because there's nothing sexy about a punter. There's nothing glamorous about special teams. Even among kickers, the punter is a supporting actor. He doesn't contribute points; he's an asterisk. He does one thing, and one thing only. Punters generally occupy the fringe of a football team. But Ray Guy never stood on the fringe of the Raiders, on or off the field. He was a Badass from the very beginning.

"People said, 'How do you draft a punter in the first round?'" says Madden. "Because every defensive guy wanted him because he helped the defense. Because every offensive guy wanted him because he helped the offense. And of course everyone on special teams wanted him."

The Raiders traditionally scoured the country for overlooked, small-program gems, but everyone in the pro game knew about Guy, if only from his nation-leading 46.2-yard average. Every scout had seen the highlight films from Southern Mississippi, which included a come-to-Jesus highlight against Ole Miss during his senior year. Guy had been standing five yards deep in his own end zone when he kicked the ball. It landed somewhere around Ole Miss's 20, then bounced through the end zone. Officially, it was a 93-yard kick. Unofficially, the football traveled more than 120 yards before it came to rest against a fence.

This was not just a punter; this was the Roy Hobbs, The Natural, of punting, although in college his talents weren't limited to kicking. As a defensive back, Guy intercepted 18 passes in three years at Southern Mississippi. It was during his sophomore year that he began to gain notice with his punts, as he grew to 6'4" and some quirk of kinetic leverage kicked in. By his senior year, he was an All-American.

But if he'd had his way, Guy would have been starting at safety for the Raiders—or quarterback, a position to which he was named all-state in high school in rural Georgia, where he grew up on a farm. Ray Guy was a stellar small-town athlete who happened to be too good at punting to allow him to pursue his dreams of being a full-contact guy.

"Ron Wolf told him he could play safety when he signed him," Madden recalls. "The first day we practice, I look up and we have Guy in at safety, and I tell him to get the hell out of there. He said, 'But Wolf told me that if I signed with you I could play safety, too.' I told him, 'Ron Wolf lied.' We never had another conversation about him being a safety."

Madden would let Guy practice with the safeties over on the side, but not in a team drill or scrimmage. He was way too valuable. "See, he was a hyper guy. He couldn't just stand around. He'd always want to jump in and help, play defense against the receivers when you were walking through practices. He *could* throw the ball farther and harder than any of our quarterbacks, so then we started letting him throw the ball, which was safe, and it got his energy out of him."

It's a good metaphor for the athlete and his relationship to his team: Ray Guy wanted to be inside the heart of this squad—a place where he naturally belonged. He may have been drafted for his punting numbers, but it turned out Davis had found a dyed-in-the-wool Raider, the ideal addition to a team where membership in the clan meant more than filling a role on the field. He reveled in the company of his brothers. He'd serenade his teammates with his Martin D-35 guitar down at Clancy's, always starting his set with Merle Haggard's "Swinging Doors"—the lament of a broken-hearted cowboy who's found his place in a "smoke-filled bar."

He tipped a few glasses, too. "Hell, you look alongside of you to see who had that pitcher of beer," says Banaszak, "and Ray was right next to you slopping them down."

"Yeah, it was Uppy's, the Grotto, Big Al's . . . from Castro Valley to Walnut Creek to Jack London Square," recalls Guy fondly of the Oakland circuit. "We'd try to get to all of them. It'd take half the night to do it, but we'd get to all of them. Then always back to the Denny's at 3 or 4 o'clock in the morning. Boy, did you feel bad the next day at practice."

Ray Guy appreciated the Badasses' feel of family, and the Raiders' distinct place in their community. That sense of community prompted him to opt for the Golden Eagles instead of the storied Crimson Tide out of high school. He took pride in his small-town, hard-work roots and put no stock in the prestige that an Alabama career might bring. "Southern Mississippi was more of a home surrounding, you might say," he told me. "With the small-town thing, you get more of a closeness with your peers. The rural life makes you responsible. You understand your roots and you have a tendency to hold on a little bit more to who you are, where you're going, what you're doing when you get there.

"I don't like complex things," he says. "Life's too complex as it is."

When Guy got the call from Wolf, there were two things he swears he didn't know: who the Raiders were and where Oakland was. "But as soon as I got to the team, there was that family sense. After the first day, it was like I'd been there all my life. They were just like me. It made me feel at home.

"And they were all kind of pissed off, which is the usual Raider attitude anyway, and then remember that I was drafted just after the Immaculate Reception. But then, we always had something to prove—to the league itself, but more, I think, to ourselves. It wasn't one or two people . . . it was the whole dad-gum team." (Yes, he really talks that way.)

After his first official punt, things could have only gone up. "I had a great preseason, but when I stepped onto the field for the first real game, I was nervous. I grabbed the ball and hit it, caught it good. I look down the field, and the ball's not there. It went about 5 or 10 yards, and about four rows into the stands. Talk about being nervous—I didn't even know which bench to go to."

He finally made it back to his own side and sat down on his helmet. "I look up, and it's George Blanda." The veteran knew that the rookie needed to be pumped up. "You messed up, didn't you?" he said. "What did they draft you for? To be a punter. Then go do it. Have fun."

"That hit home," says Guy. "I got up, got over it, and started mixing with the players." And he never stopped. "It was always like 11 guys moving at one time, and they were smoking when they did it. We were kind of like those Transformers. You keep turning all those parts, fold them in, it's one big man."

And the foot furnished an integral part of the monster. In his rookie year, Guy averaged 45 yards per kick—10 yards more than his predecessor—and was named to the Pro Bowl.

"I still don't understand why he isn't in the Hall of Fame," says Banaszak. "That's just stupidity."

You'd have to be nuts to pass up a chance to ask the master about his craft, wouldn't you? How many chances do you ever get to tap the brain (and foot) of a man acknowledged to be the best there ever was, best there ever will be? You'd ask Ali about his jab, wouldn't you? Guy is happy to oblige, as best he can. To hear Guy tell it, there was nothing complicated about punting a football. "I just learned that every part of your body has a natural process, and you just have to keep everything in a natural alignment. You have to have timing and rhythm. Specifically, you don't grip the ball tight. You drop it where your foot naturally wants it to be. Then you trust your instincts.

"Where the power comes from, I haven't a clue. Maybe it's the long legs. Maybe it's the muscles. Maybe God gave me something a little bit extra."

But, alas, He never gave Guy, once he turned pro, the chance to muddy it up as a safety, to seize the day with a key interception—just slap his foot against a pigskin a thousand times. So he naturally took the spotlight when the chance presented itself.

Celebrity and punting are not exactly the closest of acquaintances, and when people started wondering during practices for the 1976 Pro Bowl, in New Orleans' Superdome, whether Guy could hit the dome's hanging scoreboard, why shouldn't he have thought about grabbing the moment? It didn't occur to him to actually attempt the feat until the middle of the game.

"As the team was walking to the line, it just hit me right then: 'Why not?' [Official] Jim Tunney was standing next to me, and I heard him say, 'You're going to try it, aren't you?' I nodded my head. When the ball was snapped, I knew if I caught it right, and I had the right trajectory, I'd at least come close to it.

"Then when I hit it, I knew I'd done it. When the ball left my foot, it was a perfect spiral. It just started rising and rising. If I'd have been a yard farther back, the ball would have gone *over* that thing. As it was, the back of the ball hit the top of the gondola, and the ball fell straight down."

The officials ruled that Guy had to kick the ball over again. He figured he'd best miss the scoreboard this time. "I nailed the next one, too. Went just under it. All I did was lower my drop a little bit." (In a practice for the 1980 Super Bowl, "I nailed that sucker four times in a row. We come out on Sunday, they'd raised that sucker all the way to the top.")

In the second round of the 1973 draft, Davis and Wolf took Monte Johnson out of Nebraska. A smart, hard-hitting student of the game, and veteran of two national championship teams, Johnson would anchor the Super Bowl defense in 1976. Like most of the Raiders at the time, his arrival in the loose fraternity was a tad eye-opening. "Coming in from Nebraska, Bob Devaney was my coach, Tom Osborne was an assistant," he told me. "We were disciplined and structured. You said 'Yessir' to the coaches. I remember sitting in the Raider training room and [defensive back] Nemiah Wilson is on the phone cursing the person he's talking to. I asked someone, 'Who in the world is he talking to?' 'He's talking to Al Davis.'"

Johnson also recalls another moment when he realized he'd stepped into another league: his first introduction to a new kind of performance enhancer that had nothing to do with motivational speeches. "It was my rookie year, one of the first games we had. When I was in college, I had a habit of taking salt tablets. So I walked into the training room and I asked someone where the salt tablets were. 'They're on that table in the Coke cup,' someone says. I walk over there. I grab a handful. I'm moving my hand up to my mouth. I'm going to pop them in my mouth. All of a sudden someone reaches out to grab my arm. My hand opens up and those pills go everywhere. The guy says, 'The *other* Coke cup.'"

Well, remember: this was the '70s, the era of amphetamines. No one remembers what color the amphetamines were in the Raider locker room. "We had . . . what we called rat turds," says Buehler, a man as straight as they come. Buehler took one once, he says, with no discernible effect. "They were just in a jar sitting there and you could take all you wanted."

On the Badasses, any advantage was worth exploring, although it's not exactly as if they needed an outside impetus to play like madmen.

"Sure, there was some of that taken . . . I ain't gonna deny that," says Banaszak. "But steroids? Hey, our steroid came in a brown bottle. It was Budweiser we loved. Kept your weight up, too. The trainer always said, 'Instead of Cokes, have three or four beers.' We had to listen to the trainer, right?"

"We didn't use performance enhancers," says George Atkinson. "I smoked a little weed, whatever, you know, but not none of that steroid shit."

How prevalent was the weed? Consider the time. Consider the region of the country. Cast your thoughts back to your own methods of cooling out in the 1970s. And then let's let defensive tackle Korver—the cerebral Texan they called "Jethro" (he wore bib overalls), a starter in every game in 1973 whose true high was (actual) crop dusting and stunt flying—put it in perspective: "Me? I was straight as an arrow. I never even held a joint. That's saying something for being around that group."

When I relay the quote to Atkinson, he lets out long peals of laughter—and then declines further comment.

The diverse cast was assembled, from top to bottom, from Foo to Freddy to the man from Mars. As the Raiders readied for 1973, the Western Division loomed strong, but on paper the Raiders figured to be the leaders of the pack, especially with Guy on board. And they had some extra incentive: the memory of the Deception. The only way to erase it would be to climb to the top once again and hope that the Steelers would be waiting for them. A score waited to be settled.

## CHAPTER ELEVEN

# The Snake

The first three games of the season presented an extremely tough test: the Raiders would open in Minnesota, against a Viking team that would win the NFC. They would host the mighty Dolphins, who had won the previous Super Bowl to cap their historic unbeaten season. Then they'd take to the road against the Chiefs, the age-old division rival.

There also lingered the question of who would lead the team. For the record, Madden said he was delighted to have so many quarterbacks. (Blanda was about to turn 46—but was only three seasons removed from 1970, when he had figured in five consecutive wins, as quarterback and kicker.)

Lamonica had been selected to the Pro Bowl the year before. But talk on the team suggested that Snake's time had come. They were entirely different quarterbacks, and entirely different men. Lamonica had a cannon of an arm and preferred not to use it for short passes. Against man-on-man coverage, when his receiver could beat his defender and break long and free, Lamonica was unsurpassed. Stabler, on the other hand, possessed the gift that had vaulted Joe Namath to the peak: an ability to recognize and immediately exploit an opening. Stabler had been around more than long enough to serve his apprenticeship; he knew the offense well.

On opening day in Minnesota, Lamonica started. He went 13 for 30 and threw two picks, and the powerful Vikings won, 24–16, despite Siani's 111 yards' worth of receptions and a Raider ground game that churned out 200 yards, led by Clarence Davis and Marv Hubbard.

In the second week, against the Dolphins, Lamonica started again. That he threw for just 63 yards was due in part to a ground-heavy Raider game plan. But the Raiders' inability to score a touchdown took a backseat to another story line in this one: the Dolphins had come in unbeaten in their last 17 games, the entire 1972 season, and the first game of this one. They were by now a team of history, and they seemed to have no flaws.

"The Dolphins had been bragging and bragging and bragging," Gerald Irons recalls. "If they won, they'd pass the Bears for most regular-season wins in a row. They had been talking about how they were going to celebrate." The game had been moved to the University of California's home field, the old oval Memorial Stadium, over in Strawberry Canyon, because the Oakland A's, who also played in the coliseum, were in the playoffs.

That day, "Mercury" Morris, an anchor of the Dolphin running attack, was wearing black-and-white elbow pads for the first time, as he would for the rest of his career. They represented an uncommon homage. "Willie Brown had given them to me at the Pro Bowl. I loved the Raiders. They were rebels, like me. They were wild, and that's why I wanted to be one of them. They always seemed to be the nemesis of the Dolphins. We pretty much controlled our destiny over every single team we played, with the exception of the Oakland Raiders."

Morris was also convinced that Davis had watered the Memorial Stadium field; he remembers the sprinklers showering the turf.

This much is certain: the Dolphin ground game spun its wheels that Sunday. The Raider defense held Morris to 48 yards, Larry Csonka to 47 yards, and Jim Kiick to just 10. Bob Griese completed just 12 of his 25 passes. The Raiders won, 12–7, on four Blanda field goals—and a defensive game plan that muted Griese's effectiveness, cued by something that Zeman and Madden and the players had noticed on film.

"If he was going to throw to his right," Willie Brown says, "his shoulders were always turned to the right. If he was going to throw to the left or over the middle, his shoulders were squared. He did it enough for us to use it as a key." (Covering Paul Warfield that day, Brown realized that a bee had somehow flown into his pants for a few minutes, but he never came off the field, "I got stung, but I didn't get burned.")

The true star that day was Irons, the right outside linebacker out of Maryland State, another small-school Wolf/Davis discovery. Irons's consistent excellence at the position—his forte was his ability to keep his feet, stand up the block, and fill the lane—has been obscured by his lack of flamboyance; no renegade tales embellish the Gerald Irons saga. He spent his off-seasons as a Raider going to the University of Chicago to earn an MBA.

For Irons, the satisfaction of that game lasted into the next night, when he and his family were watching *The Tonight Show*. "Carson had invited Csonka and Jim Kiick to come on the show the following day," Irons recalls. "Csonka and Kiick had these somber faces. Carson said, 'Guys, we were supposed to be celebrating. What happened?'"

As Irons proudly recalls it, "Csonka says, 'A guy named Gerald Irons happened. You'd have thought we had said something derogatory about his mother. Every time we had the ball, he knocked us down.' That was definitely a high for me."

✕

Irons vividly remembers his first exposure to the team, as a rookie in 1970: a seminar in the Raider way of doing things. He'd expected professionalism. He just hadn't expected the level of commitment he encountered. "It was my first practice. Madden blew the whistle, calls the whole team up: 'Great practice, guys. Go get some lunch. See you this afternoon.' I felt good. I take off running to the locker room, and suddenly he called me back: 'Irons, where you going? Turn around and look at where your teammates are.'"

None of his teammates had left the field. They'd all stuck around to get in some extra work. "Biletnikoff had his 20 or 40 balls with Stabler, working on his timing. Tatum and those guys are working extra on pass coverage. I was the only one going into the locker room."

That was the day when Irons discovered another key to the Badass' success at their craft: they took it more seriously because they seriously enjoyed the game. Football was far more than a job. The lesson stuck with Irons the rest of his career. "After that, I was out there with them, every practice, after morning and after noon, for 30 minutes at least, working on blitzing, working on shedding blocks, on wrapping up the tackle, on covering guys out of the backfield. Little things you don't get a chance to work on during practice, right down to things like keeping your feet in bounds, tiptoeing on the sidelines. You'd always get a couple of other guys there to help you improve. That was just the Raider way."

"Guys would always help each other out," says Madden. "Branch would help Shell on speed rushes. Or if a defensive back wanted more work to prepare for a guy who had a good inside move, someone would stay after to help the DB get his inside foot up. During the regular season, you can't get a lot of repetition, so that's where they'd work on the extra stuff. Biletnikoff would stay out 'til no one was left to throw to him. Then he'd use the Jugs machine. But everyone did stuff like that. Guys would always practice after practice. They enjoyed it. They had fun doing it; that was the key. Because they were all friends. They loved each other."

Irons would be a stalwart at linebacker until he was traded to the Browns. Eventually he would be named one of the top 100 Browns of all time. But today, it's not Cleveland he wants to discuss: "Even if you go to the Cleveland Browns, you're always a Raider. Once a Raider, always a Raider. That's a beautiful legacy. We were the class of the league."

The third week, at 1–1, the Raiders traveled to Arrowhead Stadium, home of their age-old rivals, full of fans wearing the traditional Chief bright red, clouds of fragrant barbecue smoke perfuming the tailgate air. On this day, one of the signs in the stands read, "The Only Good Raider Is a Dead Raider."

"We definitely didn't like each other," says Walter White, a Chiefs tight end in the '70s. "They got after you. Everything was fair play. Clothesline, cheap shot. It was just a 15-yard penalty to them." Well, no; it was just football the Badass way, at least whenever it was the Chiefs on the other side of the line.

That third game also signaled a significant transition on the offensive line. The week before, when Boomer Brown went down in the first quarter, second-year tackle big John Vella had spelled El Boomo. That week, Madden called Vella in to tell him he'd get the start against the Chiefs. Vella's first reaction wasn't joy and elation. Nor was it nervousness. "Nope, my first thought was, 'Has Madden told Bob yet?' I didn't want to go out there with the first team at the start of the game and have Bob be there, too.

"So I ask John if he's told Boomer yet, and he says, 'Oh, no, no, I haven't told him, but I will, I will.' I didn't know if or when he'd get around to it. And I don't want to risk Bob being in the huddle with me. So I decided to tell him myself: 'John told me I'm going with the first group.' And Bob says, 'No problem. I'll help you.' And he did. He went out of his way. That was the atmosphere on the team. The feeling on that team was guys always helped you. He couldn't have been nicer."

Brown's replacement didn't go in for guns. Or gambling. Nor did he favor slugging pitchers of beer. Vella's calling card was his attitude. "He had his Italian temper," fullback Mark van Eeghen says now. "He just didn't take shit from anyone. He wasn't as big as Shell, but he had a temperament that made up for it. He had quick hands and quick feet. On the line, usually with a guy who was bigger and tougher you don't want to mess with, he'd be the guy to say, 'Fuck you.'"

Now, in the fourth quarter, the Raiders were down 9–3 to the Chiefs, and facing the unthinkable: two losses in their first three games. The offense was entirely out of sync. Lamonica had completed just 4 of 12 passes for 53 yards, with one interception, and the Chiefs were stifling the ground game.

So, with six minutes left, Madden reached for his Alabaman, as he had in the Deception game. Stabler came in and threw six passes and completed all of them. Unfortunately, two were to Chiefs. Stabler's second pass bounced off Hubbard and was intercepted by Willie Lanier, who returned it 17 yards for a touchdown.

The final score was 16–3, Chiefs, and the Raiders, at 1–2, were now a team adrift. They'd played 12 quarters without a touchdown. The next week they'd face Don Coryell's high-powered St. Louis offense, which, behind quarterback Jim Hart, was averaging more than 25 points a game.

"Looking back," Bob Moore says today, "it wasn't a team that was really settled at that point."

"We were struggling," Madden admits now. And the quarter-back position obviously had something to do with the problem. Stabler, of course, wanted the shot. He felt he deserved it. A few days after the Chief game, Stabler walked into Madden's office.

"We were struggling and he was pissed," says Madden now. "He said, 'I don't want to wait until the game is over and have to do the mop-up shit.' He thought he should be the starter.

"Well, you have to *do* something," Madden told him. "You're not going to come in here and talk me into starting you. You have to show me. You have to show the team that you should be the starter. What are you doing? You're not showing anyone."

That week, imitating Hart in practice plays, and running Coryell's offense, Stabler picked apart the Raider defense. "He started to practice with a chip on his shoulder," Madden says. "Maybe I watched him more closely after that. And I started him. And he just came in and took over. I said, 'Holy Shit.'"

Stabler finally got his chance. But the promotion was significant for the head coach, too. "Remember, as a head coach, he became my first quarterback. I inherited Lamonica. Stabler was never a starter before I was the head coach. He was my first." And his last.

The next week, Stabler led a 17–10 defeat of the Cardinals, completing 19 of 31 passes, and Gene Upshaw gave Stabler the game ball. The Cardinal win was the first of five straight Raider victories, including a game against the Baltimore Colts in which Stabler completed 25 of 29 passes for more than 300 yards, including 14 completions in a row. Stabler started the rest of the season, and most of the next seven years (barring injury), taking the Raiders to five straight conference championships and the Super Bowl.

For some Raiders, the change was a long time in coming.

"Kenny should have been the quarterback as early as 1971," says one of his teammates now. "There was a constant sense on the team that Kenny should have been playing. Daryle was a different personality. He wasn't really a Raider, and that made it hard for him. It was a situation where there was a lot of anxiety, angst on the team. Daryle liked to run around and shoot lions or something. He was a big-game hunter. Kenny liked to hang at the bar, chase girls, and have fun."

"We were lovable renegades," Ken Stabler says now of his Badasses. But he's really talking about himself.

In the spring of 1968, the Raiders' second-round pick stood smack in the middle of the Haight, in San Francisco, the Raiders' second-round pick, wearing an Alabama letter jacket. Stabler was a $50,000 bonus baby with a four-year contract for $76,000 more. There he stood, the Raider future, amid the fragrance of pot and patchouli, the forests of wild hair, the tie-dyed ensembles of the street musicians: the future of the franchise.

"That was the first time I went out there," Stabler recalls. "Wolf took me—the first stop—to the corner of Haight and Ashbury. I don't know why. Honest to god. The second stop was Telegraph Avenue"—over in Berkeley, the epicenter of the student revolution.

Wolf doesn't remember why he chose that locale, either. But isn't it logical? Wolf knew he had a fun-loving renegade on his hands, and what better way to introduce the boy to the Bay than to bring him to the capital of joyous rebellion?

He'd come a long way from rural Alabama, and while physically he'd eventually return to his beloved Gulf Coast, psychologically he would forever be a Raider—the laid-back leader, the life-long keeper of an unquantifiable statistic: he invariably knew how to find a way to win.

Six months later, in the autumn of 1968, Stabler stood in the middle of a bleachered, high-school-size stadium, several hundred miles to the north of the coliseum and Haight-Ashbury, but metaphoric worlds away, wearing the colors of the Spokane Shockers, of the Continental Football League—a team named not for its potential to intimidate but for a different kind of shocker: farmers who would gather sheaves of wheat. He was a bonus baby playing for a team named for a grain. Throwing a football in practices so half-assed, with teammates so clueless, he recalls, that he'd fade back and see offensive linemen running down the field for passes alongside his receivers.

He was playing in front of a few thousand—or hundred—people, competing against . . . well, who remembers? Was it the Oklahoma City Plainsmen? The Quad Cities Raiders? Gimping around on a post-surgical left knee, all Stabler knew was that he'd once won the Sugar Bowl for the Crimson Tide and turned down Major League Baseball offers as a high-school senior, but here he was in the minors. "It wasn't exactly the coliseum. You're in Spokane. And you ask yourself, 'What the hell are you doing here?'"

Technically, he was getting a tryout. Davis and Madden wanted to see if the kid's knee would hold up, the knee that had bloody fluid drained out of it after every game of his senior year at Alabama. He completed 17 of 41 passes in two Shocker games and returned to the Raider injured-reserve list.

By the next spring of 1969, there stood Stabler in the parking lot of San Francisco International Airport, having borrowed a teammate's car to get to his flight home: he was quitting the team. This was year two for the Crimson Tide phenom. Wasted.

By now, Stabler was mired in last place on the quarterback depth chart. In 1968, the Raiders had used their first-round pick on Dickey, out of Tennessee State, the first black quarterback ever drafted by an NFL team in the first round. Davis and Wolf thought that Dickey could be used as both quarterback and wide receiver. Other than in exhibition play, though, Dickey never played quarterback and caught just five passes before the Raiders cut him, in 1971.

How could Stabler have been available in the second round, after his stellar years in Alabama? Easy, Wolf says: "There was this belief that left-handers could not play." There was no science behind this philosophy, of course, just superstition as much as anything else; left-handers were, well, just thought to be different. "Paul Brown came out and said it. Other than Frankie Albert [in the '40s], there weren't any left-handers. But I had seen him play. Ken Stabler personified the term *accurate*. So you had to just get rid of that basic prejudice. It came down to somebody like myself saying, 'Why not? He's playing at Alabama. You don't have a higher level.'"

But in spring camp of 1969, Stabler began to have doubts about whether the strength of his arm could meet the demands of the NFL. He had lost confidence in himself, for the first time in his life. "I couldn't play the way I wanted to play," he says now. "I couldn't be the athlete I wanted to be. I got frustrated with that. I got frustrated with being separated from my wife. So I took off. I was capable back then of throwing it all away."

And then, one year later, thanks to a phone call to the Raiders made by an attorney who would become a life-long Stabler friend, there he stood in front of John Madden, asking for one more chance at the spring workouts. He was delighted to find that his coach was more than forgiving.

"Madden and I went through all the reasons I'd left," Stabler says now. "He said, 'You want to come back and make things right? Come back on the team.' And Madden was all for it."

As chance would have it, the league's players association was threatening to strike, and owners had barred vets from working out with their teams. Madden watched his only quarterback closely and liked what he saw. In this third year under contract, Stabler had finally come home to stay. The veterans returned to camp in time for the preseason, but Stabler played three quarters in the first exhibition against the Colts, taking some violent hits from the Super Bowl losers, and earning the respect of his veteran teammates.

Looking back, the fact that he was still standing at all was a little surprising. "He did live life hard," says Monte Johnson. "Kenny kept the pedal to the metal."

"Just stay in the fast lane, and keep moving," Stabler wrote in his autobiography, *Snake*. "You cannot predict your final day, so go hard for the good times while you can."

Whether it was kicking out the lights on the top of a police car as a teenager, piling up a catalogue of youthful speeding tickets, or scrambling out of a pocket on that weakened left knee, Ken Stabler always seemed to be moving—until he found his place with the black and silver. The team had found the man to personify its image: the Badass King.

Stabler grew up outside of a town called Foley, 4,000 strong: corn and soybean country. He averaged 30 points a game in basketball and he was an ace pitcher in high school. But throwing a football was his true gift. As the starting varsity quarterback, his teams won 29 of 30 games.

His athletic prowess in one particular game earned him his first car from his dad: a big-block Chevy. Ken Stabler would always be into motorized speed, whether on the highways or pushing his speedboats to the limit on his beloved Alabama Intercoastal Waterway. That particular game also earned him a whupping, a few days later, when he skipped practice to spend a little time with a local female acquaintance, and had to bend over and grab his ankles for a paddling from his coach—the same coach who'd bestowed him with his nickname: "Damn, that boy runs like a snake!"

And, like many a high-school kid, he had a taste for the suds. Blame the beer for the time he kicked out the light on top of a police car—but even that indiscretion carried a promising football subtext: to pay back his dad, who had to pony up for the damages, he was given a construction job by an Alabama alum.

Any kid can stomp on a *car* after a few beers. But a police car? Sure, it was done to exact revenge for a friend who'd been hassled by the local cops. But a squad car?

"I was a victim of circumstance," Stabler says now. "Just a victim of circumstance," he repeats.

"I don't know that I was wilder than most," he insists. "I don't know that I did what other kids don't . . . But there has to be a fire in you. I don't know if there's a wildness, but I think there has to be inside of you something that makes the fire burn harder than others."

In his junior year at Alabama, Stabler set an SEC completion-percentage record and led his undefeated team to a 34–7 rout of Nebraska in the Sugar Bowl, for which he earned MVP honors. But after tearing up some cartilage in his left knee while training that spring, he started skipping practices. He would later reflect that the injured knee, which would never fully heal, made him a savvier quarterback, teaching him the necessity of pocket presence when his instincts told him to scramble. But he had speed, he had an instinct for approaching linemen, and he could still run when he had to. Today, Ron Wolf insists that, had his legs been healthy, Stabler would have been decades ahead of today's running quarterbacks: "He would have revolutionized the game."

But that spring at Alabama, the frustration of not being able to participate on the field compelled him to run away all the same. Road trips down to Mobile to see a girl, memorialized by the speeding tickets, took the place of practice attendance, and soon he was ignoring school altogether. Of course, he was following in some pretty hallowed footsteps; four years earlier, Paul Bryant had suspended a guy named Namath for the final two games of the 1963 season for a drinking incident. "Kind of a badge of courage," Madden says now, with a laugh, of the Stabler pedigree.

Bryant suspended Stabler by telegram. Two hours later, a follow-up telegram from Namath to his fellow Alabaman read, "He means it!" Stabler was allowed to return to the team, after pleading his case before his coach, and celebrated his reinstatement with a six-pack. Three plays into the first game of the season, Bryant put him back on the field. He never left. Years later, Bryant would confide to Madden that "Stabler's better than Namath." Lifetime statistics would back it up. In his senior year, he took the Crimson Tide to the Cotton Bowl. They lost that one, but Stabler had established himself. Whether it was the nonchalant reputation at 'Bama or the left-handed throwing arm, he slipped to 52nd in the draft. But as he'd always done, he shrugged off the insult. He just wanted to play ball. He just wanted to keep moving.

Stabler had been able to familiarize himself with the Raider system over the previous three years he'd spent on the bench. But it's not as though he ever paid much attention to the playbook or the game plan. Ken always played more of a version of schoolyard ball: Get open, I'll get it there. "I didn't study in front of film, like a Peyton Manning," he says now. "I went out and played the game. But remember: it was a simpler time, and a simpler game. The

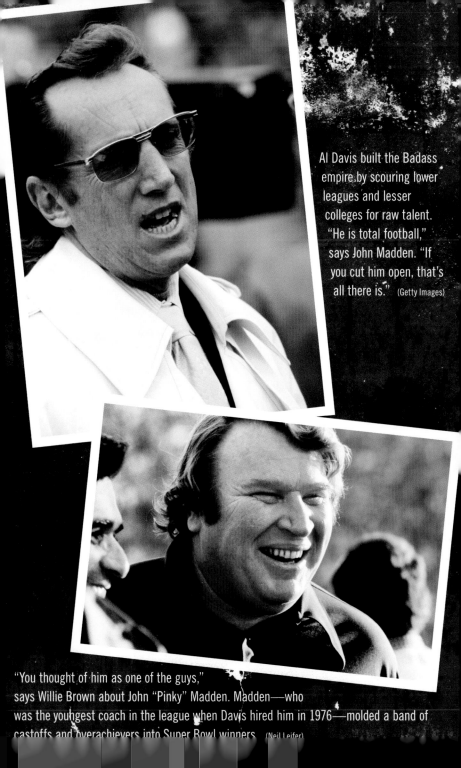

Al Davis built the Badass empire by scouring lower leagues and lesser colleges for raw talent. "He is total football," says John Madden. "If you cut him open, that's all there is." (Getty Images)

"You thought of him as one of the guys," says Willie Brown about John "Pinky" Madden. Madden—who was the youngest coach in the league when Davis hired him in 1976—molded a band of castoffs and overachievers into Super Bowl winners. (Neil Leifer)

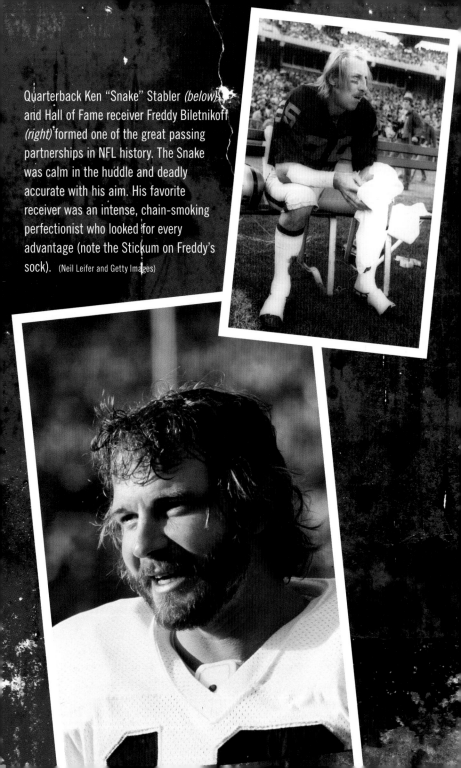

Quarterback Ken "Snake" Stabler *(below)* and Hall of Fame receiver Freddy Biletnikoff *(right)* formed one of the great passing partnerships in NFL history. The Snake was calm in the huddle and deadly accurate with his aim. His favorite receiver was an intense, chain-smoking perfectionist who looked for every advantage (note the Stickum on Freddy's sock). (Neil Leifer and Getty Images)

Fullback Pete Banaszak was a leader when it came to hitting the bars in Santa Rosa, where the Raiders held training camp. "When the Raiders were in town," says the Rooster, "the hookers rejoiced." A short-yardage specialist, the Rooster scored two touchdowns in the Raiders' Super Bowl victory over the Vikings in 1977.

(Getty Images)

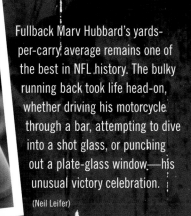

Fullback Marv Hubbard's yards-per-carry average remains one of the best in NFL history. The bulky running back took life head-on, whether driving his motorcycle through a bar, attempting to dive into a shot glass, or punching out a plate-glass window—his unusual victory celebration.

(Neil Leifer)

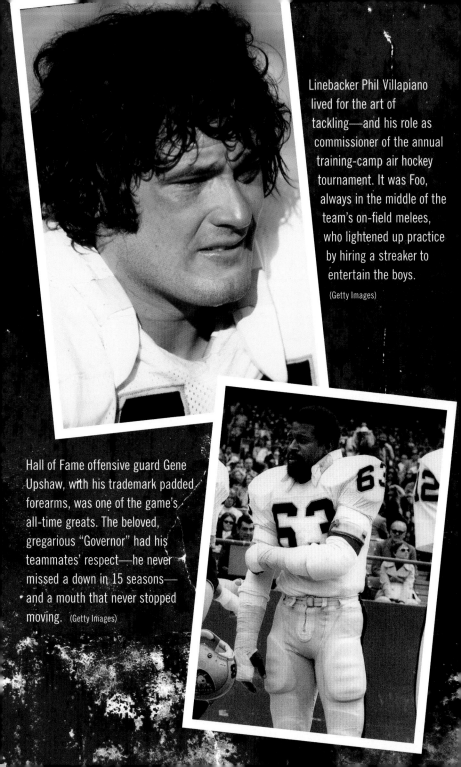

Linebacker Phil Villapiano lived for the art of tackling—and his role as commissioner of the annual training-camp air hockey tournament. It was Foo, always in the middle of the team's on-field melees, who lightened up practice by hiring a streaker to entertain the boys. (Getty Images)

Hall of Fame offensive guard Gene Upshaw, with his trademark padded forearms, was one of the game's all-time greats. The beloved, gregarious "Governor" had his teammates' respect—he never missed a down in 15 seasons— and a mouth that never stopped moving. (Getty Images)

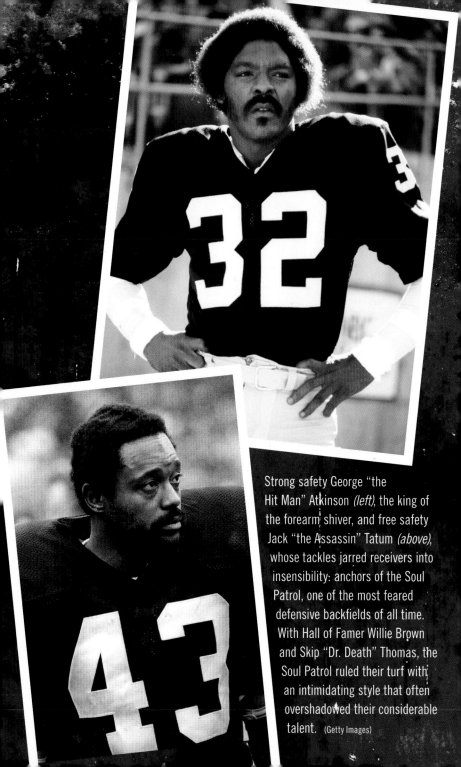

Strong safety George "the Hit Man" Atkinson *(left)*, the king of the forearm shiver, and free safety Jack "the Assassin" Tatum *(above)*, whose tackles jarred receivers into insensibility: anchors of the Soul Patrol, one of the most feared defensive backfields of all time. With Hall of Famer Willie Brown and Skip "Dr. Death" Thomas, the Soul Patrol ruled their turf with an intimidating style that often overshadowed their considerable talent. (Getty Images)

Workmanlike fullback Mark van Eeghen, the economics major from Colgate who three times put in a thousand-yard season—"the most underrated fullback in the history of the game," according to lineman Mike McCoy. Van Eeghen's blocking and running were highlights of the Super Bowl victory. But off the field he stayed out of the fast lane: "I was a choir boy compared to most of them." (Neil Leifer)

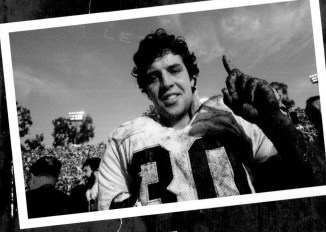

Flamboyant Hall of Fame offensive tackle Bob "Boomer" Brown: always on the attack, whether protecting the quarterback, bulldozing the training-camp goalpost, gambling on the team plane, or firing his pistols in the middle of the night.

(Neil Leifer)

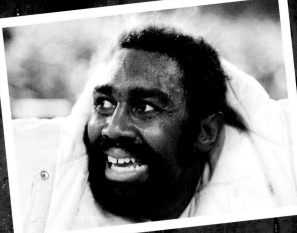

Defensive end John Matuszak provided the final piece to the Badass puzzle. The huge wildman's outrageous behavior, including his fondness for guns and his taste for various substances, ultimately overshadowed a solid career. "When people expect you to be wild, talk about you being wild, encourage you to be wild, you begin to *be* wild. It's almost as if you *become* your image." (Getty Images)

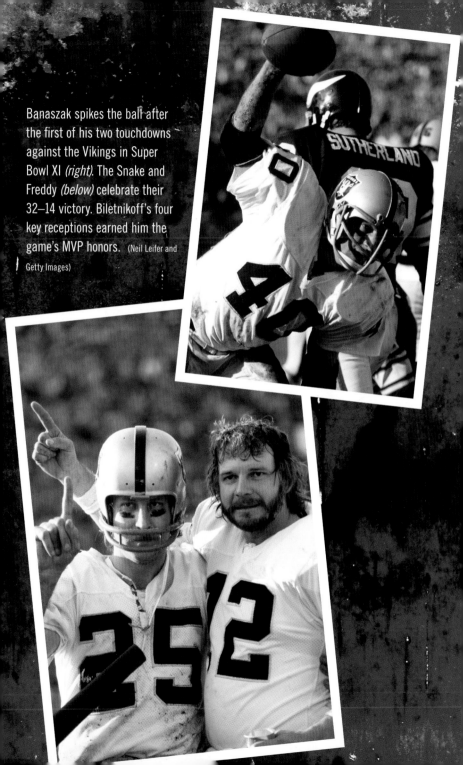

Banaszak spikes the ball after the first of his two touchdowns against the Vikings in Super Bowl XI *(right)*. The Snake and Freddy *(below)* celebrate their 32–14 victory. Biletnikoff's four key receptions earned him the game's MVP honors. (Neil Leifer and Getty Images)

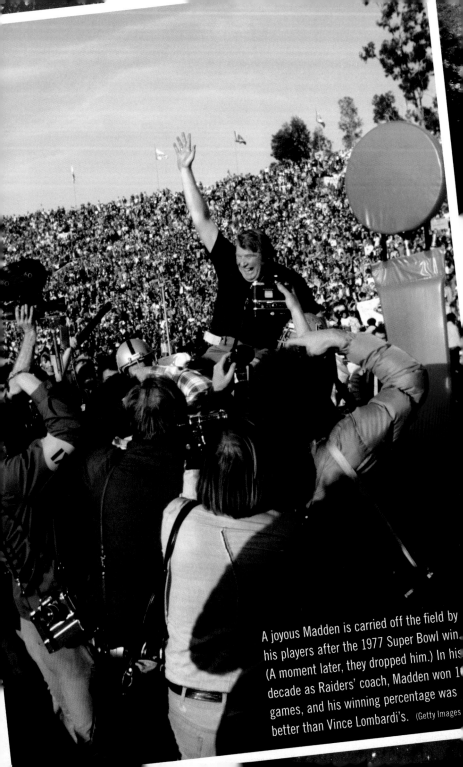

A joyous Madden is carried off the field by his players after the 1977 Super Bowl win. (A moment later, they dropped him.) In his decade as Raiders' coach, Madden won 1 games, and his winning percentage was better than Vince Lombardi's. (Getty Images defenses weren't sophisticated. John would give me the playbook at the Wednesday-night meeting. But I didn't study the game."

As for his particular skills? Start with the quick release. Any Stabler fan remembers the eyes darting all over the field, the ball held out in the left hand, poised and primed for flight; once he saw an opening, the ball would be out of there in a flash.

"The whole thing is seeing it, reading it, deciding where you're going, and getting it on its way," says Madden. "He had that quicker than anyone. He was amazing."

"Kenny," says Banaszak, "was the most accurate fucking thrower. If you wanted the ball between the four and the zero, he'd put it there. If you wanted it in the ear hole, Kenny could put it there."

"It sure didn't have a lot of velocity on it," Stabler says now, with a laugh. "But I think accuracy is the thing that's overlooked and underrated. That was my game. It's not just a high completion percentage, or quickness of release. It's where you put the ball. I had a pretty good knack of putting the ball where I wanted."

He also arrived at the right time. When Lamonica started out, defenses generally played man-to-man coverage, and a quarterback with a big arm could exploit that scheme. But in the early '70s, defensive coordinators began to turn to zone coverages, and against a zone, the strength of your arm didn't matter as much as your ability to anticipate the openings in the zones—and your ability to exploit the openings when they appeared.

"It was kind of a fun chess game between the offense and the defense," Stabler says. "The idea of calling the plays, of matching up, that's the part I enjoyed the most, and John let me go do that. There were times he'd be ranting and raving, 'I need a play! I need a play!' I'd just stand back and let him rant and rave, and then when he was done, he'd look at me and say, 'What do *you* want to do?' I'd say, 'I'd like to do this,' and he'd say, 'Then go do it.'"

But accurate quarterbacks are hardly an anomaly. Teammates

and coaches suggest that it was Stabler's almost serene demeanor on the field, in the huddle, on the sideline, in practice that distinguished him most from any other quarterback. He may have lived wildly on the circuit, but on the field he was laser-focused.

"The bigger the situation, the calmer he got," Madden says now. "Which was a great combination with me, because I was just the opposite. I was intense. If everything were normal, and we were ahead, he'd get bored. He had to have his ass to the fire to get really focused in on something. Then, when he really got focused in, instead of getting excited and tight, he'd get calm."

Madden vividly recalls a moment near the end of the memorable 1977 playoff game against Baltimore, which went into six quarters. "I was thinking of a play to call, or three plays. 'We'll do this, or this.' So anyway, he was listening to me, he had his helmet cocked up, and he was taking a drink, and he says, 'I'll tell you one thing,' he says. I thought what was coming was 'Let me throw this, I'll get you a touchdown.' Instead he says, 'These fans are getting their money's worth today.'"

Equally impressive to his offense was Stabler's egalitarian attitude: he never stepped over the fine line from teammate to commander. He never pulled rank. The most critical thing anyone can ever recall him saying in the huddle, after a brutal sack, was "That ball sure attracts a crowd, doesn't it?"

"I want to tell you what I never saw him do," says John Vella. "I never saw him chew guys out. He never once said, 'You should have run here.' Never did I see Stabler single a guy out. It was always just like 'All right, next play.'"

"He was usually the one guy in the huddle who *wasn't* talking," says Bob Moore. "In the huddle, it was always Upshaw talking, or someone else—well, primarily, Upshaw talking and someone responding to Gene. Meanwhile, Kenny is as quiet as you can be. Calls the play in the same voice in the fourth quarter as the first quarter. Same guy starting the game as he was at the end. Same guy as he was in practice. All kinds of things would be going on around him, and he'd be as calm as he could be. Strangely calm."

"I learned a lot from the way Madden would always put it in perspective," Stabler says. "He would always say, 'Don't get too high, don't get too low.' There's a calm plane, a middle plane in there. Win, lose, hurt—you can't get too low over it. Put it in perspective."

"I started my life third and long," Stabler told me. "I skipped practices. I got kicked off my high-school team. I got kicked off my college team. I left pro football in 1969. I've had third and 15 my whole life. Everybody's had rocky moments from day one. But sometimes you pick up third and long, and that's where you make your money. That's where the satisfaction comes, from the game and from life."

He was the son of a complicated, mood-swinging, deep-drinking, and occasionally violent man named Leroy "Slim" Stabler, ace fix-it and auto mechanic. According to Stabler's book, it was the bourbon that fueled the third-and-longs for the father. It was the bourbon behind Slim Stabler's desire to take on four men in a fight outside a social club over something as petty as the outcome of a high-school basketball game. It was the bourbon that lay behind the kid's awareness that physical punishment from the old man could lurk a sip away.

"He was a war veteran" was all Snake would tell me. "He didn't peel potatoes. He killed people. And those war demons . . ." He lets the sentence go unfinished, settles on something else. "He didn't have anything, he didn't make much money. I went and signed a contract for more money than he'd probably made in his whole lifetime. Maybe he felt a little jealousy. He saw my games at Alabama, but he never saw me play in the pros. He died of a massive heart attack."

I ask him what role Slim Stabler played in his youth, a youth that coupled extraordinary athletic achievement with that rebellious streak. "I don't really know how much he had to do with it," Stabler told me. "I learned how not to do some things. How not to treat family. Because of issues that I had with him, it put a lot of things in perspective."

Perhaps Slim is the source of his son's famous cool. A hint comes from a passage in Stabler's book. "I was made up of Slim Stabler's genes," Stabler wrote. "I had to guard against ever losing control the way he did. . . . Maybe that's why, from way back, going for the good times became such an important part of my life. Having fun, I could not be set upon by anything like Slim's demons."

"He was a million years old," says Betty Cuniberti, who counts herself a true Stabler fan. For all of the girl chasing, Stabler—unlike some of his teammates—treated Cuniberti like a gentleman. With a kind of age-old, innate wisdom. "He came across to me as someone who knows suffering. And he kind of understands that."

Growing up, Stabler idolized the famed late quarterback Bobby Layne, a man known for his hard-drinking ways almost as much as for his football prowess for the Lions and Steelers in the '50s and '60s. "Maybe I wanted to be that kind of player," Stabler says. "You don't have to do the conventional things the night before. It doesn't matter as long as you did it the next day, and we did it consistently."

Was he striking out at disbelievers as he grew up? Was he trying to prove a point to the doubters? "I don't know if maybe I was fighting out against everything. You just go and do it, regardless of what people think. Sometimes it's the fact that you were the kind of kid who always had issues. Sometimes that makes you play better. Sometimes it made for a chip on the shoulder, an 'I'll show you' attitude. You take it out on the field, you take it out playing sports. You think about the things you go through coming up, the hard times, the adversities off the field."

"How could he not be in the Hall of Fame?" asks John Vella. "Are stats everything? Ask the Steeler defense in the '70s. The best defense. Who would they have not wanted to face? Ask the Dolphin No-Name defense who would they *not* want to face in the clutch. That says it all. They would say to a man, 'We don't want to face Snake.'"

These are the lifetime NFL stats of Namath, his fellow Alabaman, who was inducted into the Hall in 1985: 62–63–4, with a lifetime completion percentage of 50.1, 173 TDs, and one conference championship game, and one Super Bowl. These are the stats of Snake, including his final five mediocre years with the Saints and Oilers: 96–49–1, with a completion percentage of 59.8. And 150 touchdowns. And one Super Bowl. And five conference championship games.

Perhaps we can chalk up the Hall of Fame's cold shoulder to Stabler's final years, with New Orleans and Houston, although Namath suffered an anticlimactic end-of-career, too. Or to the low-profile media town he played in. Or his team's legendarily nonexistent publicity machine.

Or maybe it was the infamous incident in 1979, after a Sacramento sportswriter named Bob Padecky had visited Stabler's hometown of Gulf Shores, Alabama, and written a series of articles examining Stabler's colorful off-season lifestyle, without Stabler's cooperation. Subsequently, Stabler had invited him to Alabama for a follow-up interview. During the interview someone planted cocaine in a magnetic key case on the writer's rental car. After leaving a restaurant where he was interviewing Stabler, Padecky was pulled over. The police found the cocaine and Padecky was arrested and jailed. Stabler has always vehemently denied any involvement in the incident and called a press conference to refute any suggestion he'd had a role in the bust. But the writers make the call in the Hall, and that asterisk will likely never fade from their minds.

Perhaps it was the team's ultimate results that kept him from the Hall: so many flirtations with greatness but not enough rings. Or perhaps the team's outlaw image has worked against him.

So I ask him: Did all the partying keep this team from greatness? Did the Badasses' renegade reputation, their unrelenting love of a well-lived life, make any difference in the long run? Did his own?

"I don't think it made one ounce of difference," he answers, quickly, with conviction. "How can you say that? Look back at the five championship games. At how I led the league three times. You're part of so many key plays. How can you possibly say, 'Well, if I didn't stay for that last call, got in earlier, do this, do that, then maybe I'd have gone to six?'

"I would never second-guess. I can't do it any other way. I did it that way. That was me."

## CHAPTER TWELVE

# Hubbard, Uppy, and the Saga of 1973

The Raiders' five-game winning streak under Stabler in 1973 came to an end in the ninth week with a 17–9 loss to the Steelers in the coliseum, in a duel between backup quarterbacks. Bradshaw was out with a shoulder injury, and Terry Hanratty played for the Steelers. Joe Greene fell on Stabler's bad left knee early in the second quarter, a blow that would lead to off-season surgery. Lamonica came in and threw for 236 yards—and four interceptions. The Raiders outgained the Steelers by a wide margin, but the four picks—two by lineman Dwight White—snuffed their scoring chances. Later reports, quoting a "friend" of Lamonica, suggested that Madden had taken off on him in a team meeting. The veteran quarterback was clearly displeased with the situation. You could hardly blame him. Lamonica was coming off that Pro Bowl year—his second—and three years earlier had been the AFL's MVP.

But this was Stabler's team now. The following week, playing the Browns with a brace on his knee, Stabler was ineffective. The Raiders lost 7–3, which meant that the team would have to win its remaining four games to make the playoffs. They routed the Chargers at home. They beat the Oilers in a close game, behind Hubbard's 121 yards rushing, and came home for the penultimate game against the Chiefs, in the coliseum, with the division title still up for grabs.

"It's still the two of us, when you get down to it," Davis said that week. "That's still our season. Oakland and Kansas City." As usual, Kansas City came into town with an intimidating defense. Madden decided that he would challenge that defense with the simplest strategy of all, straight at them: size against size.

The key to winning the Kansas City game—indeed, one of the keys to success for the next several years, until injuries derailed him—was Marv Hubbard. In a fullback-oriented running game, Hubbard was the man you loved to watch carry the ball: not with finesse, just a metaphoric bludgeon.

"He was unbelievable. He was just a street fighter," laughs Bob Moore. "When he ran the football, he was looking for a fight. Marv probably ran all of a 5.5 40 at the time—he'd start the season at 250, go up to 275—and he was going to run right over you. You'd slip off your block, and he'd be running past you, right up your nose. He's not trying to avoid you. He's trying to run right through you. I don't care how big you are."

Davis and Wolf had discovered their huge fullback off the beaten path: in the 11th round of the 1968 draft, out of Colgate, of all places, which he'd attended on an academic scholarship. But the Raiders cut him, as did the Broncos, and Hubbard spent the 1968 season playing for the Hartford Knights, of the Atlantic Coast Football League: the consummate Badass pedigree. On the Badasses, *anyone* could get a shot—if they wanted it badly enough, even if they were coming out of the minors. How many championship football teams feature two key starters who did time in the minor-league pro ranks? The Raiders did, in Sistrunk and Hubbard.

The following summer, the Raiders invited Hubbard back to camp. This time, they had the wisdom to hold on to him. Marv Hubbard would come to epitomize, like Snake, and Foo, and Rooster, the team philosophy: take life head on, with a smile and a shout of defiance—and a song or two, accompanying himself on guitar, down at Clancy's. He was the Raider renaissance man: talented, and driven, at every stage of the Badass spectrum.

"So many guys have all kinds of ability and never reach the pinnacle Hubbard reached because they don't have faith in themselves," says Ron Wolf. "They get a block in the road and succumb to that, rather than fight through it. Marv fought through it."

On the day of the final cuts in 1969, Hubbard didn't attend practice. He stayed in his room playing his guitar. He figured if he was going to get cut, why practice? But he made the team. Within two years, he was starting. By 1972, he had run for his first 1,000-yard season. A three-time Pro Bowl selection, by the time his Oakland career had ended, Hubbard had achieved a remarkable average of 4.8 yards per carry: rivaling Gayle Sayers' numbers, if achieved at a slightly different pace and in a slightly different style.

Of course, this ultimate underdog kept up his side of the bargain on Camaraderie Nights, too. "We called him Ira Hayes, after that guy who raised the flag on Iwo," Banaszak says. "Marv was always the last one to leave the bar."

"He was tough," Madden says, "and he enjoyed being tough. He enjoyed a good fight. He said where he came from you could go to a bar, have a drink, fight a guy, knock him down, pick him up, dust him off, buy him another drink, and you were buddies. He said, 'I come out here to California, go to a bar, have a drink, get in a fight, knock a guy down, they want to sue me.'"

But no Hubbard tavern habit surpasses the legendary ritual of his celebratory punching out of the plate-glass window of the dry cleaner's next to Clancy's—but not until he'd left $200 at the bar in advance to pay for the damage. "He was so proud of this technique where he could punch the window and break it and not cut his hand," says Madden. But the coach was less than pleased on the day he received a call from the store's owner, who said that the next time Marv shattered the glass, she was going to call the cops.

"And so I called him in and told him, 'You can't do that.' And he said, 'Yeah, but I pay. I'm not running away from anything.' I said, 'But you can't break the window of a business. *You just can't do it.*' And he couldn't understand why he couldn't do it. I told him, 'Just don't do it.' And he stopped doing it. But he couldn't figure out *why* he couldn't do it. Or why he couldn't fight."

What he couldn't do was dive headfirst into a shot glass. One night, Banaszak says, Hubbard bet 20 bucks he could plunge into a four-inch pool. Yes, you're right, physics would insist that this wasn't possible. Hubbard apparently ignored the logic of the deal. "He was pretty close to it," Banaszak recalls, "because he cut the top of his head."

"He played real hard and partied real hard, too," says van Eeghen. "But, then, a lot of people did." Yeah, but no one else ever rode his motorcycle through a bar, from the back door to the front. The bar? The Picadilly Pub, in Castro Valley.

"It was a straight shot back to front," Vella says. "There was a long hallway from the back door before you got to the bar. And you could go straight to the front, with no tables or bar stools in between. So Marv rode his motorcycle, back to front. I'm not saying people had to dive to get out of the way. It wasn't like he was going 100 miles per hour. Put it this way, though: he never stopped."

Straight on: the perfect metaphor for Marv Hubbard (who let it be known through a teammate that he did not want to cooperate for this book). Ask his teammates and they'll tell you that no one was ever tougher than Marv Hubbard, in any and all ways. "Marv played an entire year, in 1975," Buehler says, "with a dislocated shoulder. He had to have a belt wrapped around his ribs, tied to the belt on his pants, so his arm couldn't go any higher because it'd come out of his socket. He went to Stabler before one game and said, 'Snake,' he said, 'if you're going to throw the ball to me, it can't be any higher than this because of my arm.'

"Ken looked at him and said, 'Marv we're not showcasing you in our passing attack today.'"

Hubbard had always relished taking on the vaunted Kansas City defense, led by linebacker Willie Lanier. The two had something of a history, the bulldog fullback against the Hall of Fame linebacker. "On one play in 1970," Duane Benson recalls, "Hubbard and Lanier hit the hole at the same time. Bam! The whole stadium goes silent. I thought they were both dead. Then Hubbard jumps up and says, 'Is that the hardest you can hit?' Next thing you know Hubbard is walking toward the other goalpost. He's so knocked up they have to escort him off." But before his fog set in, Hubbard had picked up 93 yards in the first half and scored the winning touchdown in a 20–6 victory.

On December 8, 1973, in the coliseum, it was Hubbard's turn again. "Now keep in mind," says Bob Moore, "that the Chief defense was the biggest football team you'd ever seen. They were huge. So in that game John decides in the second half we're just going to run it right up their ass.

"So the Chiefs do this overshift, where they take the defensive end off the tackle and move him outside the tight end. John runs right at it. I don't know how many times we give it to Hubbard. By the middle of the fourth quarter, these guys on the Chiefs, who I thought were the toughest guys I'd ever played against, had given up. They were so tired of Marv, they just quit."

For the record, Hubbard carried the ball 25 times that day, gained 115 yards, and even rumbled 31 yards for a touchdown. The final score was 37–7, testament as much to the Raider defense as to the offense; they held the Chiefs to just 82 yards on the ground, including a total of 1 yard for Ed Podolak, the team's leading rusher.

And therein lies another story. This game lives on for more than Hubbard's steamrolling of the Chief defense. What would a Chief-Raider game be without a rumble? "That was a fun one," Foo recalls now, with not a little delight. And why not? He was, of course, right in the middle of the thing. "It was always a war with those guys. No matter who won or lost, you knew it was going to be good."

The setup: the Chiefs had the ball, and Podolak was running around right end. Atkinson hit Podolak—"smashes him in the face," according to Foo. "A total cheap shot." The runner was knocked out of bounds. In the meantime, Villapiano nailed lineman Jeff Kinney: "I blasted him so hard, I fall down, and everyone starts punching me. I'm getting *kicked*. Now I'm under the Chiefs' bench, and here's 'Trunk's arm reaching down underneath, so I grab on to him. Then the referee, Tommy Bell, he grabs me and puts me in a full nelson.

"The next thing that happens is my cousin Otto and my father and a mailman from Jersey named Red DeAngelis are there, in that part of the stands, and they see the fight, and Red jumps over the fence—he dove right over this red snow fence—and two cops grab him and throw him to the ground. And he ends up with a face full of mud."

By now, players were rolling around on the ground, in a pile of boiling fistic chaos. "One of their DBs got a Gatorade bucket, and picks it up," remembers Monte Johnson, "and dumps all this ice water on the pile, and it looked like Moses parting the Red Sea. The whole pile just sort of divides.

"But the funniest was something we didn't see until we watched the films, because they had a panorama shot. There was this guy in the stands shadowboxing while we're all fighting. Then he starts to come toward the sideline to come to the fence to get over. One of the security guards sees him. He's still shadowboxing. The guard takes out his billy club, hits him on top of the head, and lays him out flat. He's out cold."

Actually, the funniest thing was probably what Tommy Bell said to Villapiano. "You have to know the background to it," says Foo. "See, my uncle ran the recreation center in Elmira, New York, right? And every year we'd go up for his Easter-egg hunt in the rec field. So one time I'm speaking at a dinner in Elmira, and I tell the story of the Easter-egg hunt and how my uncle used to tip me off to where the eggs are. And it turns out Bell was at the dinner.

"So when he's got me in the full nelson that day, Bell says to me, 'This a lot more fun than an Easter-egg hunt, isn't it?'"

In all, the Raiders gained a remarkable 259 yards on the ground that day, averaging more than four yards per carry. If one constant ruled 1973, it was the Raiders' astounding running game: 2,510 yards and a ridiculous 4.6 yards per carry—much of it over the left side of the line, where lurked one of the game's greats, the man whose name would forever be synonymous with the Badass era. The man they called "Uppy," and "the Governor." To watch 260 pounds of Gene Upshaw spring out of his stance, padded forearms waving in front of him like clubs, pulling to clear the way on sweeps, knocking pass rushers to the ground, erasing defensive tackles, was to watch an electric, outgoing figure—wired from the very start to be the epicenter and the conscience of a football family.

✕

He grew up in rural Robstown, Texas, west of Corpus Christi, the son of a man who worked for the local oil company. The Upshaw house didn't have indoor plumbing until Gene was 13. The brothers, Marvin told me, earned $1.25 for every hundred pounds of cotton they picked during the summers, to afford clothes and books for the segregated elementary and middle school they attended. The segregation, of course, was routine for the Upshaw brothers; this was the Jim Crow '50s. "When we won the little-league championship," Marvin recalls, "they wouldn't let us sit at the counter at the drugstore for the malts and shakes they were giving the team for winning. So the rest of the team didn't, either. There wasn't anything in the newspaper, no press conference. Those were just the times."

Marvin, one year younger, was the starter in high school. As an adolescent, tall and thin, Gene was not an aggressive athlete at all. He preferred baseball, and he started on the football team in only his senior year in high school. No colleges recruited him. In fact, if one day he hadn't decided to wander up the road to Kingsville, home of Texas A&I, as Marvin recalls it, and sit in the stands to watch a practice, a very different future might have awaited the Oakland Raiders.

"He wasn't even enrolled," his brother remembers. "The coach saw him in the stands and told him to suit up. They saw him play, liked what they saw, and gave him a scholarship, but it was just a room in a boardinghouse, money enough for the books. But he just refused to not make the team. He just had that determination." A&I used him at center, at tackle, and at tight end.

By the time he was drafted, four years later, Gene was 6'5" and 265 ("I don't know how," says Marvin. "Weren't any steroids back then.") The Raiders picked him in the third round of the draft, and Rauch moved him to guard—specifically to neutralize the Chiefs' "Buck" Buchanan, who had always wreaked havoc against the Raiders. At the time, guards weren't the tractor-trailers they've become. Upshaw was relatively huge, and unusually mobile. He started his first year and, astoundingly, thereafter would play every single *down* for 15 years. He would play in six Pro Bowls, three Super Bowls in three different decades, and enter the Hall of Fame in his first year of eligibility.

But it's a funny thing about one of the greatest linemen in history: the first thing his teammates always affectionately recall is the talking. Upshaw produced mile-a-minute commentary, as if his effervescent, ebullient personality could not be restrained by mere contact sport. To a man, his friends—and they were *all* his friends—remember the nonstop monologues in two-a-day huddles when everyone else was too drained to do anything but pant. The running commentary about the game itself: who he'd just flattened, how he'd flattened him, who he was about to flatten. The pep talks in the huddle, the self-help pump-ups. The reminders to teammates about their assignments. The polite and reasoned and diplomatic discussions with the officials.

"Sometimes Gene would talk so much I'd fall asleep on him," says his roommate Willie Brown. "I'd wake up three minutes later and he'd still be talking."

"Upshaw was talking 100 miles per hour all the time, pumping you up, pumping himself up," says Banaszak, "but that was part of his leadership role. His mouth was going all the time, but he played all the time. He never dogged it. That's what a leader does. Shit—if you can walk it, you can talk it."

His voice was his motor. No filter intervened between his brain and his mouth—not in a huddle, anyway.

"He was always yelling and screaming," says Stabler. Stabler not only abided the commentary; he enjoyed it. Of course, it would behoove any quarterback to stay on the good side of the dominant figure on the line that kept him upright for so many years, the man who could clear out the entire left side of the line with tackle Art Shell, swinging those padded forearms to pave the way for Hubbard and Banaszak and Davis and van Eeghen.

But woe the newcomer who didn't understand the unwritten rules. "I made a mistake in one game my rookie year," quarterback David Humm remembers. "In the huddle, I said, 'Gene, would you shut up?' He came across and grabbed me around the throat, walked me out of there, right past the ref. He said, 'Rookie, I'll tell you when to talk.' He was shaking me like a rag doll. Madden's going crazy. I get to the sideline, Madden says, 'Can you handle that huddle?' I say, 'I'm having some problems.'"

If the team had a collective bitch about something, if Upshaw felt that the vibe was amiss, he would act as the spokesman/messenger for the squad, the channel to the big man. If Madden had a message for the team, Uppy would be his messenger.

"Upshaw would handle me like butter," Madden says. "We'd start off with a big argument. He was a great politician, not in a negative way. (In fact, he would often talk of running for political office when his playing days were over.) He knew how to manipulate and get what he wanted. He'd come in and say, 'The guys could use a day off.' I'd say, 'The way they're practicing today, they're not doing piss anyway,' so I wouldn't do it then. I'd do it two days later. But I'd do it.

"Or I'd want to talk to him: 'There's something going on, and guys are doing this or that, and if you're really the captain, get it knocked off,' and he would. We had a really good relationship, because he could get stuff done. He was such a good guy." Madden pauses. "He was *such* a good guy."

"I think he had the most generous spirit of any human being

I ever met," says Bob Moore. "Everybody who ran into Gene Upshaw thought he was one of his great friends. He honestly made
everyone feel that way."

That was the captain: layering his spirit on whoever needed it.
Mocking Madden platitudes on signs taped to the blackboard, at
which the coach would laugh before tearing them down. Lighten-
ing up the film sessions by loudly counting down the endless seconds as Stabler stood back in the pocket, unthreatened, as the line
neutralized the opposing rushers.

One film session sticks in everyone's mind. After a game in
which Stabler was sacked Madden exploded on the sideline: "Do
anything you have to! Hold them! But I don't want goddamned
Snake to get hit!" A few series later, the Snake didn't get hit, but a
holding penalty was called: Upshaw.

So two days later, Madden was playing the game film. "We've
got to cut down on the holding," he said to the room when he got to
the particular play on which Upshaw was flagged. Madden didn't
mention the player. But it was obvious. And then the distinctive,
resonant voice rang out from the darkness. "You said if we can't
block them, we got to hold them," said Upshaw out of the darkness.

"I didn't mean you got to *hold* them," said Madden.

"Oh, no," came Upshaw's answer. "I remember exactly what
you said. You said, 'If you can't block them, hold them.' You didn't
want Snake to get hurt. So I held him." Madden had no comeback.
Gene had won the argument, as he always did.

Ironically, his teammates often profess to be at a loss for the
right words when they talk about the significance of the man to
their team, for their lives: as though Gene Upshaw were too big a
subject to take on.

"It's kind of hard to put it all into words," says van Eeghen,
who would gain thousands of yards running behind number 63—
or Highway 63, as the lane Upshaw carved out would come to be
known. "You were always aware of Uppy. Even if he wasn't talking,

you knew he was there. In a good way. That's a presence. Some people just command it. On Sundays, you're standing in the tunnel, and you look around to see your teammates, and he's the one you'd like to see standing next to you. He had a swagger, and I don't mean it in a negative way. He was in charge without saying he was in charge."

"When I think of Gene, I think of his confidence," says his captain across the line, Willie Brown, his roommate for 10 years in camp and on the road, the man who, as player representative for the team in 1967, talked Upshaw into getting involved in the union, and thus spawned Upshaw's second career, as executive director of the NFLPA. "He not only had confidence in himself but in his teammates around him. He played at such a high level, had such confidence in everything, guys couldn't help but rise to the occasion with him.

"And there was no ego. He didn't think he was better than anyone. He could be in a room with 50 superstars, and claim he was the fiftieth. Not the first. The 50th. He could be the everyday Joe Blow in the barbershop."

"He couldn't have been a better teammate," says John Vella. "He couldn't have been a better player." And he couldn't have been a better holder. When I ask Marvin to describe Gene's blocking technique, he laughs: "Holding." Gene Upshaw had holding down to a science.

"Upshaw was the greatest holder on our line," says Banaszak, with nothing but admiration. "You'd have to get an icepick to get the thread out from underneath his fingernails after a game because he was grabbing so much—red thread if it was KC, black if it was Pittsburgh.

"But what he really had was speed. He was quick, real quick off the ball. Shit, he was fast. I had to run my balls off just to keep up with him on a sweep, and he knew that. He'd say, 'Rooster, we got to get out of there quick.' I'd say, 'Holy shit, I just gotta try and get behind him and try and hold on to him.'"

Upshaw's durability went beyond never missing a play. No one recalls him ever being hurt. "I never remember him even being in the training room with an ice pack," Vella says. "I'd think, 'Is this guy a bionic man?' I can think of every other player tweaking something, at one time or another. Upshaw was, like, unreal."

Not that he didn't use other kinds of packs; Upshaw is nearly as legendary for his forearm padding as he is for his chatter. Actually, when I ask van Eeghen what he remembers about the man, the first thing he says is, "Other than the padded forearms?" Let's consider Upshaw's armor as we would Freddy's Stickum, as we would remember any Badass going for a semilegal advantage. Upshaw's trademark, the two stretches of scuffed, grass-stained white tape that hugged each forearm like a second skin, sported a considerable bulge; he'd wrapped a pad beneath several rolls of tape on each arm. Not an inch of skin was visible from the palm to the elbow.

"Not only did he tape and wrap them; he'd soak them," says Korver, the defensive lineman who would come up against Upshaw's weapons in practice. "The refs would check your arms during warm-ups, right? Then Gene would come back and put them under hot water, and if you took that tape and put it under hot water, it'd set up like a cast . . . then he'd hit you with that."

"Upshaw spent hours on those things," says Buehler. "That's kind of the way he got up for the game."

"He looked like the Michelin Man," laughs Vella, "but I'll say this about Gene Upshaw. Players know when other guys are exceptional. We knew he was great. You knew he was a special guy. I'd say that if there was one constant, it was Gene Upshaw."

✕

The 1973 division title came down to the last game, against Denver at home. The winner would advance. The losers would clean out their lockers. After starting the season 1–3, the Broncos had put together a strong offensive season, behind Hall of Fame running back Floyd Little and Pro Bowl receivers Riley Odoms and Haven Moses.

True to form, the Raiders continued to pound the ball in this one, averaging four yards per carry behind Upshaw and his linemates. After taking a 14–0 lead on two rushing touchdowns, they never trailed, and won 21–17.

But this game belonged to the defense, which knocked Bronco starting quarterback Charley Johnson out of the game with a concussion in the third quarter. His backup, Steve Ramsey, playing catch-up, completed just 4 of 16 passes. The Raiders recorded five sacks and made three interceptions, two by Willie Brown. The winning touchdown came on a Stabler-to-Siani pass of 31 yards in the fourth quarter.

For Stabler, an added highlight underlined this day. At halftime, he received the Oakland Raider Booster Club Award, voted by the players, given to "the player who best exemplifies the pride and spirit of the Oakland Raiders." The ultimate compliment for the ultimate Badass. He would win the award two more times but would never delight in the award as much as he did for this one, in a season he'd begun on the bench.

It had been a long, strange trip, but by making the playoffs the Snake had staked his claim. His teammates' stamp of approval left no question about who owned this team. And the impressive victories over Kansas City and Denver, featuring the feisty brawl against the Chiefs, left no doubt that the Raiders were in fighting form for the postseason.

## CHAPTER THIRTEEN

# The Soul Patrol

The Raiders had been granted their wish: the Steelers won their division and Pittsburgh would be their first playoff opponent— at the coliseum, this time, with a healthy Stabler and 52,000 fanatic fans to cheer them on. And Pittsburgh, at 10–4, had been anything but dominant. They'd lost three of their last five games, winning against only lowly San Francisco and Houston.

An interference call against Hall of Fame Steeler cornerback Mel Blount—"I was running a hook pattern," said Siani afterward, "and Blount just threw a punch at me"—led to the first score, a Hubbard plunge, and, three field goals later, the Raiders led 16–7 midway through the third quarter. Then Willie Brown broke the game open, returning an interception 54 yards for a touchdown on a play that the Steelers had inserted during the week, a play-action to halfback Preston Pearson. Brown wasn't fooled. Brown's score made it 23–7.

The Steel Curtain had no answer for the Raiders' running game. Controlling the clock with efficiency and ease, the Raiders cruised through the Steeler defense for 232 yards rushing, led by Hubbard's

91 yards, averaging more than four yards per carry. The Raider defensive line of Sistrunk, Tony Cline, Art Thoms, and Horace Jones held the Steelers to just 65 yards on the ground—including a total of 29 yards for Harris in 10 attempts. Bradshaw threw three picks—to Atkinson and Villapiano, along with Brown's. Minus any miracles this time around, the Badasses thoroughly outplayed the Steelers. The final score was a lopsided 33–14.

And in his first playoff game as a starter, Stabler justified Madden's faith: playing a ball-control offense, he completed 14 of 17 passes, mostly throwing underneath the coverage; his longest completion was for 21 yards. Siani caught five, and three more went to Bob Moore, who, this year, had had an uneventful, hospital-free evening prior to the game.

There was no mystery to it: the Raiders were the better football team, on all sides of the ball. "We didn't have our frenzy," Joe Greene said afterward. "They had it . . . They just beat the hell out of us."

"They didn't use any dirty tricks this time," said defensive lineman Tom Keating, a former Raider. "They didn't need them."

But now the Raiders had to venture to Miami, into hostile territory—literally. The night before the game, two Bay Area reporters told Miami police that a bullet flew through their motel window and ricocheted around the room at 3:30 in the morning. It had apparently been fired from an embankment adjacent to the motel. Clearly, not the sweetest of omens. Miami had Oakland in its sights.

The next day, in the Orange Bowl, Miami's rocking, steel-boned stadium set smack in Little Havana, the Dolphins, bent on their own revenge, used the bludgeon instead of the bullet. Maybe the Raiders had left it on the field against Pittsburgh. That was Stabler's theory, anyway: that they couldn't summon the intensity they'd used to win the grudge match the week before.

On the other hand, they were playing a far better team. After losing to the Raiders in the second week, Miami had won 11 of their next 12, and coasted past Cincinnati in their first playoff game, using a powerful rushing attack spearheaded by Csonka, Morris, and Kiick, running behind an offensive line that is still considered one of the top units in NFL history.

Against the Bengals the week before, Bob Griese had thrown the ball just 11 times. Against the Raiders, he had to throw only *six* passes. This one was that one-sided: of the 60 Dolphin plays, 54 were runs. The Raider defense that had been so effective against the Steeler ground game was powerless to stop Miami's. Using the same formula that would win them the Super Bowl in a 24–7 rout of the Vikings two weeks later, the Dolphins pounded the left side of the Raider line. Double-teaming Sistrunk, taking advantage of the huge weight mismatch between speed-rushing defensive end Cline and the Dolphins' two-time Pro Bowler tackle Norm Evans, the Dolphins pushed the Raiders all over the field.

The key, Villapiano says now, lay in the Raider defensive ideology of the day: to keep Morris and Kiick from getting to the outside. So the Dolphins ran straight through the Raiders' gut: Csonka finished with 117 yards rushing and three touchdowns. Even Griese picked up 39 yards on three runs, including a long ramble up the middle to key the first of Csonka's three touchdowns.

"It wasn't Csonka," says Villapiano of a game in which he provided one of the few highlights, with 14 tackles. "It was their scouting. The Dolphins just kicked our ass. It was the same defense we used against the Steelers in '72. Three times in that game, we finally got them third and long, and we'd keep two linebackers on the field and make them go man-to-man on the backs. But all three times they'd send the backs out and the two linebackers would go out with them, and three times Griese would run right up the middle. We didn't catch it until the next day on the films. They scouted us. They took advantage of us. Even Freddy dropped one, and he never dropped one. Just not a good game."

The final was 27–10—the most frustrating loss, Madden would say, of his entire career. The Dolphins had seemed to have a blocker on every Raider defender, all day long.

"It always meant a little bit more to me to beat the Raiders," Manny Fernandez told me. "We just didn't do it often enough."

And the Raiders were left with the same old feeling of also-rans. "We fought hard to get to this title game," Madden said, "and we're going to come back."

The local press was less optimistic: "The world knows that the Raiders always come up short in their final game," wrote a *Tribune* sportswriter. "It's as if every season is four quarters too long."

"By then," says tackle Vella now, "I think the Raiders were close to having the reputation that Minnesota and Buffalo would eventually have: looked at as a playoff team, they'll be right there but lose in the playoffs and not be able to do the whole thing. I think that was something that we were starting to feel. We took it for granted we were going to the playoffs. Now it was a matter of getting to the Super Bowl."

But their time had not yet come. The doldrums of the next two years were of a predictable sort: during the regular season, the wind in the pirates' sails took them everywhere they wanted to go—until the prize was tantalizingly close in sight but ultimately unattainable. Convinced that they were among the class of the National Football League, for the Raiders to perennially glimpse the finish line and not be able to touch it was like some infinitely cruel dream.

The fourth quarter of their games, the players believed, always belonged to the Raiders. "'You never beat us' is what Gene used to tell me," says Marvin Upshaw. "'Time might run out, but we never lose a game. If time goes on, we would find a way to win.' I'd say, 'Shoot, you're crazy.' But I came to believe it. The fourth quarter always did seem to belong to the Raiders."

The last game of the season, it was beginning to appear, did not.

On paper, 1974 would be much of a repeat: a dominant 12–2 regular season—and another loss to the Steelers in the AFC Championship game. But in Raider lore, 1974 was the season of the formation of the Soul Patrol, the most famous—and infamous—defensive backfield the game has ever known, and easily its most entertaining: two great cover guys and two safeties who just wanted to hit anyone who moved.

No group of men epitomized the Badasses like the defensive backfield. Their legend would range from adulatory to scathing, but on one thing all of their opponents agreed: theirs was terrain you didn't want to spend a whole lot of time in. On the other hand, for a fan, they were the unit you'd love to watch. Think about it: how cool was it to want the other team to complete a pass, just so you could see Tatum or Atkinson blow someone up on a pass route?

In the '70s, before receivers became so rules-protected that defenders today have to ask them permission to cover them, a defensive backfield was usually the most anonymous squad on a team. Not the Soul Patrol. They played original football: Ray Guy's "whoever hits harder, wins" football. They established intimidation and aggression as a way of life on the field. They spoiled a lot of receivers' sanity.

The roster in 1974, and for many years to come: Willie Brown, the captain, at right cornerback and Skip Thomas ("Dr. Death") at the left, two adept coverage corners who were larger and more physical than convention had allowed for in the past. Cornerbacks had traditionally been cover men, selected for fleetness. Brown and Thomas packed more power. Lurking behind them were Jack Tatum ("the Assassin," a.k.a. "the Reverend") at free safety and George Atkinson ("the Hit Man") at strong safety. It was a unit on which, as Tatum insisted, every player would have been an all-star if he'd been playing on another team.

Strip them of their aura of intimidation and they were skilled enough to cover anyone; from 1974 to 1976 the four of them collected a not-too-unrespectable 46 interceptions. But the lasting impression remains of a group of men whose weapons were as psychological as they were physical. No one liked to line up against the Soul Patrol, a hirsute bunch with madness glimmering in their eyes.

"That beard, the hair, that was part of our persona," Atkinson says. "Part of our makeup. It was saying, 'Fuck you,' more or less. 'We're here. We don't care. We're going to kick your ass and walk out of here, and we don't care whether you like us or not, but you're going to respect us and you're going to fear us.'"

It is a little ironic that the cornerback with the most sinister name—the man whose gifts have been lost in the shadows of his more famous and infamous peers—was not an intimidator, quite simply because Skip Thomas, Dr. Death, didn't have to play such games. The Raiders had picked up Thomas in the seventh round out of USC, and, in the weeks before the 1972 draft, Atkinson traveled down to Los Angeles to work Thomas out. "I saw tremendous athletic ability," Atkinson says now. "I saw good foot-change direction, and good explosion to the ball. I saw good bump-and-run skills. It all seemed to come to him effortlessly."

Thomas played physically. He liked to crowd the line of scrimmage, and his tackles were throw-them-to-the-ground fierce, but his real strength lay in negating the receiver at the line, tangling him up, daring his man to try and find a way to get past him.

"He was the size of a linebacker," Villapiano says of Thomas, "and he could run like the wind. I thought 'Tiger Nemo' [Nemiah Wilson, whom Thomas replaced] was good, but he was so small he'd get outmuscled. When Skip came around, that was the end of the outmuscling. Because Willie [Brown] had so many All-Pros behind him, people would keep throwing at Skip, which was just stupid. Skip was as good as Willie."

"Shit, he was a hell of a cornerback, Dr. Death," says Atkinson. "And he was different. From his own world."

"A unique individual," says Mark van Eeghen.

"I wouldn't mess with Skip Thomas," Villapiano says, "in a million years."

"They told me I was the piece of the puzzle that they needed," Thomas says now, smiling as he signs autographs over the din of a fete being thrown southeast of Oakland by Angela and Fred Biletnikoff's anti-drug foundation. Inside the ballroom of the luxurious hotel, videotaped highlights entertain fans who have donated to the foundation, scenes of Stabler and Biletnikoff and Branch and the rest of the offense.

No Skip Thomas highlights grace the screens. Thomas doesn't care. Thomas avoided the spotlight, seldom giving interviews to the press—though when he did, his interviewer invariably found him thoughtful and polite, as eager to talk about the book he was reading as the men he was covering. But Thomas had never felt the need or desire to promote himself, ever since his high-school basketball coach back in Missouri— he never played football in high school—told him that bragging only brought more pressure on yourself; performance itself was enough—if you could pull it off.

In this, Thomas shared at least one thing with others of his black-and-silver fraternity: he never let the game get in the way of his unusual style of life. It's a good thing he was drafted by the Raiders. But if his off-field routines were out of the ordinary, he told me, "I played every game. That's all that counts. Right or wrong?" If Thomas's name hasn't resonated through history, it's only because of the fame of the men who surrounded him.

The oft-repeated legend that Boomer Brown gave Thomas the nickname when Skip looked particularly cadaverous after a tough practice is apocryphal. For one thing, Thomas was never known for taking practice too seriously. "I used to mess around, because it was so boring," he told me. "Sometimes in practice I'd kick the ball like a soccer ball, like a soccer player flipping his leg up and kicking it away. They'd throw a pass, I could jump up in the air and kick it down."

And Madden allowed this? Thomas flashes a smile. "Sometimes John would just laugh and say, 'Catch it in the game.' Or sometimes he'd bawl me out. He'd say, 'Catch the damn ball.' I'd say, 'Pay me.'"

But why the nickname? Skip's response implies something a little more sinister. "I was wild, man. I could flip on you in a minute." He says this as though it's an admirable character trait. Of course, for a cornerback, it was. The Skip Thomas stare, glowering at you from just a few yards away, was the look of a boxer staring down his opponent just before the bell. "That was basically why they called me Dr. Death, because I was so wild. They didn't know what I was going to do one minute to the next. *I* didn't know what I was going to do."

He laughs. "I knew one thing: if I did something wrong, Willie was going to get on my ass," Thomas says. "George was going to get on my ass. John was going to get on my ass. John was going to send Gene and Art after me. They went all the way to make sure I did what I had to do. So I kept it where it needed to be."

In Thomas's case, where it "needed to be" included several locations. The field, where he picked off six passes in his first starting year, and six more in '75, was only one. Midair on his motorcycle was another. It was John Matuszak who once called Thomas "the Black Evel Knievel." "I *was* that," Thomas says now. How good was he on the bike? Good enough never to spill one, he says, when he was drag-racing with other players' cars in the El Rancho driveway.

"Then I built a ramp so I could jump over some cars. But John said, 'Nope,' and took it away from me."

"I hear all this hootin' and hollerin'," remembers Madden. "I go out there and they got this big ramp up, he was going to jump over a fence into a field next to the practice field. Skip was revvin' this goddamned thing up. I wouldn't let him jump the fence. I made him take the motorcycle back to Oakland."

Soon, Thomas upgraded to a larger Harley: "I wasn't going to lose that one. I took that one to the hospital with me." And therein lines the ultimate Skip Thomas legend. Dr. Death seemed to spend nearly as much time in various hospitals, even if he wasn't hurt, as he spent with the rest of the team. "He'd check himself in on Sunday night after the game to make sure he's rested," Atkinson laughs. "He'd do that after every home game. With his motorcycle. Can you imagine that? He had his motorcycle with him in his room."

"That was the Harley, 1200 cc's," Thomas says now. "I'd ride it through the front door of the hospital, right down the hallway, ride it to the room, push the bed over and put it to the side. See, I'd go to the hospital after the game because I wanted to be ready to play the next Sunday. And I knew that once the game was over with I was going to do my thing. I was going to have fun. So if I go to the hospital, and then if I'm back for practice on Wednesday, I'm good to go. So I'd stay in the hospital 'til defensive day on Wednesday. On offensive day, John might even say, 'You look bad. Go back to the hospital.' They wanted to keep me out of trouble."

They didn't succeed entirely. Part of Skip's rehabilitation process was fairly unique. "I had a bunch of nurses down there I'd play strip poker with," he says, laughing at the memory. "They'd have my liquor for me. They'd have a fifth of Crown Royal or a fifth of tequila, and they'd have it waiting for me."

I have to profess amazement at his routine. What other team would ever allow a player to miss practices so he could spend a few extra days in his own unusual spa? What kind of player carves out his own bizarre schedule? What kind of coach would sanction it?

"I liked Skip," Madden says. "Skip Thomas had no one to take care of him at home. So he'd go to the doctor. Like if he had a cold or something, they'd just put him in the hospital. He started to enjoy it. 'Cause he was getting, like, service. So the doctor said, 'I don't think there's anything wrong with Skip. But he wants to be in the hospital.' I said, 'I'd rather have him be in the hospital than anyplace else he's gonna be. So just put him in the hospital. I don't give a shit.'"

"John was the greatest person I ever met," Thomas says. "He was great to me. He put up with me. No one else would. I didn't listen to other coaches. Madden I listened to. He was like a father to me." That's not merely the cliché that it sounds. Dave Rowe recalls a light Saturday morning practice before a trip to Kansas City that's often reminded him of the unusual rapport between Skip and John: "Madden comes in and says, 'Get your helmets on.' Skip is looking at John. John says, 'Come on, put your hat on, Doc.'

"Skip says, 'I'm not putting my hat on. It's going to make my head look terrible. I just got my hair fixed.' Now, Skip's hair looks pretty good. He turns around, shows us. And it *does* look pretty good.

"'Everyone listen up,' Madden said. 'Skip just got his hair done. Skip, don't put your helmet on. We don't want to mess that hair up. Everyone, be careful. Don't run into Skip.'"

And so Skip practiced without his helmet. "There's not any other NFL coach who would have done that," Rowe says. "He would have walked right off the field. But that was John. And that was Skip."

Dr. Death's counterpart Willie Brown provided the perfect counterpoint, in both alignment and demeanor: Brown was never elected captain, mind you, as far as any players remember, but there was no question about who was going to lead the defense. Brown had just come off his fourth Pro-Bowl selection at the start of '74. Like Upshaw on the other side of the line—but with far fewer words coming out of his mouth—Willie Brown's title of stewardship was simply a given.

"Willie was the stability back there when the others were lethal and crazy as bedbugs," Stabler says. "He held everything together. Willie kept order. When Willie had something to say, we listened. He always backed it up on the field. So much ability, so much class, so much credibility."

His eventual Hall of Fame induction and career 54 interceptions attest to Brown's supremacy at his craft. But it was the work ethic, say his mates in the backfield, that merits as much praise as his displays on the field.

"This is the truth," said Tatum, who played behind him, the man who cultivated an image of ferocity when his captain cared to cultivate no image at all. "When I first got here, I saw Willie Brown working after practice, and I thought, 'This guy is All-Pro, and he's still out here working after practice? I'm not going to let this old man outwork me.'"

Today Brown is a quiet, proud, serious, self-effacing man with an easy smile but still possessed of a degree of confidence that helps explain why he's universally considered one of the supreme cornerbacks of all time. "They talk about how good I was, but I didn't see it that way," he tells me in the dining area of the Raiders' office complex. Just inside the entrance hangs a black-and-white photograph of nothing but a lineman's left forearm and hand, holding a helmet. The hand is wrapped in torn tape and the tape is splotched with blood. Other teams hang photographs of former heroes in their headquarters. The Raiders hang shots of bleeding limbs.

"The things that happened in my career," says Brown, "I attribute to the Raiders, number one—my teammates. They're the ones who helped me get into the Hall of Fame. I didn't look at it in terms of how great I was; I always wanted to be *better* than how great they think I am, you see? I wanted to be the guy on third down where if you threw the ball to my man, I know it's going to be incomplete: 'Try it. I'm going to pick it off or knock it down. One of the two things is going to happen.' I didn't worry about how hard I hit them, because chances are I'm not going to have a chance to hit them anyway, because the ball is not going to be complete."

Brown savored his role of captain, but more important to him was his role as the leader of the quartet. "I wasn't a drinker. Didn't chase girls. I was captain. I had to be at a higher level. I had to reel them in once in a while, because they'd get out of hand on certain days. But I didn't care what they did off the field. Come game time, my job was to make sure those three guys were focused. That's the way the secondary took it: that I wouldn't stand for any bullshit.

"You try to keep them calmed down some, make sure they're in compliance with the rules. But that's the thing about the Raiders: 'Hey, we're not going to break the rules, but we're going to bend the rules as much as we possibly can.'"

Willie Brown came undrafted out of Grambling in 1963, where he'd played tight end and linebacker for Eddie Robinson. He was cut as a walk-on by the Oilers, who first tried him out as a defensive back, and signed on with the lowly Broncos. By his next contract he was an all-star. In part because of his revolutionary style of play: he liked to crowd the line, go face-to-face, at a time when, by and large, cornerbacks gave the receiver space to begin his route.

"The bump and run had never been seen," Brown says. "I had used it at Houston, then I took it to Denver. They couldn't believe it, that a guy could stand toe-to-toe with a guy. But I knew they couldn't outrun me. And I was as big as most of them [6'1", 195 pounds]. I could beat 'em up on the line."

How did Denver let him get away? Stupidity. According to Brown, Bronco coach Lou Saban was not a man who abided an opinionated player. When Brown joined the boycott in New Orleans in 1965, he believes, the seed was planted for his trade to the team that would welcome a man who backed down from no one.

"They wanted to get rid of me," Brown says now. "They said I was a troublemaker because I spoke my mind. You have to remember, this was the '60s. You didn't question a coach. When Lou Saban said that any of his players boycotting that game would be traded, released, or cut," Brown recalls, "I said, 'Hey, OK.'"

He got the call from a teammate after the 1966 season, asking if he'd read the papers. He'd been traded to the Raiders. Davis believed that Brown was the single best defensive player in the league, and would sidle up to Brown before Bronco games and say, "You're gonna be a Raider." Willie Brown was delighted when his new boss greeted him with this advice: "Just be Willie. Be a football player."

✕

The sounds of silence. That's what George Atkinson wants to talk about one sunny day, in his backyard in Livermore, a half hour east of Oakland, a yard ringed by cedar and poplar trees, with a pool and a Jacuzzi. Inside his home, in his living room, bracketed by a photo of him and Tatum and a plaque commemorating the Soul Patrol, sits a cabinet full of replicas of ancient Egyptian figures. ("I collect Egyptology," he explains, apologizing for the absence of his most prized item: a solid-gold depiction of King Tutankhamen. His ex-wife got that one.)

Not that he isn't willing, happy even, to revisit those days of violent victory. It's just that, in his early sixties, and looking far younger (no facial hair, no glower, only a hint of a stomach), Atkinson would prefer we rather talk about, well, the nature of the universe and its infinite unfathomability. George Atkinson wants to wax philosophical.

"The universe is an intelligence," he says, with a deep, slow smile. "You got to plug in to it. Plug in, man. Once you start getting plugged in, you can hear the sound of a crack in the woods, the sound of a bird . . . You can hear an ant piss on cotton." These are not the thoughts usually associated with the Hit Man. It's a little disconcerting, this Buddha stuff, coming from the man about whom Villapiano told me, "George Atkinson would pull your face off . . . now there's a guy you better not turn your back on. If I were a receiver, George was the guy I would fear."

I hadn't expected the Hit Man to be the resident intellectual of the Soul Patrol. Atkinson, after all, *is* the guy who once said, "This is not a contact sport; this is a collision sport." He was the Badass of badasses. But no trace remains of the strong safety whose image remains among the meanest in the annals of the '70s game. No trace of the wilder days, in which he took full part. Only a surprising sense of peace.

"Yeah, we all liked to party," he says, ". . . but we drew the line when we had to. There was a point, come later in the week, you've got to gear down. To be human encompasses the whole being, you know what I'm saying?

"You exist through a process you don't understand," he says, as our conversation veers sharply from the subject at hand—the marauding aura of the Patrol. "You don't even know what's inside of you. And to not humble yourself and realize you were given a gift makes no sense—a gift not to be made a mockery of but to be displayed."

There are those who would argue that it wasn't a gift that lay behind Atkinson's patented forearm-shiver displays, that his propensity for borderline-legal hits is what gave George Atkinson his place in history. But they'd be overlooking the athlete inside the competitor, the man who collected 30 interceptions in nine years. He wasn't just a predator; he could cover his man.

And to hear Madden tell it, he was a leader—"one of the best I ever had. George was the type of guy, if you needed something done, you could just call him in and say, 'Get this straightened out.' And he would."

He was the classic off-the-radar acquisition from Davis and Wolf: a seventh-round pick, a speed machine from the South, from tiny Morris Brown College, in Atlanta, in 1968, where he pursued a double major in psychology and social studies. In his rookie year as a Raider, he set the team's single-game record for punt-return yardage—205 yards—and made All-Pro as a returner. What he lacked in size (he weighed 165 when he got to the Raiders) he made up for with the speed.

It was only after a few years that the Hit Man evolved into the intimidator who was playing two games at once: the psychological one, wherein the fear of being cold-cocked could make a receiver think twice about testing him, and the physical one, wherein he would relish giving a taste of his arsenal at the expense of a gift completion.

"Yeah, we had fun," he says now. "We rattled other teams. Teams didn't rattle us. We had 'em scared. Especially after the first quarter. We'd let guys catch a pass and jack 'em up. We intimidated people. We didn't sit back and wait. We initiated shit. We made shit happen."

And not only to opponents. Woe to the uninvited visitor to the Soul Patrol's special corner of the locker room: "The Ghetto. That's what we called it. You couldn't come down to our end of the locker room. We had a stripe of tape laid down on the floor. Colored it black on one part, and part of it was white. If you crossed that line, we'd put you in a trash can, upside down."

The high-pitched laugh spooks a couple birds from a nearby tree. George Atkinson watches contentedly as they flitter off into the infinite blue sky.

Jack Tatum said he probably would have been a farmer. The Assassin, whom I met four months before he succumbed to heart failure at the age of 61, thought all along that he would have been tilling the land. It's a little difficult to picture him behind a couple of oxen, isn't it? Unless you envision him hitting one of them chest-high, and the bovine collapsing in the dirt. The Assassin as tiller of the fertile land: the mind reels.

"My grandfather was a farmer," Tatum told me. "I spent all my summers in North Carolina, a little town called Crouse. I just liked the peace and the serenity. I liked being outside all the time. I didn't mind the hard work."

In conversation, Tatum was quiet and funny, eager to give credit to his teammates, offering up soft chuckles and a sharp, ironic sense of humor. History seems to have forgotten the reflective personality that belied the ferocity of which he was capable. "Believe it or not," says Pat Toomay, "Jack Tatum was quiet and soft-spoken. He looked like Genghis Khan—he had an Asian feel to him, and he had a big Afro, and he looked fearsome—but he was a gentle presence."

"He was quick to smile, and so relaxed," says van Eeghen. "Quick to giggle and laugh. Then he'd put the helmet on, and, Jesus, the switch that would turn. It was hard to think it was the same guy. Jack used to count KOs on the field. Anyone who didn't get up in eight counts was a KO."

"You can't be off the field what people see on the field," Tatum said. "That's a whole different world . . . It was a different person when you take the field."

One of Tatum's nicknames was "the Reverend" because he seemed so pensive. "Both my dad and grandfather were quiet and reflective guys, but they were real men," he said. Clearly, in Tatum's mind, the two were not mutually exclusive concepts. The nickname that stuck, of course, was "the Assassin," coined in a club press release soon after Tatum had separated the immortal Baltimore Colt tight end John Mackey from his senses.

"The Assassin" rang a little more loudly than "the Reverend," and it stuck—not without reason. "Tatum?" says the Dolphins' Jim Kiick. "He hit you with all he got, every time. Everybody respected him." On the field, what receivers feared was the distinct Tatum hit: torso to torso, mano a mano. He didn't dive for the legs, he didn't bother trying to strip the ball. He'd just freight-train his man, wearing a distinctively intense expression across the line: "That's the way I learned to play from Woody [Hayes]," he says now. "He said, 'You never make a tackle with a smile on your face.'"

"Pound for pound," says Mike Siani, "he was the toughest football player I've ever seen. The only guy I could ever compare him to is Butkus as far as being ferocious. He would rather have a receiver catch the ball and drill him than try and knock the ball down. John had to tell him in practice, 'Don't hit your own players. Don't hurt your teammates!'"

Apparently, though, Tatum had little tolerance for getting hit himself, especially if he perceived it to be a questionable shot. To hear John Vella tell the tale of one particular practice down at Sonoma State, reflective thoughtfulness wasn't the only facet of Tatum's personality. The man backed off from no one, and the menacing attitude made for a most uncomfortable incident that Vella recalls in detail. It was a running play, and Vella was knocked around and bumped into Tatum: "Now, I definitely wasn't going after a safety in practice," says Vella. "That was something none of us ever did. So we collided."

Words were exchanged. Vella insisted the collision had been an accident. But on the next drill, Tatum confronted Vella again. "He says, 'I'm gonna get your ass, man.' I said, 'Man, just forget about it.'

"So we go back to the showers in Santa Rosa, which is like this tiny 10-by-10-foot cement room, and there's six or seven of us in there, and all of a sudden I feel a presence behind me. Tatum is standing six inches from me. He kept repeating the same thing: 'I'm going to get your ass, man.' I said, 'Will you just forget it?' I turned my back on him. No way do I want anything happening in that cement shower room."

It happened a third time, in the cafeteria. Vella had had enough. He went to Madden—not to squeal, just to let the coach know that a fight was looking on the horizon.

"Madden gets all fired up: 'Don't do anything! Don't get into it with him! I'll take care of it.' I don't know what Madden did. I never asked him. But Tatum didn't confront me anymore. But we didn't talk again the rest of the year. Not a word. I saw him one time in the off-season and we ignored each other. And then the next year, in training camp, I thought, 'You know what? I'm going to see if he's ready to move on.' I asked him how his off-season was, extended my hand; he shook it, and we moved on"—as did the hard feelings.

"Put it this way," Vella says now. "You were glad Jack Tatum was on your team, and that's the highest compliment I can give any player."

"Yeah, John was a little concerned," Moore says of that particular feud. "Because Jack is quiet, but you don't know what's underneath it all."

Is it any surprise that as a kid growing up in Jersey Tatum idolized Jimmy Brown, the man of steel? His coach (a Woody Hayes fanatic) at Passaic High School ran the Ohio State offense, and that's exactly where Tatum ended up. For the Buckeyes, Tatum was a unanimous All-American pick in his junior and senior years, playing that hybrid "monster": on any given play, he could act as cornerback, safety, or linebacker. Whatever the Buckeyes needed, Tatum could fulfill the role of three men in one. But when the Raiders took him with their top pick in 1971, Wolf says, they had only one thing in mind: a tackler who would control the middle of the field.

"He was a great player," says Wolf. "When you talk about guys, people use that word a lot: *great*. But Tatum really was great at what he did. There were stories that he could have been a better running back instead of a defensive player, but that he was so outstanding as a defensive player, Woody didn't want to make the move. He definitely had an aura. He's the only rookie I know who never had to get up and sing his alma mater's fight song. No one wanted to challenge this fellow."

The aura didn't need a uniform to make its point. Bob Moore recalls a day during the week before the 1970 Rose Bowl when both Stanford and Ohio State were taken to Disneyland. The buses pulled up side by side in the parking lot.

"Now, we have a receiver named Randy Vataha (who would go on to a stellar career with New England)—a little guy, looks like he's 15 years old. So Jack gets off their bus, he's about 215, big head, huge shoulders, and he's pretty gnarly looking. Randy gets off our bus, Tatum gets off that bus, and Randy gets back on our bus and says, 'I'm not going to that fucking place with this guy.'"

Tatum expected to be drafted by the Browns. The Raiders had never contacted him, and he was nonchalant enough about the whole process to be driving to the beach on the day of the draft, taking a spring-break road trip with a couple of Ohio State buddies. It was a full week before Tatum contacted anyone from the team that took him with the 19th pick of the first round. The man clearly did not stand on ceremony.

The player who followed him in the Raider draft already had a relationship with Tatum, albeit a distant one. Villapiano felt as if he'd been following in Tatum's footsteps forever. "He was a Jersey guy like me," Foo says now, "and the whole state had heard about Jack. I thought, 'Who the fuck *is* he?' I'm jealous. Then he goes to Ohio State, I go to Bowling Green, and I'm still Little League compared to him. I get drafted, and I'm *still* behind him. Then once I got to play with him, I immediately understood why I'd been behind him." Today, there is no man of whom Villapiano speaks as highly; Jack Tatum may have been the only Badass to hit harder than Foo. "When you're a pro, you look for guys you can learn something from, guys you can say about, 'Wow. That's what I want to be like.' I had my own way of hitting, he had his, and I liked his better.

"When Jack hit someone, it was a different sound. It was like a blow. I knew it was him just from the sound of his tackles. There was a different sound between everyone else's hits and Jack Tatum's hits. It was much more solid. Put it this way: it was like a pro golfer hitting the ball, compared to a guy like me hitting a golf ball."

Echoes of the collisions resonate in teammates' memories. "He was rock-solid," Ted Hendricks says. "I had a few occasions to survive the hits I was close to. I remember one time when he had Earl Campbell on a fourth-and-one at the goal. To this day Earl doesn't remember scoring. I thought for sure that somebody was really hurt. Bad.

"Another time Atkinson was getting beat by [Denver tight end] Riley Odoms. Odoms was running slants, and Atkinson couldn't get there in time. They talked about it in the huddle. Tatum says, 'Let's just switch. Take my guy. I'll take care of him.' Tatum knocked him out of the game."

The play that stamped Tatum's name forever on the NFL's marquee was a tragic one. It took place in the second quarter of a meaningless exhibition game in the coliseum, on August 12, 1978, between the Raiders and the Patriots. Steve Grogan threw to receiver Darryl Stingley on a crossing pattern about eight yards deep. As the ball sailed high, and the two men converged, each prepared for the hit. And despite history's magnification of the play, despite Tatum's well-deserved reputation for hitting hard, replays show, and teammates insist, that this one was completely legal. He had been backing up to cover another receiver, and when he changed his route to head for Stingley he'd had little time to anticipate the throw and ready the hit.

Tatum lowered his head to the left, so as not to go helmet to helmet. Stingley, on the other hand, lowered his head straightforward. When Tatum's right shoulder slammed into Stingley's head, two of Stingley's vertebrae were crushed.

"My shoulder pad hit him," Tatum told me, reluctant but willing to discuss the play. "It wasn't head-to-head. And, yes, it was legal."

It was a horrid confluence of events, just tragic physics. "The Stingley collision was a total fluke," says Toomay, who was on the field for the play. Tatum wasn't penalized. Nor should he have been.

After the game, Tatum went to the hospital to visit Stingley but was denied admission: "When I got there they told me only the family was allowed to come that day." Cowed by the ensuing national press coverage, he did not return. He retreated.

"Maybe Tatum thought he had to live like the guy he wanted everyone to think he was," Stingley's son Derek told me. "Maybe Tatum thought, 'I got to do it on my time.' But his time never came around."

Up until his death in 2007, Stingley never professed any anger for Tatum. "For me to go on and adapt to a new way of life," Stingley, a quadriplegic who would die of complications from the injury, said in 1983, "I had to forgive him. I don't harbor any ill feelings toward him. In my heart I forgave Jack Tatum a long time ago."

"I wanted them to know that I was in control of the field from the middle to the hashmarks," Tatum remembered. "If you wanted to play in that area, you had to pay. You had to pay me."

Three decades later, a *Sports Illustrated* poll named Tatum one of the top five defensive backs of all time. Does it bother him that the reputation of the Soul Patrol resonates more with the violence of the hits than the multiple interceptions? That his three dozen interceptions have been obscured? That the Soul Patrol lives on in memory as the occupants of a land of unbridled mayhem?

"I guess that's the image we got to keep . . . It doesn't bother me. A lot of the time a receiver we played would change their game because they didn't want to come across the middle. Staying away from me and George played into Skip's and Willie's hands. Either way, the receivers got no breaks."

They were the team within the team, a paradox worthy of an afternoon with Atkinson: four distinct personalities playing as one proud collective. Thomas, Brown, Atkinson, and Tatum comprised a tightly bound quartet who not only anchored and inspired the defense but whose attitude epitomized the personality of the team—and bolstered the offense's confidence. In 1974, the Badass defense limited opponents to 16 points a game, backed by the demonic foursome.

"The Soul Patrol: I wouldn't trade them for any secondary in the league," Stabler says now. "It's as simple as that."

## CHAPTER FOURTEEN

# The Sea of Hands

I n week three of 1974, the Soul Patrol kickstarted a nine-game Raider winning streak that would sew up a weak division and see the Raiders ease into the playoffs again. A satisfying 17–0 shutout of the Steelers in Pittsburgh featured picks by Atkinson, Thomas, and Tatum and 96 yards of rumbling by Hubbard. Atkinson picked off three more passes the following week in a rout of the Browns, using his forearm on this day only to cradle the ball, the team's third victory in its first four games.

By week eight, the Raiders' first game against the mediocre Broncos, the team felt nearly invincible. Davis had put the team up at Denver's Continental Hotel—described by Stabler as roach-infested and bare of lampshade. Saturday night, he and Biletnikoff, who was single at the time, were joined in the room by a couple of local women and multiple bottles of wine. The evening ended somewhere in the early hours of the morning.

Monte Johnson remembers a slightly different hour, and a different liquid. "I couldn't sleep the night before." So the linebacker decided to get a soda. On his way to the vending machine, he ran into Stabler and Biletnikoff. "They were just walking in. This was probably about three in the morning. I can't remember what Fred had in his hand, but Kenny had the small portion of a bottle of Wild Turkey, I think. I thought, 'Oh, my God, we're not going to have a very good game this week.'"

On the contrary. In the first quarter the next day, Stabler hit Biletnikoff with a 23-yard touchdown pass and Branch for another one of nine yards. He finished a four-touchdown afternoon with a 61-yard bomb to Branch for a final touchdown, one of Branch's 13 touchdowns for the season, and the Raiders won 28–17.

"After the game," Johnson remembers, "we're cleaning out our lockers. Kenny walks by me and goes, 'That's not too bad, right?' He knew I'd seen him. It was like 'I can do what I can do: I can drink, and I can throw touchdown passes, and I can win.'"

As Stabler said, one of the game balls should have gone to Bobby Layne. As it is, the game balls went to Biletnikoff and Branch, who had reached his stride, literally and figuratively. In the three years from 1974 to 1976, the slight but speedy receiver would catch 157 passes for more than 3,000 yards and 34 touchdowns—earning first-team All-Pro honors in each season.

Branch was well known for his legs, ever since he'd set the Texas-schoolboy record of 9.3 in the 100-yard dash. But Siani was the better possession receiver and earned the starting spot, until he tore a hamstring in training camp in 1974. "That's where Cliff took over my job," says Siani now. "And as soon as he stepped on the field, he became a superstar. He gave us something we needed. Here we have two slow white guys, Freddy and me, and we needed an explosive guy, which Cliff was."

Or as Ron Wolf puts it, "When Cliff got even, he was leavin'."

Despite his speed on the track, there was little question which sport captured Cliff's imagination. Houston's Evan E. Worthing High School alumni included the great Otis Taylor, of the Chiefs, an AFL all-star while Branch was still in high school. In Houston back then, Branch was intrigued by the glories of the NFC receivers he'd see in the storied Cowboy-Redskin games that were broadcast locally: the Cowboys' Bob Hayes and the Redskins' Bobby Mitchell.

After earning All-America junior-college honors in his home state, Branch transferred to Colorado, where, in his senior year, he averaged 25 yards a catch for the number three team in the nation. He earned an invitation to the Hula Bowl, which turned out to be the future-Raider Bowl: Vella, Siani, and Dave Dalby were in the same game. They might as well have called it the Badass Bowl and served beers on the bench.

A few months later, Flores, Madden's quarterback and receiver coach, showed up in Boulder and worked with the receiver for a week, drilling him on techniques for beating the bump and run, for releasing on his routes. "He was so fast—this sounds ridiculous—I almost had to slow him down, convince him that he didn't have to run full speed until certain parts of his routes," says Flores now. "I kept telling him, 'You can glide faster than most guys run.' You had to slow him down and make him learn to control his feet. Of course, Cliff gets and deserves the credit—he had to want to do it, and he did. And obviously he had a pretty good guy to watch in Biletnikoff."

Studying under the master, "Branch improved tenfold as a receiver after he got there," says Ron Wolf. "Bob Hayes is in the Hall of Fame and Cliff Branch isn't? Ridiculous."

Kind of a recurrent theme, isn't it?

"I was so lucky being in Fred Biletnikoff's shadow," Branch says now. "Watching his work ethics. He was the kind of guy who was never satisfied. I said, 'Wow. If I'm going to be any kind of receiver in the future, I gotta be Freddy's shadow.' He was my mentor. He was my role model."

That's where the similarities end. Biletnikoff lived for the 15-to-17-yard square-in or square-out followed by a scamper, the money ball. Branch was known primarily for the bomb—which Cliff more or less called for on every play. "In that era," Branch says now, "Madden gave Stabler free rein to call his own plays, so Kenny would check with me and say, 'Give me a feel for what you think you can do.' Well, I was always looking for the deep pass. Kenny says I was always *begging* for the deep pass. 'Gotta get it out there early,' he'd say"—because Stabler knew as well as anyone that if he waited too long, Branch wouldn't just outrun the coverage; he'd outrun Kenny's arm.

If Stabler saw a cornerback crowding his receiver, he knew they'd have a play, and would check off to an audible: Red 24. "If a guy was playing five or six yards off, man-to-man, I could run by him easily," Branch says.

"See, Kenny was such a pure, pure passer, and it's not just about communication, it's about location. He was a phenomenal pitcher in high school, right? So if he could locate the ball for a catcher, he could locate the ball for us. We were his catchers, and he was the pitcher."

The four weeks after the victory in Denver became the Cliff Branch Show. Branch averaged more than 100 yards a game, including five touchdowns. In a defensive battle against the Chiefs, in the 13th game of the season, he scored the game's only touchdown in a 7–6 victory.

Stabler-to-Branch had developed into one of the game's great tandems. Lest anyone doubt that they had a special on-field relationship, consider Branch's ultimate endorsement of the Snake: "Look at it this way: after he left the Raiders, neither of us were All-Pro again."

The final regular-season game of 1974 brought a meaningless victory against the Dallas Cowboys, a contest best remembered by Atkinson for the ruse he played involving Cowboy receiver Hayes. Atkinson and Hayes had run track against each other in college, and they were chatting before the game. Tatum spied them in conversation. "Man," he said to Atkinson a moment later, "what the hell you doing talking to Bob?"

"Then it hit me," George says now. "There's something I can do here. A little agitation. So I say to Jack, 'Bob was talking about you. He said you ain't shit. He said you can't tackle.' Jack said, 'What?' So as I'm leaving Jack, Bob is coming toward me. I say, 'Bob, don't go near Jack today. Jack said he's going to jack you up. He says he doesn't like you.'

"'Why?' says Bob. 'What did I do to him?'

"'Man, I don't know,' I say, 'but you need to stay away from him. He's pissed with you about something.'"

The act had so angered Tatum that he pushed Hayes in the coliseum tunnel as they were coming out for the introductions. "Man, what's wrong with him?" Hayes asked Atkinson. "George, whatever it is, tell him I didn't mean it."

On the game's first play, Tatum laid Hayes out. The Raiders won the game, finishing 12–2. Hayes caught a single pass. Afterward Hayes asked Atkinson for an explanation. "I finally broke it down to him," says Atkinson, "told him what I'd done.

"He said, 'Man, that is messed up.'" Just a simple Soul Patrol mind game.

The first round of the 1974 playoffs brought a chance to exact revenge on Miami, the defending Super Bowl champs—this one in the Raiders' home, where this particular game hangs in the Badass hall of history. "It was the most significant win for the franchise—ever," says Bob Moore.

He knows, of course, that it wasn't a title game. He knows that the Raiders would come up short, again, at the end of the season. But how could you not bow in respect, whether you loved the Raiders or not, after the Sea of Hands?

This year the Dolphins had proved relatively human, losing three games in an average division. With Mercury Morris limited by a knee injury, taking away some of the outside running threat, Csonka, coming off three consecutive 1,000-yard seasons, had averaged under four yards per carry for the first time in five years.

On the other hand, the arrival of rookie wide receiver Nat Moore gave Bob Griese an added weapon to complement the immortal Paul Warfield, who—despite now being a senior citizen, at 32—was coming off a stellar first-team All-Pro season. Griese had completed 60 percent of his passes for the first time in his career. The Dolphins had won eight of their last nine games, including a four-game streak in which their defense had surrendered all of 15 points.

The Dolphins were still the on-field class of the National Football League. They had the rings from the last two years to prove it. They also had the Rushmore-profiled Shula, who had led his team to an astounding record of 43–5 over the previous three years.

This one was not only a good football match, it made for good theater: Madden's black-robed, crossboned crew against a team that decked itself in white and vacation-tropical aqua with orange trim, a hot-weather team that played a cold-weather game to a backdrop of white towels and hankies waved by fans scented by sunblock.

Now they had to play in Oakland, in a stadium where they had never won a game, with an evil, spying eye perceived to be lurking in every corner. Shula was so paranoid about Al Davis that every time a small plane flew over the field in practice, he'd tell the offense, 'Mill around, mill around, don't line up.'"

"Csonka looks at me and says, 'Is he serious?'" recalls Morris. "I told him, 'You heard the man.'"

The coliseum crowd, remembering the defeat of 1973, was amped. "When we came out for that game," Madden would later say, "there was more excitement in the stadium than I've ever heard anywhere, or felt anywhere. From the pregame warm-ups, they were wired."

As the players ran out for introductions, a sea of waving black handkerchiefs provided a dramatic backdrop, a Homeric wine-dark sea. The coliseum shook from the noise—until, on the opening kickoff, Nat Moore broke through the wedge, cut left at the 30, then sprinted down the sideline and took it all the way for a Dolphin touchdown. Madden turned to Stabler and said, "This could be a long day."

That score held up until Stabler hit backup running back Charlie Smith down the middle of the field for a 31-yard touchdown in the second quarter. A Dolphin field goal made it 10–7 at the half, but the Raiders were having success stopping the Miami run.

During halftime, the Raider coaches decided to concentrate on getting the ball to Biletnikoff. And halfway through the third quarter, the strategy paid off, in a sequence that still defies belief: in the span of a minute, the tightly wound "mess" of a man made two catches, one of which counted, both of them remarkable, and both speaking of Biletnikoff's powers of concentration.

On the first, an underthrown 40-yard lob by Stabler from just inside midfield, Biletnikoff and Dolphin defensive back Tim Foley, running down the right sideline, both met the ball on the Dolphin four-yard line, popping it into the air, where it arced slowly toward the goal line. Biletnikoff followed it, Stickum'd and focused, and cradled the rebound in the end zone. But the official ruled, despite Biletnikoff's protest, that one of his feet had touched out of bounds, rendering the catch incomplete.

A few plays later, Biletnikoff simply did it all over again. From the 13, Stabler looked left, then turned to the right, saw Biletnikoff, and lobbed the ball just inside the end zone. Once again, Foley had the coverage, and as both men went up for the ball, and Foley thrust his right hand in front of Biletnikoff, the ball once again bounced into the air. Foley hooked Biletnikoff's right hand and pulled it away from the receiver's body.

As they both fell out of bounds, Biletnikoff had one hand to use—his left. He cradled the ball into his hand and chest, and managed to keep both feet in bounds as he fell over the sideline: touchdown, and a 14–10 Raider lead. The endless hours of post-practice fine-tuning, trying to anticipate any and all circumstances under which he might have to snatch the football, had paid off.

"That play," Stabler would later say, "was the best catch I've ever seen."

"The ball's not always going to be perfect," Biletnikoff says now, shrugging it off. "The whole thing about being a receiver for me was . . . you gotta keep going. You may not be successful that one time. You may have to wait to make up for a mistake. Being a success and a failure in a matter of seconds was always intriguing for me."

Had that touchdown been the winning score, it would have been immortalized. As it was, a game with four more lead changes in the last 20 minutes was more or less just getting started. Warfield scored a 16-yard TD, but the Dolphins missed the extra point, making it 16–14 after three quarters. A Dolphin field goal made it 19–14. But then Stabler got the lead back, this time thanks to a phenomenal reception by Branch. From his own 28, Stabler barked

"Red 24" at the line, calling for Branch deep—and woefully underthrew the ball. As cornerback Henry Stuckey kept running, Branch doubled back five yards, dove flat out to his left, and picked the ball just off the ground at the Dolphin 30 before hitting the turf. Regaining his feet, he went the rest of the way down the sideline, outrunning the cornerback and the safety.

"My greatest catch," says Branch today.

Now the Raiders led, 21–19. But the Dolphins answered with a long drive, topped by a 23-yard sweep—a play the Dolphins called Flow 30—to the right by halfback Benny Malone. Shedding some uncharacteristically poor tackling by the Raider secondary, Malone gave the Dolphins a five-point lead with 2:08 remaining in the game—more than enough time, the Dolphins knew, to give the Raiders a chance to rebound. "I was thinking, 'Don't go in yet,'" says Dolphin lineman Bob Kuechenberg of Malone's run. "I knew Mr. Stabler was waiting. Now, I know Roger Staubach had a lot of great comebacks. Montana, too. But if you ask me, if you're up by two or four points with a minute and a half left, for my money the man who you do not want to see in the opposite huddle is Ken Stabler."

The Raiders returned the kickoff to the 32. And Stabler went to work. A minute and a half and a string of completions later— a six-yarder to Moore, two to Biletnikoff, of 20 and 18 yards, a square-out to Branch, and a juggling catch across the middle to backup Frank Pitts, who'd caught one pass during the year—and the Raiders were on the Dolphin 14. Clarence Davis, ducking his head and twisting, ran the ball to the eight with 35 seconds left.

Today, Stabler refuses to take credit for that final drive. The comeback was made possible, he says, by his line, which kept him safe while he picked apart the soft zone defense. "They put the prevent in, and we worked with it," Stabler says. "Freddy made a big third down in that route over the middle." Stabler is being modest: on the 20-yarder, Snake threw the ball perfectly, a foot over the outstretched arm of a linebacker, dropping it in front of the deep coverage; Biletnikoff was wide open.

The Raiders took their final time-out. What followed was one of the most dramatic playoff catches of all time. Not that you've seen it very often. How many times have you seen "the Catch"? God Montana to Dwight Clark? A hundred? Or Eli to Tyree, "the Helmet Catch"? So why is it that the Sea of Hands catch is a piker on NFL history's scale? Could it be because it involved the Snake and an undersung running back, buoying a Badass squad that somehow doesn't fit the right mold for historical highlights? Just a thought.

"It was supposed to go to me," says Moore, the tight end, who'd lined up on the right side. "It was a tight-end delay. I bang against [linebacker] Doug Swift, but he just grabs me—a very smart guy. I'm trying to slap him, get rid of him, fight him off, but he figures it out. So Snake has to go the other way."

Biletnikoff and Branch were both covered. Now Stabler was under pressure and scrambled to his left. He'd danced a couple of yards when Dolphin end Vern Den Herder chased him down and wrapped his arms around Stabler's legs from behind: big John Vella's man. "I decided to get too aggressive on that play, for whatever reason. Den Herder slips my block, he's on the chase for Stabler, and that's Ken's blind side. Stabler senses it somehow, and moves away from the pressure. How he senses it, I don't know. But my heart is in my throat: my guy is going to sack Stabler to end the season. I'm yelling at Stabler, 'Look out!'"

In the meantime, running back Clarence Davis, the man with legendarily bad hands, was simply supposed to circle left and clear the zone. As Davis drifted through the end zone, right to left, covered by linebacker Mike Kolen, Den Herder was pulling down Stabler from behind, but the quarterback was facing the end zone. He had to throw it—anywhere.

"The play seemed to take so long," Stabler recalls. "You see a black jersey, you get a glimpse of that black jersey, you try and make a play. You just try and find a way."

"He was well covered," says Kiick, who was watching from the sideline. "It was one of those freak things. I was sure that Stabler was going down." Stabler *was* going down when he flung it—"and there wasn't much on it," says Snake now. As Den Herder wrapped up the Snake's legs, the quarterback had about a millisecond to flick the ball with his wrist. The ball wobbled, but the pass was not a fluke; it was on target or, at the very least, in the general area where Davis was running—surrounded by Dolphins, surrounded by a Sea of Hands.

Kolen, on Davis's left shoulder, had good position. In fact, he could have made the interception, with his right hand stuck out in front of Davis. The ball actually hit Kolen's hand, which deflected it up to Davis's left shoulder. The running back didn't have possession until a frontal hit from defensive back Charlie Babb, running at full speed, which should have popped the ball away. Instead, Babb, colliding with Davis, lodged the ball firmly between the two of them, whereupon Davis managed to wrap both arms around it, wrench it away from all the scrabbling hands of the two Dolphins, and fall to the ground.

Touchdown: 28–26, Raiders. By the man whose hands, in Stabler's words, were "pure wood."

"It was miraculous" says George Buehler.

"I think that play represents the attitude of that team," says Stabler now. "You find a way to win. It doesn't matter how, it doesn't matter who, as long as you get it done. You trust that somebody will make a play."

✕

Befitting any Raider landmark moment, this one included a comical coda: a brawl in the coliseum end zone. One overzealous and obviously overfueled Oakland fan, perhaps angling for a tryout, jumped on the field and ran through the end zone, punching Dolphin linebacker Nick Buoniconti in the stomach. The guy kept running but turned back to look at Buoniconti—which is when he ran into a left forearm shiver from Dolphin Manny Fernandez. The fan is lucky that Fernandez's separated right shoulder was tethered and harnessed beneath his jersey. Otherwise he might not have survived. With his one good arm, Fernandez took out all of his frustration, clotheslining the guy, who immediately went down, as other Dolphins joined the scrum, taking their shots at the intruder.

"Well, somebody had to do it," Fernandez says now, with discernible glee. "He was continuing to run right toward me with his head turned looking at the damage he'd done. God bless him, he turned around just in time to catch it in the face. He got what he deserved."

By the time order was restored, 24 seconds remained—time enough for the Dolphins, with luck, to drive for a winning field goal. With 13 seconds to go, on second down from his own 20, Griese threw a 30-yard pass to midfield, but Villapiano had dropped back into coverage—on the opposite side of the field he was supposed to be patrolling—and picked it off. Foo ran over to Madden, gave the ball to his coach, and watched as Madden joyously thrust the ball into the air.

Twelve seconds remained. And this being an era when playing a football game meant playing a football game, Stabler didn't take a knee. He handed off to Hubbard—twice. On the final play, Marv ran around the blocks of Shell and Upshaw to the left and broke three tackles, gaining 12 yards as time expired. The Raiders had won it, 28–26.

"You'll never see a better game than this one, ladies and gentlemen," said NBC announcer Curt Gowdy. "I'm sure you'll agree."

"Frankly," said his partner Al DeRogatis, "it was maybe the greatest football game I've ever seen."

In the Miami locker room the tears flowed. Even *Shula* was crying. Kuechenberg, too. "It was the most bitter loss ever. It's the game I sleep with almost every night, and will forever. All their touchdowns were freaky—Branch falling down and getting up, Davis on that last one. And it would have been our third-straight Super Bowl that year, but with Csonka, Warfield, and Kiick going to the WFL, we knew that was it for us." (The Dolphin offensive triumvirate bolted for the Memphis Southmen, of the newly formed World Football League, which would fold before the end of the Dolphin contingent's first season.)

"That was the toughest game I've ever been in, and the toughest loss I've ever been through," says Dolphin offensive lineman Jim Langer. "It was a kick in the balls."

"We were stunned and disappointed," says Kiick. "They were like enemies. Everybody disliked them as a team. They were basically disliked by everybody. But we had mutual respect for them. Yeah, they were all crazy, but I guess that's why they were so good."

The opponent in the championship game—of course—would be the Steelers, who had won their division easily, with 9 victories in their last 11 games. The week before, they'd routed the Bills, putting the game away by halftime and winning 32–14. They'd amassed 253 yards on the ground, including 48 on five Bradshaw scrambles.

This one would be played at home. But the Steelers had Pro Bowlers by the bushel. They had the healthy and rocking Franco Harris–Rocky Bleier duo, both heroes in their own right—Harris for his quiet, dignified dominance, the scrappy and revered Bleier for the shrapnel he absorbed in his foot and leg from a grenade in Vietnam. They had emerging rookie receiver Lynn Swann and the now-maturing Bradshaw. And the immortal Mel Blount in the defensive backfield.

On game day at least one of the Steelers was supremely confident. Reclining in a chair in a coliseum hallway near a television hours before the game, defensive end L. C. Greenwood was watching the Ram-Viking game. Asked by a passerby what he was doing, Greenwood replied, "Just watching to see who we're going to play in the Super Bowl."

The Steelers' Andy Russell had noted to reporters that the way to rattle Stabler was to force him to pass. Ordinarily the Raider game involved using the running of Hubbard and Davis and Banaszak to set up the play-action pass. The way to force Stabler to pass was to stuff the run, which on this day the Steelers did with stunning ease, using stunts, shifting around on the line—defenses that Stabler would later call the most complex he'd ever seen.

On this day, there was to be no tipping point, no fluke intervention. The battle in the trenches resulted in a good old-fashioned ass-whupping. The Steelers ran at will against a Raider line that featured Bubba Smith at one end, in his final of two years with the team and, because of injury, far removed from his glory days, and Horace Jones at the other, with Thoms and Sistrunk at the tackles. The Steelers had noticed that the Raider defensive line could be trap-blocked in certain alignments, and, calling audible traps all day, they rushed the ball 47 times for 224 yards. Harris rambled for 111 yards, Bleier for 98—and a game ball.

The Raiders, meanwhile, were running into a wall, all day long. Considering that the Steelers had held O. J. Simpson to 49 yards the week before, it should hardly be surprising that they'd challenge the Raider running game. But this contest was comically one-sided: Oakland rushed 21 times and gained all of 29 yards, averaging 1.4 yards per carry. On their first play, Clarence Davis gained four yards. It would be the Raiders' longest rushing gain of the day. They didn't earn a single first down on the ground all afternoon. Hubbard managed only six yards on seven carries.

"People just don't do that to us," Hubbard said afterward. "We let them control the line of scrimmage. That's it."

But what a line of scrimmage. Up front, the Raiders were facing "Polite" Dwight White (who had a tremendous day at right defensive end, against Art Shell), "Mean" Joe Greene, Ernie ("Fats") Holmes, and Greenwood. As that foursome neutralized the Raider front line, the Steelers' tremendous linebacking corps was free to clean up: Russell, future Hall of Famer Jack Ham, who played one of the best games of his life, and Jack Lambert, in the rookie year of a dominant Hall of Fame career.

But the Raider offensive line was hardly made up of slouches. In the third game of the season, they'd run all over the same defense, with Hubbard gaining 96 yards. How to account for the difference? "Instead of being ferocious and vicious, we were thinking," was Buehler's post-game assessment. "We were trying not to make mistakes. We might have gone out there afraid of losing."

In fact, for the first 30 minutes, it was still anyone's game. The teams traded first-half field goals before the Raiders took the lead in the third quarter. Tatum recovered a Bleier fumble; Stabler gave it right back on a terrific, diving interception by Ham. Then Stabler put together an 80-yard drive, completing four of five, including a sweet 38-yard reception down the left sideline by Branch, who would beat Blount all day. The TD put the Raiders up, 10–3.

But on the ensuing drive, the Steelers answered with a Harris touchdown run of eight yards after a long, grinding drive. The touchdown run, Tatum would later say, came when the Raiders had the wrong defense called; the safeties weren't in position to stop Harris's run up the middle.

A few moments later, Ham again picked off another Stabler pass, at the Raider 34, and returned it to the nine, leading to a Swann six-yard touchdown. Skip Thomas had been covering and fell for Swann's first move to the outside. The rookie slanted back to the middle, gathered the ball in, and the Steelers held their first lead of the day: 17–10. The tide had turned. Stabler hit Branch with a 42-yard pass, the touchdown saved by a Lambert tackle. Had Lambert not caught Branch, Cliff appeared to have clear sailing the rest of the way. On third down, Stabler had to throw it away from the six in the face of a blitz, forcing the Raiders to settle for the field goal: 17–13.

By now, with his backs finding nowhere to run, Stabler had nowhere to hide. He threw another pick, to J. T. Thomas, at the Raider 40, leading to the Steelers' third touchdown of the quarter, a 21-yard Harris touchdown run. The final was 24–13. On this day, the Badasses were nowhere near as bad as the Steel Curtain.

"They played right into our hands," said Joe Greene afterward. "We knew we could stop their run and that their only chance to beat us was with the pass. By the time they went to the passing, we knew it and could tee off for a good rush."

Hurried all day, Stabler was sacked only once, but he threw

the three interceptions and completed just 19 of 36 passes—almost half of them to Branch. In truth, the only reason the Raiders were in it at all was Branch's vibe with Stabler that day; the emerging receiver enjoyed the game of his young life: nine receptions for 186 yards—many of them against Blount, the only matchup the Raiders managed to exploit.

Blount was so ineffective that defensive coach Bud Carson pulled him out of the game. "You've seen that happen to a quarterback," Branch says now, "but to have a defensive back yanked was a very rare thing." It didn't matter. In every other category, the Steelers ruled.

If one play epitomized the flow of this game, it was the fumble that got away in the fourth quarter, with the Steelers leading, 17–13. Bradshaw, rolling to his left, simply dropped the ball. Irons, Tatum, and Villapiano had a shot at the ball, and Tatum looked ready to scoop it up for an unimpeded touchdown—but Bradshaw, pursuing, came over Tatum's back, jarred the ball loose, and recovered it.

"We had the lead, we were on top," bemoaned Villapiano. "All we needed was 15 more minutes of solid play. We just didn't come through. There's no crying this year. We just got whipped."

It was uncharacteristic of the Raiders to lose a fourth quarter. They'd left it on the field in the Sea of Hands. "I think we just figured, 'We beat the Super Bowl champs from the year before, and with Pittsburgh coming here, we're going to kick their ass,'" Siani says now. "We didn't."

It's not as if they'd been upset. History would regard this Steeler team as a dominant one. The Steelers would go on to beat the Vikings, 16–6, for their first Super Bowl, the start of a dynasty that would bring Pittsburgh four championships in the decade. For the Raiders? Another disappointing, tantalizing might-have-been. Camaraderie, fellowship, and Badass good times made for a unique atmosphere off the field. But in history, it's the standings that ultimately count. The frustration continued to mount.

"Every damn year it's like this," said Hubbard. "We had everything in our favor. We had them in our stadium. We had them on grass, coming off that great game last week. It just wasn't in the cards this year, again. When will it be?"

Madden was a little more succinct. "Defeat," he said, "is a bitch."

## CHAPTER FIFTEEN

# The Ice Bowl:
# Coming Up Short Again

"In the off-season, there's only one thing in the back of my mind," Stabler would say the following summer when he arrived at camp: "the Super Bowl . . . To get that close every year, and get kicked out, over and over, it gets to you. I don't think anything needs to be changed on this team . . . We're not a choke team. We may have gotten that reputation, but we know what we can do."

Well, everyone knew what they *had* to do: take it over the hump. Find a way to keep the penultimate game of the season from draining them of all of their playoff emotion after a now-typical dominance of their own division. And while the 1975 season would prove to be a gridiron version of the movie *Groundhog Day*, changes on the field would lay the groundwork for the ultimate powerhouse finish the next year. This season signaled the emergence of three new nicknames: "Kick 'Em in the Head Ted" (nee "the Mad Stork"), "Double-D" (a.k.a. "Piggy," a.k.a. "Bubbles"), and "Van" (a.k.a. "Bundini"). They were three entirely different personalities, but Ted Hendricks, Dave Dalby, and Mark van Eeghen each fit the Raider mold perfectly. Dalby would start on opening day. Van Eeghen would get his chance in week two. And the astoundingly talented Hendricks, the man who would make the biggest difference of all, arguably the most cerebral and naturally talented figure in Badass history, had to wait his turn until the end of the season. But when he got his shot, he seized it.

In the meantime, off the field, Al Davis's legal machinations had finally won him complete control of the team. When Wayne Valley had brought Davis back in 1966 and allowed him to buy into the team, he'd made Davis one of three general partners, but their relationship had deteriorated drastically over time. In July of 1972, Davis, looking for a contract extension, had persuaded the largely irrelevant third general partner, Ed McGah, to sign an agreement that would go into effect on January 1, 1976, giving Davis a 10-year extension as managing general partner—and, in effect, reducing McGah and Valley's role to consultantship. By the terms of the Raider bylaws, only two of three partners had to sign any agreements regarding club policies. And why wouldn't McGah sign a document giving Davis all the power he wanted? The man had taken a laughingstock team to perennial dominance. Better yet: he'd given them a national identity. He'd configured a football team into a treasure for a benighted town.

When he came to understand the full implications of a document he himself had never signed, Valley sued to have Davis removed from the team and the contract nullified. The case went to court. Under oath, McGah testified that he had never fully read the contract he'd signed. But in June of 1975, in a California courtroom, Judge Redmond G. Staats ruled that while certain parts of the contract were not valid, the contract as a whole was sound. Davis would remain in his position, as managing general partner and principal owner. As Ribowsky put it in his biography of Davis, "He all but devalued Valley and McGah right out of existence." Defeated in his attempt to oust Davis, Valley soon relinquished his share of the team, and the only man in charge of the Oakland Raiders was now Allen Davis. As, in effect, he always had been.

One month later, a far more significant transition took place on the field: the changing of the guard at the center position. Jim "Pops" Otto had been with the team since its inception, never missing a game during his 15-year career. Madden called him "the greatest center who ever played," and no one who knew the game would ever argue the point. But time had caught up with him, and both of them knew it. He'd had two knee surgeries in the nine months prior to the 1974 season. That year, Otto had had to have his right knee drained four times a week, and Dalby had spelled him in games. Following the season, he had a bone graft in his right leg, and in training camp in 1975 it came loose. But he still wanted to prove he could play. He still wanted to fill his spot at the Bamboo bar.

"I like to think I'm the toughest guy who ever lived," Otto told me (and the nearly 70 surgeries he has endured on various parts of his body attest to the fact). But the knees, the back, the whole body couldn't take the battering any more. In the 1975 preseason, Davis offered him a front-office job if he wanted it.

But Otto insisted on trying to play, starting a preseason game against the 49ers, and taking part in a 12-play Stabler drive that produced a touchdown. Madden then replaced him with Dalby on the next series, and Otto's playing career had officially come to an end. (He would eventually have both knees replaced, twice, and a decade after the last one, a series of life-threatening infections resulted in the amputation of his right leg. It was replaced with a carbon-fiber prosthesis decorated with the Raider emblem.)

"Dalby certainly was more than ready to take over," Otto wrote in his autobiography. "He was a scrapper, just like me." The Raiders held a press conference to announce Otto's retirement. "That's all I got," he told the worshipful crowd. The Bamboo Room would be losing a Hall of Famer who would never wear a Super Bowl ring.

The undersung Dave Dalby, an elemental, hardworking man, would start every game of the 1975 season. He would play in 205 consecutive games. He would start (and win) in three Super Bowls. But if some of his teammates are baffled that he's not in the Hall of Fame—how many centers ever started and won three Super Bowls?—the answer may lie in this: to be in the Hall, someone has to notice you, and the man known as Double-D seemed intentionally to play his position in a vacuum, to avoid attention and the press with as much purpose as he'd chug his beers—an activity for which he was famously renowned. Otto owned one of the largest personalities in the locker room. But no one ever sought publicity less than Dave Dalby, and no one of his level of accomplishment ever fulfilled a wish as fully.

Dalby wasn't a public person, but he enlivened the team like nobody else. He didn't like to draw attention to himself for his play, but he had no problem with his "Piggy" nickname, or dressing up in full pig regalia, from the nose to the ears to the pink tights, at the team Halloween party. Or, if you want to revisit a more adult-oriented version of a Dalby Cactus Room escapade, picture a 6'3", 260-pound fellow with a smile on his face hoisting himself onto the bar and dancing nimbly down its length, avoiding the patrons' glasses, as he sheds his clothes—perhaps to his underwear, perhaps further, depending on the storyteller.

(It couldn't have been easy for him to work them off. He had 19.5-inch Popeye calves, and frequently had trouble finding pants to accommodate them.) That was the night that Dave Dalby earned the third nickname: "Bubbles."

"That was just Dave," says Kathy London, his former wife. "He just loved being with the guys. He was a man's man. He just frigging loved having fun. *Fun* was his favorite word."

Kathy wasn't there on that particular Camaraderie Night, and not just because Thursday nights were men-only affairs, either: "That was part of my wedding vow: that he would have Thursday night out every night of his life. And it was OK with me. Those guys just had so much fun—good, clean fun. It was amazing. *They* were amazing."

The highly intelligent kid from UCLA, entrusted with calling the offensive-line plays, with facing men considerably larger than he, presented something of an enigma: he showed no aggression off the field. "He never hurt anyone on purpose, ever . . . he couldn't stand to hurt someone's feelings," says London, speaking from a home that still contains some of the porcine paraphernalia the couple collected from friends and fans over the 13 years of their marriage. "He did not like any confrontation with people whatsoever of any kind, which is so weird, because he kicked butt on the football field."

He was quiet, shy, ultra-modest, and self-deprecating. When people would ask him why his degree from UCLA was in geography, he'd answer, "Because I like coloring maps."

On the field he was unflappable. He never retaliated if he thought he'd taken a cheap shot, just turned around and went back to the huddle: let's get on with it. He never had an argument on the field, no matter how savagely a tackle or linebacker might have tried to maul him. No one recalls Dave Dalby ever getting into it with anyone across the line. He didn't yap on the field, and he didn't yap off it.

But it's not his football talent that his teammates remember. It's the little-kid personality. Surrounded by Badasses, Dave Dalby was the ultimate Goodass. "If you had to vote for the most popular guy on the team, Dalby wins hands down," says John Vella. "There wouldn't have been a close second. That's how much he was liked, how much people liked being around him." Vella roomed with Dalby for nine years in training camp and at road games, and lived with him in Oakland when both were bachelors in 1972 and 1973.

The Vella-Dalby room in Santa Rosa was nearly as legendary as the Stabler suite, if a bit more innocent. No women's underwear festooned the walls. Dalby's pinball machine and foosball table furnished the allure, forever attracting a crowd—as, of course, did the refrigerator well stocked with beer and Mexican food, regularly delivered from the owner of their favorite Mexican place down in Oakland who, in return for his efforts, would be allowed to sit in on practice—and drink at the Bamboo.

One thing Dalby shared with his predecessor, of course, was his love of his beer. But Dalby took the passion to a whole new level. Vella remembers the first time the two roommates went grocery shopping. "We're going to split the cost," he says. "We're picking out groceries, and he picks up a case of beer. I didn't say anything. I'm not a big beer drinker. A case would have lasted me a month at home. Two or three days later, it's gone. And I've had one. He had 23. I said, 'Double-D, we're not splitting beer anymore.'" When it came to competitions involving beer, Dalby was the acknowledged champion.

"Fifteen minutes before practice was over," Vella says, "he'd always start going around to his best buddies and saying, 'Bamboo Room? Bamboo Room? Gonna have a beer?' He was already recruiting for the next good time, the next time for some camaraderie. The look on his face was like a little heartbroken kid if you said no, so you always wanted to say yeah, because you didn't want to see that look on his face if you said no. You couldn't say no to Double-D."

But Double-D could say no to the press—and always did. Dalby would be out of the showers, ready to hurry out the locker-room door, before his teammates had undressed. "He didn't want to explain himself," Vella says. "I remember a couple of times where he'd be upset when the writers were inaccurate talking about us, putting blame on me or George for something: 'That wasn't even your assignment,' he'd say.

"Double-D was the prime example of the guy who really understood that linemen don't get attention, and a guy who didn't care to have it."

As to what went on underneath the good-time surface of a small-town Minnesota boy, what void he might have been trying to fill with the drinking, this remains a matter of speculation. "Dave probably didn't realize how talented he really was," George Buehler says. "Out on the field he could be the football player, but when practice is over, and now you're off the field and you're just you . . . I think partly he just wanted to maintain that party-animal type of thing."

In the end, the drinking took the ultimate toll; he surrendered to alcoholism. In the summer of 2002, Dalby died as a result of internal bleeding after an accident in which he drove his car into a tree, possibly after suffering a heart attack or stroke, his wife believes. No one knows for sure. He was 51.

"The drinking all started out innocently. It all started as having a lot of fun," says Kathy London. "Then he had to drink to feel good. I think he drank to hide any pain—emotional or physical pain. He was an alcoholic. But he was just a beautiful man," she says.

Whether the overindulgences of the Badass years planted the seeds of the alcoholism is a question that must go unanswered. Perhaps there was a price to pay for the Badass atmosphere of excess, and Dave Dalby paid it. On this all will agree: as a Raider, Dave Dalby's pursuit of a good time, as well as his love of his teammates, was unrivaled. This man just wanted to have fun—in the end, perhaps, too much of it.

The Raiders opened the 1975 season on a Monday night in Miami, and this time no shots were fired. It was Oakland who had the Dolphins in their sights, and they beat a Dolphin team that, despite the absence of their famed defectors, would go on to win its division. Banaszak, the short-yardage king, led the way in this one, with consecutive touchdown plunges from the two and the one to open a 14–0 lead, and a van Eeghen touchdown in the third quarter made it 24–7. The final was 31–21. The Badasses had opened in style.

But during the game, plowing into the line in his inimitable style, Hubbard separated his shoulder. A few days later, Madden called his fullbacks together. It was Banaszak, the veteran, who suggested that van Eeghen, the second-year man, get the start. A Colgate guy would replace a Colgate guy.

Van Eeghen rode no Harleys, danced on no bars. The new kid hardly fit the outrageous mold. He figured to spend his life in the financial world, analyzing numbers, not compiling them. "I was a choir boy compared to the most of them," van Eeghen told me. "I mean, you couldn't have had a more bizarre group of people. Dr. Death. Ted. Foo." But in a family where a curly-haired Rhode Island kid who had played his ball in the Eastern Collegiate Athletic

Conference could bond with a shaven-headed veteran of the Norfolk Neptunes, he found an immediate home.

He was, according to Mike Siani, "the last true fullback." To Mike McCoy, who would be his teammate in 1977 and 1978 but would first have to face him as a Packer, he was "the most underrated fullback in the history of the game." Van Eeghen would be the team's second-leading rusher in 1975, behind Banaszak, in a year when the Raider running game was third in the NFL. Today, the guy who plays the fullback position is a stocky, faceless man known and recognized only for his blocking. On the Raiders, fittingly enough for a highly physical team, he was the prime weapon out of the backfield. In the Badass years, the Raiders used their fullback to run the ball more than half the time, a strategy that fit nicely into the overall DNA of the team: full-on physical, the winner simply wanting it more.

"Mark wasn't going to run around anybody," Siani says. "He wasn't going to put a move on anybody. A stiff-arm and he'd just run over you, pound you, get up and do it again." Occasionally leaving a little Stickum in his wake.

He had been the third Oakland selection in the 1974 draft, the first two being used, in a reflection of Davis's priorities, to take cornerbacks Neil Colzie and Charlie Phillips. But Davis had scouted van Eeghen during a practice for the East-West Shrine Game, on a day when rain had moved the workout indoors and the players were practicing without pads, and seen something intangible. The owner had once said that he could tell within 10 seconds whether a player was going to be good. This time, he could apparently tell during a noncontact practice.

"I've got your next fullback," he told Madden. No matter that the kid came from a school where the football program was more or less an extracurricular activity: two weeks of summer camp and a 10-game schedule against powerhouses like Lehigh. "I was hardly a sought-out commodity," van Eeghen laughs now, perhaps forgetting that on draft day, Falcons coach Norm van Brocklin was desperate to trade for him. "He's Dutch," van Brocklin said to Madden. "He's got to be great." But Madden would not let the kid go. Forget the ECAC pedigree; he was a natural, possessed of what modern commentators like to refer to as the "motor."

And he was hardly among the neon names at the Shrine Game: "Too Tall" Jones and Mike Webster, a future Hall of Famer and nine-time Pro Bowler, were on the field with him. In the days before every mid-size stadium in the country got a bowl game, the handful of college all-star games provided true auditions, attended by dozens of scouts. "I felt like a fish in a fish bowl," van Eeghen says now. But van Eeghen discovered something that week. He could play with the big boys. He decided to put the financial career on hold. You can always crunch numbers. But how many people get the chance to run into people for a living? For one of the elite franchises in sports?

But when he got to Santa Rosa in July of 1974, van Eeghen was dismayed to find himself at a camp devoid of veterans. Nineteen seventy-four was a potential strike year. "No freedom, no football" was the cry from the more militant players; the union was asking for the moon: an elimination of the option clause, free agency, and the waiver clause. The owners weren't budging. On July 1, the veterans went out on strike. And Mark van Eeghen found himself playing football on a confused team of rookies and free agents. This wasn't pro football the way he'd envisioned it. This was everyone for himself, grappling for a roster spot, playing schoolyard ball.

"That first training camp couldn't have sucked worse," van Eeghen recalls. "Whatever I thought it was supposed to be, it wasn't what I was doing on the field. It was just a battleground with rookies and free agents. It was chaos.

"So one day I'm sitting there in the shower, and I'm think-ing, 'I don't have to do this. I didn't go to school to do this. It was never my goal to play professional football. It was never my dream.' Sometimes life leads you by the nose. And it did me. But in that moment, my nose wanted the hell out of here."

But the moment passed, and he's grateful it did. He'd started something, he figured, and he'd finish it. Down the line, he didn't want to wonder if he could have competed at the top and had turned his back on it. When, in mid-August, the vets came back, and he began to watch the Badasses coalesce, he was glad he'd stuck it out. "*This*," van Eeghen thought, "is a football team." Fellow Red Raider alumnus Hubbard immediately took him under his wing, as did the versatile fullback Banaszak.

Davis and Wolf had noticed Van's unusually good set of hands. Just as intriguing was the speed of his first few steps. "He was quicker off the ball than the other [fullbacks]," Stabler says now. Van Eeghen had a way of canting forward at an angle as he lowered his head to hit the line, so much so that he probably left a lot of yards on the ground. "There were times," he says, "when I hit the hole so quick and hard, with the body lean necessary for the antici-pated impact, that if it didn't materialize I would lose my center of gravity and end up falling after gaining eight yards, instead of 18. That was my style, and I guess it served me well"—well enough for him to record three consecutive, virtually unnoticed, thousand-yard seasons, from 1976 to 1978. Colgate grads don't attract a lot of attention.

He was never a fumbler and insists the Stickum had nothing to do with it. But he will 'fess up to using the stuff—or overusing it, if you listen to his teammates. "My first look at Biletnikoff, and I was sold," van Eeghen says now. "But it was just a crutch. I can tell you this much. Stickum wasn't half as good as the gloves that today's players wear. I personally tried on Randy Moss's gloves one day. I wish I'd had them when I played."

But where would the fun be in that? It would have deprived his teammates of watching Van when he rose from the ground, taking half the field with him. "He put it on his arms," says Rowe, who came over in a trade with the Chargers in the second week of the '75 season, "'cause he thought it'd be better to hold the ball. By the end of the first two series he looks like a Chia Pet. He has grass all over him."

"We called him 'Grass Monster,'" says Siani.

If Mark van Eeghen didn't fit the rebel role, if his name never pops up in the catalogue of storied anecdotes and Santa Rosa escapades, the team nonetheless embraced him, and Hubbard would introduce him as "my heir apparent." On the defense, his mentor was Tatum, who called van Eeghen "Bundini," for the curly dark locks. The brutal Assassin and the cerebral Colgate kid, side by side on the bus to the game: a typical Badass family snapshot.

By season's end in 1975, a season in which he'd missed a few games with his own shoulder separation, he'd gained almost 600 yards, averaging 4.5 yards a carry. Today, he is thankful that he decided to get up from the shower stall that day and put the uniform back on, to discover that, "if you're inside the Raider family, there's no better place to be.

"It's hard to explain and harder to achieve. What the Patriots recently had, a few years ago, was what we had: the ability for veterans and new players to mesh for a purpose. We squeezed as much as we could get out of us. We got a lot out of the talent we had there. We were a hell of a football team."

After defeating the Dolphins, the Raiders traveled to Baltimore—and trounced a Colt team that would win its division. But during practice of the third week, Stabler twisted his right knee in practice. The good knee. The Raiders beat the Chargers in San Diego that week, 6–0, but Stabler threw seven interceptions in subsequent losses to Kansas City and Cincinnati over the next two weeks. Stabler's professed remedy to the achy knees: Ace bandages, codeine, and Darvon. "I never took a shot of Novocain," he wrote. " . . . I had a fairly high threshold of pain."

He rebounded for a 25–0 shutout of winless San Diego, and the Raiders, now 4–2, flew into Denver for a critical contest, one game ahead of the Broncos in the standings. True Raider aficionados remember this as the day when Ted Hendricks finally took the field and got a chance to show his stuff: not his physical assets (he wouldn't make a tackle all game); no, the gangly, unusual man who counted William Blake among his favorite authors would be put to a different kind of test in his brief inaugural Badass appearance. A mind game.

The Broncos were leading, 17–7, when starting middle linebacker Monte Johnson went down with a back injury in the third quarter and had to leave the field on a stretcher. Madden sent in second-year man Mike Dennery. Dennery proved ineffective, and so Madden decided to experiment. In Hendricks, acquired as a free agent that summer, he had a three-time Pro Bowler riding his bench—albeit not a middle linebacker, an outside one. But he threw Hendricks into the fray. There was only one problem: in the Raider system, the middle linebacker called the defensive signals, after they were sent in by Madden, via Zeman. And Hendricks didn't know the signals.

"In the first huddle, I asked if anyone else knew them," Kick 'Em recalls now. "Everyone shook their head." So, surveying the offensive alignments, going on gut, he stuck to the basics, calling only two defenses for the rest of the entire game: man-to-man or zone. With Hendricks calling it blind, the Raiders completely shut down the Bronco offense. Denver didn't score again. Numerous three-and-outs gave Oakland ample time to recover and score five second-half touchdowns for a resounding 42–17 win. And while the stats didn't show it, Hendricks was the hero. He'd helped win the game by his wits and his instincts.

The following week, Madden said that Hendricks would get the start. When Johnson heard the news, he confronted Madden and received one of his most memorable lectures from his coach. "I stormed into his office," Johnson recalls, "and I said, 'Is it true?' He says, 'Sit down.' I started to turn around and storm out, pouting like a two-year-old. He said, 'I'm going to ask you to come back and sit down. If not, I'm going to fine you $1,000 for every minute you're gone.' That got my attention, so I sat down. I pouted and slumped.

"He asks me, 'Do you have a quarter? Hold it up.' I pull out a quarter. He says, 'What do you see?' 'I see a quarter.' 'No,' he says, 'that's what it is. What do you *see*?' I tell him I see George Washington and a date. 'I don't see any of that,' he says. 'I see a bird and some branches. There's always two sides to every story, and it'll help you to realize that. I told [Hendricks] he was going to start. My "yes" has to be "yes" and my "no," "no." I can't renege. But nothing would give me greater joy to know you'd be ready to play.'"

Johnson wanted his position back. So that next week against New Orleans, Madden kept his word: Hendricks started—for a single play. Then Madden yanked him, and Johnson played the rest of the game. The move simmered within Hendricks. Some logic lay behind Madden's personnel choice, of course. The starting linebackers—Villapiano and Irons flanking Johnson—were playing very well; the team was now 6–2 and building a seven-game winning streak.

On the other hand, the team had given Hendricks a three-year no-cut contract, at a very hefty $150,000. This was a big investment to be sitting on the bench. "I made a mistake there," Madden admits now. "But we didn't know exactly where to fit him in. Once you have something established, it's harder to break it."

Flash forward to a Monday-night rematch at home against Denver in week 12, the final game of the seven-game winning streak. No one remembers that the Raiders won it, 17–10, to go 10–2. What they remember is an ABC cameraman capturing a most unusual sight on the Raider bench: the bottom half of Ted Hendricks's face wearing a grinning harlequin mask after the game, his left hand flashing a peace sign at the camera.

At first glance, it seemed a wonderfully Raider-esque goof, a typical moment of showmanship spontaneity in a sport known for anything but. In fact, it was a mask with a message, a statement from private Hendricks Land: "It was a smile, to show that I was sad underneath that I wasn't playing," Hendricks told me, as if this should have been the most obvious thing in the world. Leave it to Ted Hendricks to make a statement with a harlequin mask worn on a football field in front of a national television audience of millions. He'd bought the mask at a renaissance fair: the kind of event where people in costume ride horses and pretend they're living in a different time and place—a most fitting environment for an equestrian history buff. That year was the first time Hendricks had visited the fair. For Hendricks, it would become an annual event: a yearly visit to another time and place.

The next week Kick 'Em was back on the bench, sans mask, and the week after, too, as the Raiders finished their 11–3 season with a defeat of the Chiefs. The future Hall of Famer, the archetypal Raider, was being forced to bide his time.

One week later, in the opening round of the playoffs against Cincinnati, Hendricks would finally get a legitimate start, but only because of an injury to Tony Cline, the right defensive end who tore up his right knee in the Chiefs game. The Raiders would now go with a semi-3-4, putting an upright Hendricks out on the right side of the line. He was possessed of a season's worth of pent-up energy.

The wild-card Bengals, the fourth seed in the AFC after going 11–3 behind Pittsburgh's 12–2, were listed as seven-point underdogs. But this was the best team in Cincinnati's eight-year history, and they had beaten the Raiders in the regular season, 14–10, at Riverfront Stadium. That day their defense, anchored by Pro Bowl cornerback Lemar Parrish, had produced one of Stabler's worst career performances: 8 for 24, four interceptions.

On offense, the Bengals were led by the accurate, unflamboyant Ken Anderson, throwing most of the time to Isaac Curtis, who'd amassed the most receiving yards in Bengal history that season. Cincinnati had averaged more than 25 points in its final six games, and no wonder: while they were coached nominally by league icon Paul Brown, in his 41st and last year as a head coach ("We'll be a snootful for the Raiders," predicted Brown, in words that only a man who'd been coaching since Eisenhower could have used), Cincinnati's offensive coordinator was a man named Bill Walsh, then in his eighth and final year as Cincinnati's offensive guru. Walsh called all the plays. As he would later prove in San Francisco, this lover of classical music knew how to run an offense.

Walsh was most concerned with Oakland's pass rush, which had produced 45 sacks during the year, including 4 against the Bengals 10 weeks earlier. His concerns were justified: the Bengals were next to last in the conference in rushing and would no doubt be letting Anderson air it out. The game would clearly hinge on whether the Raiders could get to Anderson. But with Cline out, that pass rush was now, on paper, significantly crippled. No one could anticipate how Hendricks would perform in his place. And with Willie Brown hampered by a thigh pull, rookie Neal Colzie would be starting at left corner.

The Raiders had a little added incentive: the Steelers had beaten the Colts the day before, ensuring that another Pittsburgh-

Oakland championship game would grace the football landscape if they could get through the Bengals. Franco Harris had rushed for 153 yards, and the Steelers had reduced the Colts to rubble. Pittsburgh was in traditionally fine form.

Three-quarters of the way through the Bengal game, so were the Raiders, who until then had played a near-perfect contest. Stabler had been given all the time in the world, and with 13 minutes left, Oakland was coasting, 31–14, behind Stabler touchdown passes to Siani, Moore, and Dave Casper. After their final score, a run by Banaszak, Executive Assistant LoCasale was asking the writers in the press box how many of them would be accompanying the team to Pittsburgh the next week. It looked like a sure thing. All minds were now on another journey of revenge to the Three Rivers house of horrors.

But now the Bengals caught fire, and the Raiders, no doubt looking ahead, completely lost their cool. A Stabler pick to cornerback Ken Riley led to one Cincinnati touchdown—Anderson to Charlie Joiner for 25 yards. A rare Guy punt of a measly 38 yards led to another quick Bengal score—Anderson to Curtis, covered by Colzie, from the 14. A Banaszak fumble on an exchange on the next series gave it back to the Bengals on the Oakland 37.

The score was now 31–28, and with 4:19 left the Raiders' dreams of a Pittsburgh rematch were now beginning to look like a fantasy. Then Kick 'Em stepped up, as he had all day, and took control. On first down, Hendricks eluded "Boobie" Clark's block and sacked Anderson for a loss of six yards, putting the Bengals out of field-goal range. Three plays later, with Anderson passing ineffectively out of a deep hole, the Raiders got the ball back and held on for the victory.

It had been off-the-bench Ted Hendricks's *fourth* sack of the day. He had more than made the most of his first full game as a Raider. One of the most peculiar men to ever wear the uniform had saved one of the more important games in Badass history.

"He earned his entire season's salary," said Paul Brown afterward of the final sack, "with that one play." Hendricks also blocked a punt and diverted several Anderson passes. Lined up as a part linebacker, part lineman, part Stork, the big man had been virtually unstoppable. The Bengal linemen's cry of "Here he comes!" became the mantra of the afternoon. It was as if, simmering and frustrated on the sideline all year, he'd decided to show Madden what the coach had been missing.

"He played like a madman out there" was Al Davis's entirely accurate assessment to reporters. "He kept coming," said Bengal guard John Shinners afterward. "He was brilliant."

And thus had another weirdsmobile taken his place on this weirdest of lots. "He fit in immediately," says Monte Johnson. "He was a scoundrel in arms. He looked good in silver and black." No, he *defined* silver and black.

He was born in Guatemala—his father, a Texas native, was stationed in the country as a mechanic for Pan Am; his mother was a Guatemalan of European descent. He was raised in Miami and gifted with a mind that found Blake, Keats, Joseph Heller, John Steinbeck, Herodotus, and Thucydides as intriguing as the game of football, thanks to a high school English teacher who had instilled in him the love of reading. The love has obviously endured. Today, Hendricks would just as soon discuss the Druids as his technique at linebacker.

"I didn't want to be one-dimensional, to be only an athlete," Hendricks says now, quietly. There is no trace of iconoclast to be found in the man who once symbolized the Badass ethos. "There's a lot more worldliness out there than just being a football player."

At Miami, where he played stand-up defensive end most of the time, the love of literature took a back seat to "math equations and

physics phenomena," he says; pursuing a possible career in engi-
neering, with an eye toward work in the booming space industry
to the north, in Cape Canaveral, he was going for a physics degree,
when he wasn't being picked three times for All-America status on
the football field. "No one who ever played defensive end on the
college level ever played it better," his Hurricane coach, Charlie
Tate, once said.

But Hendricks fell to the second round of the draft, where the
Colts picked him up, the low selection thanks in large part, no doubt,
to the unusual physique, the elongated morph. ("Like a series of
toothpicks," Colt Bill Curry once described him, "with long, whippy
macaroni arms.") Standing 6'7" and weighing 215 pounds, looking like a power forward, it was apparently thought that Hendricks
might have difficulty fitting in on a professional defense. Once again,
mainstream professional thinking had it all wrong. As the Raiders
would prove, you don't mold a man into a preconceived figure if you
want to excel as a team; you mold the team to fit each individual on
the roster. In an interview with *Sports Illustrated* in 1983, Hendricks
bristled at the notion that his unlikely physique would have hampered his ability to play the game well. Today, though, there is no
trace of a bristle or boast of any kind in the man.

"I had some athletic ability," he says, almost begrudgingly, almost apologetically. "If you were a tight end you wouldn't want to
see me over the top of you during a game. If you were a running
back, I don't think you'd like to see me just standing there waiting
to hit you. I was naturally strong, and I had the long arms to keep
people away from my legs. I had quite an extensive range. I wasn't
at the top of the speed spectrum . . . but I studied the game. When
I was at Miami I used to steal the practice plays from the coach all
the time, so I knew every play that was being run at me."

It's all completely matter-of-fact to Hendricks, as if he's talking about someone else. He speaks as if his singular history—an
unofficial-record 25 blocked kicks, 26 interceptions, a thousand

plays disrupted—merely made for a routine career. I goaded Ted
Hendricks countless times over several conversations to puff him-
self up. He never once took the bait. It's enough, perhaps, that the
Hall of Fame judges him to be one of the greatest linebackers ever
to play the game. Badass lore judges him to be one the oddest, too.
But the team accords him universal respect.

In Baltimore, Shula inserted him into the starting lineup as an
outside linebacker in the seventh game of his rookie year, in 1969.
By 1971, he was an All-Pro, a member of the Super Bowl team
that had to go through the Raiders to beat the Cowboys. It wasn't
just his tackles that George Buehler remembers of Hendricks as a
Colt. It was his unusual facial expression. "He always looked like
he was smiling. In my mind I always see him on the field with this
big grin on his face."

After the 1973 season, he signed to play in 1975 with Jackson-
ville of the WFL, so the Colts traded him to Green Bay, where,
in 1974, with five interceptions and a remarkable seven blocked
kicks, Hendricks was an All-Pro selection again. When Jackson-
ville failed to pay him on time in the spring of 1975, he became
a free agent. And while it would be tempting to think that Hendricks was salivating at a chance to join the band of renegades out
west, the truth is, his arrival in Oakland was a strictly mercenary
decision. He wanted a no-cut guarantee, and he was shopping for a
buyer. Green Bay, Miami, and Atlanta all passed. In retrospect, it's
astounding, if predictable, that no one wanted to commit to one of
the greatest players ever to play the game. He was too far outside
the conventional mind-set. Or *lack* of a mind-set, for it was his
mind that made all the difference.

And so, of course, Al Davis called, and flew him to Oakland,
midway through camp. "The thing I couldn't figure out was why

they wanted me when they already had Irons and Villapiano," says Hendricks. To Raider scholars, it was obvious: he was a perfect fit. When there's a great athlete available, no matter what your position needs, you go for him. If he's the kind of guy who thinks for himself, who favors the insanely comical gesture, all the better.

They all met at Davis's favorite restaurant, Vince's. Davis was concerned that he didn't seem strong enough. Hendricks's answer was apparently convincing: "Al, when I grab 'em, they stay grabbed. I don't need weights." He was signed that evening to the three-year no-cut deal that no one else had been wiling to offer, and arrived in camp 16 days after it had started.

"It seemed like when I was elected to go to the Pro Bowl [which happened eight times in his career], there was nothing but Chiefs and Raiders on the team. Me getting there was just adding another element to an already formidable team. They were a powerhouse. And they had people from all walks of life: all different sizes, all different personalities, all pure football players.

"I just added a little bit of attitude. The main thing is that I don't think there was a weakness inside the heart of any of those players. They just wanted to win. Instead of teams pretending like they're the team to beat, they *were* the team to beat."

He never got the physics degree, by the way, if even in Madden's words, "Hendricks was brilliant." This was a brain that could recite the next team's plays in meetings before the game plan was passed out; then, according to Villapiano, Hendricks seldom had patience for ceremony in the linebacker meetings, led by the beloved late coach Shinnick, himself a cerebral sort, and a hero of the 1958 championship Baltimore Colts.

As Villapiano recalls it, Ted would rather discuss larger issues. "With us, linebacker meetings weren't for strategy; they were to get to know each other better. So in our meetings, since [Al and John] liked what we were doing on defense, they didn't implement anything new. In the meetings we'd talk about five minutes' football. Then Hendricks would look at his game plan, saw nothing had changed, rip it up, and toss it in the garbage.

"Shinnick would go, 'Ted, what the fuck you doin'?' He'd say, 'Well, if you're not going to show me anything new, I don't need to see this thing.' But our meetings always became discussions about other stuff anyway. We'd do some kind of world-concept shit. Or current events. Or ask each other how we grew up. One night Hendricks brought up the Big Bang Theory. We talked about that for a week. Then Shinnick would look at his watch, say, 'OK, it's been 20 minutes,' and we'd be out of there."

Hendricks swears he tore up the game plan only once. "It just so happened we were playing Kansas City twice within a couple of weeks. So it was the same scouting report we had from before. So I tore up the scouting matter. I'd just memorized everything. I'd already seen the same thing from two weeks before."

He never made it to Cape Canaveral. He never left the ground, except, occasionally, on the football field. Hence the etymology of the nickname "Kick 'Em in the Head Ted," or simply "Kick 'Em." He'd been christened "the Mad Stork" at the University of Miami, when a nose tackle known as "Mad Dog" decided to bestow a "Mad" prefix to the rest of the squad. "Stork" referred to the wingspan: size-37 arms. With the arms held high, Hendricks was about 10 feet tall: a whole new species of linebacker.

So a new moniker was called for in a land where "Mad" was taken to a whole new level. Hence "Kick 'Em." "We're having a scrimmage," Monte Johnson recalls. "Ted is trying to vault over Hubbard's block, and he hits Hubbard in the head. Hubbard's lying knocked cold. Then Ted kicks him in the head with his cleat. Not maliciously."

Hendricks insists that Johnson doesn't have it quite right—that myth, as usual, has eclipsed reality. Dan Conners, the linebacker who would be cut at the end of camp that year, he says, bestowed the nickname. It wasn't even an original nickname. "The original Kick 'Em in the Head Ted was a guy who played for Georgia Tech named Ted Davis," Conners told me. "I just called Hendricks that because it seemed to fit him."

Nor, insists Kick 'Em, did he actually kick Hubbard in the head that day. "Actually, three of us hit him at the same time," Hendricks says now, "and he got knocked out. It wasn't really hard, the hit just caught him just right. It wasn't a hard hit. But I didn't kick him in the head. I shoulder-padded him in the head."

"Kick 'Em" was a little more catchy than "Mad Stork." And the truth is, Hendricks wasn't crazy mad, just spontaneously whimsical, a trait that didn't manifest itself until he donned the black and silver. Something about the Raider uniform liberated the true essence of the man. Today, he insists that he'd much rather be known as the guy who improvised on the field, led by instinct, who could swat a kick out of the air, or stunt and rush and cause a fumble, or dominate a tight end, than as the guy known for the mask and the horse and the umbrella and the pumpkin helmet.

"No, I didn't do any of that stuff in Miami," he concedes. Nor in Baltimore or Green Bay; it *did* take the decidedly rare petri dish of the Raiders for the man's impish side to emerge. It would probably do him an injustice to let the oddities outweigh the skill, but how can you not love a man who showed up for a practice on Halloween wearing that pumpkin for a helmet—replete with Raider insignia? Today, Hendricks, trying to mute his eccentric history, insists the whole idea was Dick Romanski's. Romanski disputes that version: "No, he brought the pumpkin himself and had the carving done on the side. That was pure Hendricks." Why would a man want to deny his peculiar past? For a man who appreciates historic legend, you'd think that Hendricks would want to celebrate the age of high antics. On the other hand, for a man of the mind, perhaps the clownish aura cuts too acutely across his adult grain. But Badass history is as historic as it gets, and Kick 'Em deserves to be remembered for *all* of his dimensions.

"He was such a smart guy, and he knew the game," says Atkinson. "After one quarter, he'd have the other team down. He could recognize their tendencies immediately, because he had such great instincts, and he could recognize theirs. He had this ability to immediately be on the same page with the other offense and know what they were going to do all day."

"Teddy Hendricks brought the Miami spirit to the Raiders," says Villapiano. "Now, you try not to live by this, but you have to in a way: the Miami spirit is 'Help yourself and fuck the rest.' And what you mean by that is taking care of your own fucking job. And then help wherever else you can. And when you fucking dominate somebody, then you can help the lineman. But help yourself first. At the end of the day it's very true. And he should know. He dominated."

As for the personality? "He was a person that didn't let you in," says Monte Johnson. "He had a fence up. He was guarded. He was really checking things out."

"He was . . . different," says Atkinson. Well, what Badass worth the title was ever anything *but*? Still, there's also no question that, at the time, Hendricks valued being part of the crazy quilt that he'd helped make so colorful—and there's no question that, in his mind, his own storied individual exploits should be a subplot when we're discussing his team.

But ask a half dozen teammates, and you'll get a half dozen different answers about Kick 'Em's persona. *"Irreverent* kind of fits, for a start," says Buehler.

"Ted was my thorn in the flesh," Monte Johnson says, with a laugh. "I was a Christian, and if I'd been out on a Saturday night, he would say things on Sunday like 'Monte, I see you found it today but lost it last night.' I now know he meant it jokingly, but I would be hooked by it emotionally."

So who, really, is he? I ask Hendricks: Describe Ted Hendricks for me.

He pauses, then answers, "A normal human being. A human being has many facets. I'm certainly not the greatest athlete who ever played, but I guess there's something inside of me that wants to win all the time."

And how do you want to be remembered? More silence. Then, "As one that knew how to play that position pretty well."

End of conversation. Pretty good at his position? We'll give him that. For starters. Maybe we should listen to Russ Francis, who told *Sports Illustrated* in 1983, "There isn't another player in the NFL like him, and maybe there never was." And most certainly never will be. In the NFL, whimsy has long been extinct.

After the win over the Bengals, another rematch with the Steelers beckoned. "We've known from the start of the season it would come down to this," said Upshaw. "They beat us last year and it still hurts. They did a job on us last time, and they're the same guys now as they were then. They're the world champions, and we want to be."

For the fourth consecutive year the Raiders would meet the Steelers in the playoffs; their postseason tilts had become widely anticipated annual rituals. And this time the game would be played back in Three Rivers. The Steelers were six-point favorites going in. A few days before the game Davis, only semi-sandbagging, chose to accentuate the negative: "We're in trouble. We've had one injury after another, and we're still banged up." (That was no lie. Biletnikoff was out with a bad knee, and Colzie would have to start for Willie Brown again. The captain would play only in obvious passing situations.)

"We always thought Miami was the best team in the last 20 years, but now I'm not sure if the Steelers aren't better than Miami was," Davis said. "They've got a tremendous advantage at home. And they know it."

The key to the game, Bill Walsh predicted, would depend on the Raiders being able to harass Bradshaw as much as they'd flummoxed Anderson. "If Bradshaw is pressed," said Walsh, "he tends to make errors. Oakland's line has to give the quarterback a fierce rush, and he will make mistakes. Right now Pittsburgh is the best team in pro football. But if the Raiders can get to Bradshaw, the picture could change."

On the Saturday before the game, after 1,500 fans sent them off in an airport ceremony, the Raiders watched *Jaws* on their charter flight. The idea, apparently, was that they'd be the hunters, the mayhem from below.

Madden shrugged off the Three Rivers angle: "It doesn't mean anything that we have to play them back there. We'd play them in the parking lot at Macy's if we had to."

But as it turned out, asphalt would have been preferable to the surface they actually played on. This time the gods didn't have it in for the Raiders by conjuring a freakish play, an occult manipulation of any kind. This time, they used the simplest elements at their disposal: the elements themselves. All of them.

NFL annals celebrate the Cowboy-Packer championship game of 1967 as the true Ice Bowl. Don't suggest this to the Raiders or Steelers today. At game time on this championship Sunday, January 4, 1976, the temperature was 17 and the wind-chill somewhere between minus 11 and minus 14. Even the Stickum froze on that day. (Yes, Biletnikoff was out, but van Eeghen and Banaszak were healthy, both Stickum aficionados.)

"It was unbelievable," says Siani now. "The worst conditions I've ever played football in—ever. Field conditions *and* weather conditions. It wasn't like playing on an ice-skating rink. It *was* an ice-skating rink." The snow on the sidelines, thankfully, was out of play. Three Rivers was a winter palace. Or dungeon. And the Raiders preferred warm weather.

It wasn't the cold, the snow, the sleet, or the freezing rain that wreaked the most havoc. This time, the God of Winds had been at play. The night before the game, with snow falling and temperatures in the single digits, Madden had inspected the field and seen that the Steelers had put a tarp in place—stretched across the field, raised a foot on stanchions, with warm air blowing beneath it to keep the field from freezing. All seemed ready for this latest chapter in the ongoing championship saga.

But when the Raiders showed up the next day, ice coated the whole perimeter of the playing field. "And we thought that was *really* strange," Branch recalls, "because we were a team that basically ran sideline patterns. We ran the outs and comebacks, and that day every time you tried to plant, you'd be coming back on sheets of ice." As for long routes? Out of the question for Branch— and for the fleet Morris Bradshaw, the third receiver that day.

"The tarp collapsed or something," Madden says now. "So I go out the next day, and they were trying to get rid of the ice by hosing it down on the sidelines." This tactic, of course, given the temperatures, just made the surface more treacherous. "It didn't make any sense. I guess they thought it'd loosen things up."

Groundskeepers did the best they could to overcome the conditions. They not only wet the ice, they used snow shovels to try and crack it and scrape it to the sidelines. They also sprinkled chemical pellets to try and melt the ice on the edges of the field, which only made things worse; as the ice melted it only added to the slippery conditions.

"Hey," says Madden now. "That's just part of football. It didn't bother me." So he says. Siani's memory is slightly different. "John was pissed, as soon as he walked out on the field during the pre-game warm-ups, and so was Al. I saw Al and Rozelle in a very heated discussion." The subject? That this was no longer a level playing field. "Our game was to throw the deep ball," Davis said later. "So that with that ice, we had to move those receivers in, and that narrowed the field for us. I'll never forget what Pete Rozelle said to me: 'It's the same for both sides.' I said, 'Damnit, Pete, I don't understand what you're talking about. It's not the same for both sides.'"

"As physical as we were," says Siani, who started for Biletnikoff that day, "we depended more on the pass than the Steelers did. And there was no way Cliff could take off. He couldn't even run. Cliff became ineffective simply because of the field, and he was having a great year that year."

"Ten to 15 yards on each sideline was frozen," says tackle Vella. "So we were playing on a field that was 30-some yards wide. The receivers couldn't get their traction. So that game was just 'Pound it, and pound it, and pound it.' It was the most brutal game that I ever played in. You had 22 guys on a 30-yard-wide field. So the defenses knew what was going on."

The result? One of the most primal, sloppy football games ever played. The teams committed 13 turnovers between them, attributable partly to the frozen football, partly to the frozen players, partly to the slippery conditions, and mostly to the pounding each team was giving out on half of a football field. This much is certain: a game played in the trenches favored the ground-heavy Steelers—when they could hold on to the ball, anyway.

"The game itself was a very, very hard physical game," Siani says, "because you couldn't do what you normally do. You couldn't avoid people, and Pittsburgh's defense knew that. As soon as you come off the line, Blount is trying to clothesline you, the linebackers are hitting you everywhere. It was an extremely, extremely physical game."

Two Tatum interceptions in the first quarter should have given the Raiders an advantage; slipping and slithering and dropping passes, they could only muster a field-goal attempt, which Blanda pushed wide. Even if the middle of the field was playable, the Raiders' running game couldn't gain traction against the same impenetrable defense that had won the championship game the year before.

But neither could the Steelers do anything when they had the ball. The only scoring in the first half was a Roy Gerela field goal, after a diving Mike Wagner interception of Stabler, who had trouble gripping the ball and would complete just 18 of 42 passes. Stabler's vaunted accuracy was diminished by the driving, gusting wind. "Kenny's passing," says safety Wagner, "was more effected by the wind than Bradshaw, who could drive the ball."

The 3–0 score held up at the half. The Raiders had had their chances, but Clarence Davis dropped two third-down Stabler passes in the second quarter: "This was my worst game in five years," Davis said afterward.

The third quarter was scoreless, too. The linemen kept butting heads, the ball kept squirting out, the snow was mixing with the sleet and freezing rain. On the narrow field, it was as if the always-physical rivalry had doubled in intensity. The only moment of significance for the Raiders in the third quarter came when tight end Moore slipped, pulling a muscle, and Casper came in to replace him. And therein, as we'll see, lay another story. Casper, the big man from Notre Dame, would never go back to the bench again. And Moore would never play another game for the Oakland Raiders.

It was beginning to look as if the game would belong to the last team standing. The Raiders squandered a chance at a touchdown on a Banaszak fumble. "Pete was breaking free right down the field," recalls Siani. "Suddenly, he drops the ball. But he kept running, because he thought he had the ball in his hand. He was so cold he couldn't feel the ball. He didn't realize the ball was 10 yards behind him."

The Steelers recovered on their own 30, and Franco broke loose from Colzie's tackle for a 25-yard touchdown run at the beginning of the fourth quarter (discounting that run, Harris would average two yards per carry on the day). That score was aided, as Siani recalls, by the Soul Patrol's obsession with containing the dangerous Lynn Swann. "Franco busted right up the middle for that touchdown. I don't know if Phil had a chance to make the tackle, but he told me afterward he was thinking, 'No big deal, Atkinson or Tatum will get him.' Then he sees both of them chasing Swann. They wanted to beat up on Swann the whole game. They forgot who had the ball."

Swann caught just two passes that day—and took a memorable hit from Atkinson that would subsequently send the receiver to the hospital with a concussion. "He caught a low pass," Atkinson remembers, "and I drilled his ass. Joe Greene had to pick him up off the field. It was a good hit. I hit him and drove his ass to the ground." On the other hand, making up for his horrid day of a year before, Blount held Branch to just two receptions, both in the last minute and a half of the game.

With the Raiders trailing 10–0, Stabler settled down. The ground game had been completely neutralized. (For the day, the Raiders gained just 93 yards on 32 rushes. Banaszak, with 33 yards, was the Raiders' leading rusher.) But Stabler answered the Steeler score with a 60-yard touchdown drive that featured three straight short completions to the suddenly effective Casper over the middle, capped by a 14-yard Siani touchdown reception. "It was an in-route," Mike recalls. "I planted and turned toward the middle of the field, and the defender [J.T. Thomas] couldn't cut."

When the Raiders got the ball back, now trailing 10–7, the game was still winnable, especially with the prospect of a turnover on just about every other series. Unfortunately for Oakland, the next turnover was the Raiders', when Lambert recovered a Hubbard fumble. On the ensuing drive, Pittsburgh drove to the Raider 20, where Bradshaw threw one up for grabs in the end zone. Both John Stallworth and Colzie slipped as Stallworth made his cut. But Stallworth recovered his footing and pulled the ball in for the touchdown.

Befitting the old-time battering-ram nature of the contest, after the extra-point snap was muffed, kicker Gerela picked the ball up and tried to drop-kick it through the uprights. He missed. The score was 16–7. A touchdown and a field goal could still win it for the Raiders. But they still couldn't move the ball, and, at the two-minute warning, the Steelers had possession.

But there was surely a turnover yet to come, and it was Hendricks who made it happen. At the Steeler 35, with 1:18 to go, Kick 'Em hit Harris, forced a fumble, and recovered the ball himself. Now, though, three factors were working against the Raiders: the elements, the time, and the crowd, a good number of whom had already crowded the fringes of the frozen field. When Stabler tried to hit Morris Bradshaw down the slippery right sideline, the receiver looked down the field to see, first, a teenage fan edging to the field and, second, the ball slip through his fingers.

On third down and two, from the Steeler 24, Madden decided to go for the field goal with 18 seconds left, opting for the prospect of an onsides kick if Blanda converted. Before Blanda kicked the ball, Madden was jostled on the sideline by another fan. Things were getting weird out there. Steeler fans were anxious, delirious, and itching to celebrate.

Blanda's kick from the 41 was good, to make it 16–10—his final field goal in a four-decade career—and the onsides kick worked perfectly. The Steelers' Stallworth got a hand on the ball but couldn't hold on, and Hubbard recovered on his own 48. The Raiders had one last shot, with seven seconds left. They'd use it, they hoped, on two passes.

In the Steelers' huddle, Lambert warned his defensive backs to stay behind the receivers, let them catch the ball and not risk an interference call. Stabler, squinting through the now-falling snow, hit Branch for 37 yards near the left sideline. But before Branch could step out of bounds, Blount grabbed his legs—"The best tackle I've ever seen," Steeler linebacker Andy Russell said afterward.

"I was trying to scramble to get out of bounds," Branch remembers now, "but it wasn't the ice that kept me inbounds—Blount had a hand around my leg, and the sideline was too far away. The next thing I know, I'm surrounded by Steeler fans rushing the field." One was trying to rip his chin strap off.

And that's where it ended: 16–10. Every Steeler score had resulted from a Raider turnover. The gods of Three Rivers—and a Steeler squad that would subsequently win its second consecutive Super Bowl, two weeks hence—had proved too tough.

"We had practiced outside that whole week," says Wagner, "and so we were ready for it, and so I think it helped us that we were used to the conditions. It made life for the Raiders very difficult."

The game had been too physical and too exhausting for either team to talk up the rivalry afterward; each side was remarkably civil in their postgame comments. Joe Greene gave the Raiders their props. "These are rugged people," he said, making the Raiders sound like some exotic species, which was fairly accurate. "Our offense was never shut down the way the Raiders shut it down. Those guys played well enough to win.

"Now they'll go back to Oakland and get the flak that they didn't win the big one. Baloney! This was the toughest kind of football played in the worst possible conditions. The Raiders don't have to be ashamed of anything. We're just a better team . . . even on the ice and in the snow."

Noll was almost as generous, calling it a "viciously played game . . . between two great football teams." (He did manage to rip Tatum for some "cheap shots.")

For Madden, the epilogue grew even more sour. In Madden's post-game press conference, a writer called him Al.

"That's a hell of a thing at this point," Madden observed.

Like he'd said exactly a year before: defeat was a bitch. Especially at the hands of the Steelers, on an ice-skating rink. Especially in a game where the weather conditions had reduced the contest to football at its purest, trench warfare, and the other guys had proven to be the better physical team. The Raiders had coasted through their division. They'd compiled a seven-game winning streak. But once again they were an historical afterthought.

"It was a very heartbreaking situation," says Branch now. "Back-to-back years. Maybe we were a little overconfident, I don't know. All I know is that I was thinking, 'What do we have to do to beat these guys?'"

In the Pittsburgh airport, waiting for the charter, Ted Kwalick bought a Steeler stocking cap, sat at a table, put a match to it, and watched the hat, like the Raider season, go up in smoke.

The movie on the flight back? A Gene Hackman–James Coburn western that would immediately vanish from the cinematic landscape. It was called *Bite the Bullet*. Whoever selected it must have had a hell of a dark sense of humor.

## CHAPTER SIXTEEN

# The Tooz Arrives

"For a week or 10 days, after we lost," Stabler said in training camp in 1976, "I would wake up in the morning and the first thing that would pop into my mind was Pittsburgh. Then I replay the game in my head. It really wears at you. Why do we lose? I wish I could give you a good reason. One year they said it was our rushing game. Another year they said it was the weather. Another year they said it was one freak play. That's all [bleep]. I don't know what it is. Maybe it's in the stars."

Once again, the Raiders convened in Santa Rosa committed to a season that wouldn't end as the last one had. And the one before that. And the one before that—ad, seemingly, infinitum. Of course, it's not as if they'd been bowing out against fluky teams. The 1973 Dolphins were an acknowledged powerhouse, as were the '74 and '75 Steelers. Each team had two rings to show for its efforts. By now, for the Raiders, anything short of a ring represented failure.

But in training camp, more immediate concerns loomed, like

the rebuilding of the defensive line. Cline, the quick defensive end whose knee had blown out in 1975, had been waived. Art Thoms— "King Arthur," the goofy tackle who merited his own wild cheering section, "Thoms' Territory"—was out for the season with a leg injury. Horace Jones, the starting defensive end, blew out a knee in the first preseason game. The intellectual Kelvin Korver, the dependable backup, was on injured reserve. The defensive line was decimated.

Korver managed to make his presence known, nonetheless: on a day in the final week of camp, the notes of "Taps" could be heard from the players whistling on the practice field, as they watched Korver's stunt plane—he was a crop-spraying pilot who flew his planes to camp each year—skate precariously close to the nearby hilltops. (Korver knew his flying. He'd once single-handedly pushed a stranded airplane a mile across a sticky Utah desert on one of his cross-country flights, until he found a dry riverbed that allowed him to take off again.)

Now Madden and Zeman made a radical decision: to go with the 3-4 lineup, the Orange Defense, which they'd put together for the Bengal playoff game the previous December. Now Dave Rowe would start at nose tackle, with Sistrunk at right end. On the left side they'd have to try their first draft pick: the gigantic Charles Philyaw, out of Texas Southern. Philyaw stood 6'9", weighed something near 300, wore size-17 shoes, and was gifted athletically. He would become an instant legend, if not a particularly gifted football player. He would play just four years in the league, all with the Raiders.

The myriad stories about Charlie Philyaw describe a delightful, slightly confused little kid trapped in a man's body, and this image would soon outstrip his on-field exploits, which never amounted to a great deal. Like the day he closed the moon roof on his own head in his Lincoln Mark IV, or went to the wrong line meeting. Like the day Banaszak told him to go see the doctor; he knocked on Dr. Death's door and was summarily dismissed.

"I was sitting on my helmet one day," Mark van Eeghen recalls of the singular classic Philyaw moment. "Charlie comes by and says, 'Can I ask you a question?' 'Sure,' I say, 'what's on your mind?' He says, 'How come you get both names on your jersey?' I explain to him that van Eeghen is my last name. My first name is Mark. I'm dying to tell Madden, but I don't. But I tell Banaszak, who tells Madden. All of a sudden you see this big belly laugh coming out of John."

Whether Philyaw's answer to a pre–Senior Bowl question about what he took in college—"Some socks and underwear"—is apocryphal or not, it gives you a good sense of the aura he's left behind in the "character" subsection of Badass history.

"Charlie was a really nice guy," Dave Rowe recalls. "He had a world of talent. He just had a difficult time learning defenses."

To make the 3-4 work, linebacker Willie Hall, a backup since 1973, would take Gerald Irons's place. The beloved Irons had been traded away in the off-season for the draft pick that brought Philyaw to the team. Hendricks was going to anchor the right outside from his freelance linebacking position. The trade was a stab through the heart for Irons, who got the news in the middle of his final exam for his macroeconomics course at the University of Chicago. He was told that he had a phone call. And that it was an emergency. He'd been exiled from the family.

"I stop taking the test," Irons recalls, "get to the phone, and it's my wife. 'I just got some bad news,' she said. 'We just got traded.' 'Not Chicago,' I say. It was about 30 below that day, and the Bears had won four games the year before. 'No,' she says, 'but it's just as bad: Cleveland.' They'd won three."

He finished the test, got his MBA, and later attended law school—but not before a rude awakening on a new team that seemed to share none of the work ethic of the Raiders. "When I got there, I noticed that after [head coach] Forrest Gregg called practice over, everyone ran into the locker room. I'm used to six years of finding me an area on the field to work out with other guys after practice. It bothered me. I didn't say anything for the first two days. Finally, on the third day, I couldn't take it. I went to Gregg and said, 'I would like to address the team.' He says OK. Everybody got quiet. I said, 'I'm not accustomed to coming to practice every day and not working hard to get into the playoffs. On the Raiders, we'd always talk about the championship. I'm not used to going into the locker room right after practice. We have to stay out there, because we are not working. We are not working hard enough.'"

That year, the Browns went 9–5. The following year, Irons was elected defensive captain by his teammates. He had successfully exported the Badass way of doing things.

There was a new running back in camp, too. Madden had already told Stabler that the team was going to ramp up the passing game, which was fine with the Snake, but in Carl Garrett, Davis had picked up a kick-return man and halfback to back up Clarence Davis. Garrett had played for three different teams in his last four years. Named to *The Sporting News* all-rookie team for the Patriots in 1969, out of Texas Highlands, the sheen had been stripped from his young career. He was cut from New England in 1972 under interim coach Phil Bengtson for missing workouts, and was traded to the Bears, who shipped him after two years to the Jets, who released him after 1975. Davis signed him in July of 1976. The perfect Raider pedigree.

"Why he'd bounced around, I don't know," van Eeghen says. "But he was great for us. He reminded us that if you're on the inside of the Raider family there's no better place to be. As usual, we were all bitching that summer—camp was so fucking long, and one day we'd asked Madden to move meetings up so we could get the air-hockey tournament in, and he'd said no, and we're in the warm-up circle, bitching about how we're going to have to change the date or sneak out to finish it, and Garrett says, 'Listen, guys, can I tell you something? I've played a few places. You got no idea what you have here.'"

"He came with a reputation as a troublemaker if he doesn't carry 25 times a game," says Banaszak. "On our team he was the best team player that ever was. Like every player today thinks it's a mark against them if they play special teams, right? Not Garrett. Then, on the Raiders, *everybody* wanted to play special teams. For me, that was the greatest thrill of my life. Hit them and knock their dick off."

But the team had lost a very reliable and popular tight end. It had been a dark day for the Junior Board, playing a round out on the Alameda golf course during the off-season, when word came that Madden wanted to talk to Bob Moore immediately. Moore left the course and took the call—to receive the depressing and unexpected word that he'd just gone to Tampa in the expansion draft.

"I had no idea where the hell Tampa Bay was," Moore says now. "I had no idea where they played." Nor had he seen it coming. Casper, in his first two years, had been used sparingly, but after his stellar playoff game against the Steelers, it was obvious that the man who would come to be known as "the Ghost" possessed extraordinary athletic abilities.

"I had to do something I didn't want to do," Davis says now of letting Moore go. "But Casper was ready."

"I made a mistake with Casper," Madden admits now. "I waited too long to start him."

Moore went back out to the links and shared the depressing news. "Then we had to come in and commiserate over multiple rounds of drinks. I think we commiserated most of that evening." His tone is only half in jest. Leaving the team hurt. Leaving the board was a blow. But, as we'll see, Moore's friends would not forget him.

What the team lost in a beloved Board member from Stanford it gained in an immortal if enigmatic and complicated football player from Notre Dame. Lineman Steve Sylvester, who played with Casper at Notre Dame and on the Raiders, calls him "the best tight end who ever played the game . . . the best blocking and receiving tight end I've ever seen"—even if the game never really seemed to matter to the man. Dave Casper was a future Hall of Famer who, by all accounts, did not live and breathe for the game of football. "I would have just as much fun plowing a field," he once said, "as I would playing football." (Casper declined to be interviewed for this book.)

If he could never replace Moore in his teammates' hearts, Casper and Stabler would immediately establish an on-field vibe that the lefty never had with Moore. As Stabler's favorite receiver in 1976, with opposing defenses often double-covering Branch or Biletnikoff, Casper's 53 receptions would lead the team and earn him first-team All-Pro honors; his 13-yards-per-catch bested Biletnikoff. In his four full years as a starter, he'd average more than 50 receptions per year.

"He was a very precise route runner," says the Snake. "He ran good, sharp out routes and good, sharp in routes. He knew when to sit down in coverage and when to keep going." (Casper's most memorable catch was the famed "Ghost to the Post," in the 1977 playoff game against Baltimore: asked how he'd made it, Casper answered, "I caught it with my fingers because my chest does not have very good fingers.")

Stabler also appreciated Casper's blocking ability and the mismatches he was able to create on his routes. "Because of Freddy being so great, and because of Cliff being a dangerous world-class speed guy, teams would try and cover Casper with safeties. We'll take that. Or with a linebacker. We'll take that."

At Notre Dame, Casper played offensive tackle before shifting to tight end his senior year, 1973, when the Irish won the national championship. He earned All-America honors and served as a team captain. A cum laude economics major, known to assist friends on papers and test preparation, he strummed the guitar, drank Pabst by the quart bottle at Corby's Irish Pub, in South Bend, and fished for catfish and trout in the St. Joe River. He was a big fan of Willie Nelson and Crystal Gayle.

On the Raiders he'd party with the rest of the team, playing his guitar down at Clancy's with Hubbard and Guy. "Sometimes he was one of the guys," says Sylvester. "He played golf on Tuesdays, and he was involved in all the tournaments." On the other hand, as Stabler recalls, "after games when we would go hang out, sometimes he would go down to the estuary and get his fishing rod and fish. Hey, on that team everybody beat their own drum."

Teammates remember him as a man who took delight in mystifying everyone else with his off-the-wall repartee. "He'd frequently say things that you sort of wondered about," says George Buehler. "If you walked up to him and asked him a question, he'd ponder for a second. Then he'd give you a series of confusing answers."

"Casper would say these things to John and get him started," Dave Rowe recalls. "Odd things. One day we're about to go on the field for practice, Madden is all pumped up, and Casper says, 'Hey, coach, did you ever notice that if you lost something, you find it in the last place you look?'

"Madden looks at him and says, 'Well, yeah, that's just stupid. It's the last place you looked because after that you stop looking.' So Casper says, 'Coach, one time I found something in the last place I looked, but because I didn't want it to be in the last place I looked, I kept on looking.'

"Madden goes, 'What?' Then he goes, 'But you found it, right?'

"'No,' says Casper, 'I kept on looking.' And he just walks away. Madden is dumbfounded. With Dave everything he said was sort of rhetorical. There were no right answers."

"Madden loved Casper," says Sylvester. "He loved his weirdness. He's off the wall. Casper would draw up these crazy plays on the blackboard: 'This is what we gotta do!' It'd be something like a tight end around double reverse. Madden would love to watch it happen. But he'd never use the plays."

"El Strange-o" is how Atkinson sums up a man who few, if any, teammates professed to understand. "A deep man. From a different world. Trust me. Different world altogether."

"I don't really know how to explain Dave," Bob Moore says now. "I don't think anyone does."

"Dave was with us," says backup quarterback David Humm, "but not really with us."

"He was part of it all, but he could also leave it all behind him," says Monte Johnson. "In practice, traveling, playing . . . he always gave you the impression he *had* to do it. It was an obligation. His love for the game was muted. . . . He was torn between being a professor and happening to be a really good football player."

The most dramatic change on the roster that summer came at a position that, on the Raiders, had been stable and sacrosanct for almost a decade. The Raiders had drafted a kicker named Fred Steinfort in the fifth round, and there was only one way to interpret that move: 48-year-old George Blanda, in his fourth decade in professional football, was finished; Blanda's field-goal percentage had been declining through the years, and he'd missed one of every three in 1975.

Although the grizzled Blanda's legendarily bristly demeanor had not endeared him to everyone, he commanded universal respect. To many of the players, he'd been a mentor and stabilizing presence, and a tangible link to the true past. He'd played his first pro games in 1949, during the *Truman* presidency. No one enjoyed seeing him sitting on the bench for every exhibition game that summer. Blanda would not play a single down in the preseason.

"It's been embarrassing," Blanda told a writer that summer during the preseason, in a lounge chair by the El Rancho pool. "It's like waiting to be beheaded. I'm like a cancer out on that field. The players treat me like I have leprosy. I wish I'd known what the situation was before I got here. I never would have come. I have no animosity toward Al Davis or John Madden. I just don't care. Have you ever gotten to the point where you don't care? I don't care."

Before the final preseason game against the Rams, Blanda was cut. He left camp during one of the final practices. Players came off the field to see a disarmingly empty locker.

"It's kind of sad," said Biletnikoff that day. "They owe you something. There should have been some way of having him leave that would give you a good feeling. There should have been something to bring a tear to your eye . . . it's like the guy going to the electric chair."

"I thought there'd be a big press conference and he would go out with glory," said Stabler. "He deserved it. As cold and hard as he was, I enjoyed being around him. He would tell you what he thought. If you liked him, fine. If you didn't like him, the hell with you."

*San Francisco Chronicle* columnist Herb Caen's spin reflected the sentiments, no doubt, of the Raider Nation at large: "Raider boss Al Davis's ticker has to be as hard as the [granite] 'Banker's Heart' sculpture outside the Bank of America headquarters."

"This is the first game in a 14-game schedule, and nothing more," Madden told reporters before the first Sunday of 1976. "OK, so they are the World Champs. But it's just another regular-season game." He was kidding no one. The ratings-savyy schedule makers had given the Raiders a chance for early redemption. The Steelers were coming to town for another chapter in what had become the league's most compelling rivalry.

"The two Super Bowls they went to were through us. They beat us both times. We couldn't take it anymore," says Villapiano now. "Here come the Steelers all cocky. We were going to leave it out there. If we don't win that day, forget the season. We put it all on the line."

By now, two things were certain. First, that the Raiders would make the playoffs again. The postseason was now part of the regular schedule, especially with a weak AFC West that year. Despite the injuries on the defensive line, no one doubted that the Raiders would be standing come the end of the regular season. They were just too consistently Bad.

Second, to get to the Big One they'd invariably have to go through the Steelers in the postseason. "I knew we were going to take care of the West," Stabler says now. "You know you're going to beat San Diego and Denver. The question was: Where are we going to play Pittsburgh?"

On opening day, Sunday, September 12, the gods seemed to be favoring the Raiders, at least weather-wise. With the Santa Anas blowing, the temperature at the coliseum was balmy. The crowd was bloodthirsty, the players hyped.

And George Buehler was . . . greasy. On this day, line coach
Ollie Spencer had devised a new strategy for Fog to try and elude
Mean Joe's mitts. "Before the game, Spencer comes up to me with
Vaseline, and he starts putting it on my chest," recalls George. "I
say, 'Ollie, they don't grab me here. They grab you on the back.' I
go in the bathroom. Van Eeghen is there. He wipes the stuff off
the front, puts it on my back."

You have to admit: the Raiders never lacked for coming up
with a new creative edge. "After the first couple of plays, Greene
goes over to the ref. The ref comes over, looks at me. Wipes my
chest, says, 'There's nothing here! Play ball!'"

A 30-yard Stabler-to-Casper touchdown opened the scoring in the
second quarter, but Bleier tied it at 7–7 with a two-yard touchdown
run, and touchdowns by Stallworth and backup receiver Theo Bell
gave the Steelers a 21–7 lead midway through the fourth quarter.
It was at that point, John Vella recalls, that the tone on the team
subtly shifted: they were in Raider time now. "The Steelers acted
like they had it won. In our huddle we just said, 'Keep doing it,
keep doing it.'"

Stabler's 21-yard touchdown pass to Biletnikoff drew the Raiders within a touchdown. But Harris ran in from the three to restore
the Steelers' two-score margin. The Raiders trailed 28–14 with
less than seven minutes remaining, and after a Stabler interception, the Steelers were deep in Oakland territory. But Monte Johnson—"he had the game of his life," Villapiano says now, "he was
everywhere"—recovered a Harris fumble, and Stabler, the fourth-
quarter fire now lit, took the Raiders 76 yards, capping the drive
with a 10-yard pass to Casper, his second touchdown of a seven-
reception day: 28–21.

The defense held on the next series, and backup tight end and special-teams captain Warren Bankston blocked a punt. The Raiders took over on the Steeler 29. The Steelers stopped the Raiders three times, forcing them to go for it. On fourth down, Stabler ducked under Greene's swipe and found Branch at the 15. Cliff took it to the two, and on the next play Stabler scrambled in for the tying touchdown.

On the Steelers' first play after the kickoff, Dave Rowe tipped a Bradshaw pass, and Willie Hall gathered it in and took it to the 12. Steinfort, the rookie playing in his first regular-season game, punched in the field goal and the Raiders won it, 31–28. First blood drawn, in classic fashion: a 17-point come-from-behind rally to topple the reigning champions.

But as dramatic as the game had been, it became an historical afterthought compared to the long-term legacy created by a single play in the first half, when Atkinson cemented his reputation with a single blow that would resonate for months, whose repercussions would reach beyond the coliseum, into a San Francisco courtroom. The Hit Man had laid out the most notorious blow of his life.

Lynn Swann, lining up on the right, cut across the middle about 15 yards deep into Atkinson's turf. Bradshaw, under pressure, scrambled and threw a pass to Harris, who cut up the middle for a sizable gain—a wide-open middle, because Atkinson had other things on his mind. Atkinson had trailed Swann to the other side of the field, cocked his right arm, and drilled the back of Swann's helmet with his forearm.

The receiver slumped like an inflatable doll with all the air let out of it, collapsing to the infield dirt. Atkinson turned to watch Harris run by him. The safety was out of the play. But he'd made his point. In the second quarter, Swann left the game with a concussion, never to return.

The officials didn't see the blow. No penalty was called. But the play had been caught on NBC's cameras. The replay revealed the most ugly of attacks: the Soul Patrol at its unholiest.

Afterward, giddy hysteria enveloped the Raider locker room. "It did look dark for a while," deadpanned Stabler. A few hours later, he and Banaszak partied hard: "about a bottle of Johnnie Walker Red apiece," recalls Pete.

Down the hall, though, Chuck Noll wore a decidedly different expression. He and Swann were incensed about the Atkinson hit. Asked why he'd taken Swann out in the second quarter, Noll answered, "I took him out because he kept getting hit in the back of the head. He has a concussion."

"There should have been a rule against slapping a receiver years ago," Swann said. "Maybe they're waiting for someone to get killed."

A reporter pressed on: which teams are most flagrant?

"If you don't know," Swann answered, "you haven't been covering the Raiders very long. Sure, it happened last year against the Raiders. How do I know who did it? I'm running with my back to the defender, watching the ball, and somebody smashes me in the back of the head with his fist. . . . There's one Raider, Skip Thomas, who's never given me a cheap shot. I can't say that for the others."

The next day's *Oakland Tribune* featured a fan quote that spoke worlds: "The Raiders and Steelers should throw away the rest of the schedule and play each other 14 times a year. Those guys hit."

The Steelers found nothing glorious about the Raiders' play. On the other side of the country, discussion still concerned the

Atkinson blow to Swann's head. Given a day to think it over, Noll gave full vent to his anger at a Pittsburgh luncheon. "I'd like to see those guys thrown out of the league," he said. "It's football with the intent to maim, and that's not football. We have a criminal section in every aspect of society, and apparently we have one in the NFL."

Madden responded with a metaphoric shrug. "All I can say is that it was a very physical game, a tough game, a rough game," he said, "and there were a hell of a lot of incidents on both sides. . . . Chuck Noll is probably mad because they lost."

A week later, having reviewed the films, Pete Rozelle fined Atkinson $1,500 for the hit—and Noll $1,000 for the "maim" quote. He also shot off a letter to Atkinson: "In sixteen years in this office, I do not recall a more flagrant foul than your clubbing the back of Swann's head."

Today, George remains firm in his belief that the hit was justified: he had acted out of retribution. A few series before, after Branch had made a catch, Blount had hoisted the Raider receiver, a key to their offense, turned him over, and planted him headfirst onto the turf. "OK, you're not going to come into our house and do that," Atkinson says now "You want to try and treat our receivers like that? OK, watch this. Receiver for a receiver, you know? [Noll] saying what he said was so fucking hypocritical."

Cliff Branch confirms Atkinson's account of the series of plays. "George was always looking after my back, because we were roommates," Branch told me. "He'd seen when I ran a hook pattern right in front of Blount, caught the pass, and Mel picked me up, carried me five yards, and dumped me on my head. The whistle was already blowing, and he dumped me on my head.

"And that all started because Noll benched Blount because he couldn't stop me the year before. Mel always remembered that.

George just said, 'An eye for an eye. You're going to do that to our receiver? Let's go after the Steelers guy.' He went after Swann."

Why did Atkinson focus on Swann out of all the Steeler receivers. "He was soft," he says. "The guy got all that publicity for making one catch a year, two catches a year. He was arrogant along with it. It just rubbed me the wrong way, you know? So every shot I got, I took. Hey—when we hit the field it was about kicking someone's ass."

One month later, Atkinson decided that Chuck Noll's words carried more power than any of his own hits. In October he sued Noll and the Steelers for slander. The football world assumed that the suit was Davis's idea, perhaps another way for the man to duel with nemesis Pete Rozelle—a suspicion voiced by one of Atkinson's lawyers, in court, who stated that one impetus behind the suit was to establish "a conspiracy on the part of the Rooney-Rozelle establishment to get the upstart Oakland crowd led by Al Davis."

Atkinson demanded $2 million in damages. The following July, the suit was heard in U.S. District Court in San Francisco— not the kind of black-eye notoriety that the NFL was anxious to receive. On one level, the trial offered a microcosm of the friction between Davis and Rozelle. On another, it provided a futile exercise in airing dirty league laundry.

Six attorneys, more than a dozen players, Madden, Noll (himself a former law student), Steelers president Dan Rooney, Davis, and Rozelle were in attendance for the 10-day affair—Rozelle, as *Sports Illustrated* reported, attended to "deny under oath that his game was fraught with criminal players and brutal plays."

Atkinson lead attorney Willie Brown (not the Raider; the California assemblyman) called the Steelers "the leading cheapshot artists in pro football." Atkinson testified that Noll's words had given him the kind of publicity afforded the likes of Charles Manson and Sirhan Sirhan.

Amid the hubbub, Madden tried to defend his player's actions with an explanation that more or less skirted the issue. "There's a difference between how a cornerback covers a wide receiver and how a strong safety covers a wide receiver," he said. "With a cornerback, a forearm is more likely to be premeditated because he's always covering that wide receiver. With a strong safety, who usually covers a tight end, that wide receiver is suddenly in his area, and he reacts."

Endless hours of film of violent hits—including Steeler blows—and forests of verbiage produced an anticlimactic result. After a few hours of deliberation, the jury decided there was no slander, no malice, no nothing. Atkinson lost. Noll was judged to just be a frustrated coach who'd taken off on a player with a reputation and used the wrong word: "criminal."

But it didn't take a federal case to certify what the football world already knew: the game at its best relied on licensed brutality. And no one practiced it better than the black and silver.

In the meantime, a more innocent type of violence lurked, announced in a seemingly innocuous headline in the *Chronicle*, four days after that glorious opening victory over the Steelers: "Matuszak in Raider Bid." The huge journeyman defensive end, recently released by the Redskins, had been invited to try out in Oakland. Philyaw was playing decently, but Matuszak's résumé seemed to cry out for a shot with the Badasses. Too many also-ran seasons in Oakland called for drastic measures. Davis was bringing in every available body, from wherever he could find them.

As Mike Siani put it to me, "We came from all different parts of the universe." "The Tooz," from his very own planet, was about to find his home at last, and provide a final piece to the championship puzzle.

Despite his size, the heretofore underachieving Matuszak had not overly impressed his opponents in his three years in the league. "Madden asked me about Matuszak," Art Thoms recalls with a laugh. "He asked if I thought he was any good. I said, 'Every time we see him play, we laugh at him. He just can't do anything.' I didn't recommend him. They signed him anyway. He didn't have a lot of moves, but he definitely had a lot of power."

"At this point, we really needed a defensive end, with all the injuries," Villapiano says now. "Al keeps bringing in these other people, and I kept saying, 'Al, they're horrible. I got a guy in Bowling Green named "Mad Dog" MacKenzie. He's selling for Carnation Foods. He's as good as these guys. Can we bring in Mad Dog MacKenzie? Give me someone who can fuckin' play! I'm out there on an island!' So one day Al calls me and says, 'I got your guy: John Matuszak. But I'm going to get him a house next to your house. And I want you to watch over him. He's fucking wild.'

"And then we start playing some fucking football. And now we had a fucking defense. He was perfect for that team."

It had started with a phone call from the Redskins' George Allen to Madden, three weeks before the season opener. Allen was seeking the opinion of a coach in the Chiefs' division about the 25-year-old, 6'8" 280-pounder whose résumé was littered with behavioral asterisks. Madden advised against getting him.

In retrospect, it's somewhat remarkable that the straightlaced Allen was even considering trading for Matuszak, who had spent his rookie year in Houston before being traded to the Chiefs. "Allen was so anal," remembers Monte Johnson. "We had a scrimmage against the Redskins in a training camp. He made this comment, 'You guys can't be a football team. You're so disorganized and undisciplined.'"

Allen must have known about Matuszak's trip to the intensive-

care unit at a Missouri hospital, brought on by an unwise inges-
tion of a combination of barbiturates and alcohol that resulted in a
straitjacket, convulsions, and Paul Wiggin, his head coach, pounding on his chest to keep him alive. The four-day stay in the hospital
made the news (although doctors wouldn't comment on specifics,
and the Tooz chalked it up to a bad diet, which, when you think
about it, was refreshingly accurate). Matuszak's pot-possession bust
in Houston, after his car had been impounded when he hit another
car (the auto's contents also happened to include a .44 magnum),
had made the wires, too.

"I'm the kind of guy who's all or nothing," Matuszak once told
an interviewer, prior to taking the writer to 13 different bars in one
evening. "I mean, if I'm going go out and get screwed up, I do it
all the way."

He'd started his career at Fort Dodge Junior College, then played
for Dan Devine at Missouri—the first of many, many coaches with
whom the Tooz would not exactly bond. (Devine slapped him once
in front of the team.) He transferred to the University of Tampa
and was the first pick in the '72 draft by the Oilers, but before he
could suit up for a single game in that strike-shortened preseason,
he walked the picket line wearing a shirt that read, "On Strike for
Freedom and Dignity." He'd announced the arrival of the Tooz.
After the strike ended, according to his book, *Cruisin' with the
Tooz*, he prepared for his first professional game by sleeping with a
different woman every night of the preceding week.

The Oilers started the season 0–5, and general manager Sid
Gillman stepped in to coach Houston. This was not a good fit
either, and Matuszak decided to play for the Houston entry in the
WFL, which led to a cool piece of NFL history: he became the
only player to ever play for two different professional teams in two

nights, in the same stadium. He played only seven days for the Texans before a sheriff served him on the field with a restraining order from the Oilers. He waved it at the fans as he walked out of the Astrodome.

Manny Fernandez, in town with the Dolphins in January 1974 to play the Vikings in the Super Bowl, remembers Matuszak's distinctive welcoming gesture when the boys hit town. "Me and a couple of other guys walk into a bar called the Sports Page," Fernandez recalls. "We walk into the darkened part of the bar, and the second we walk in: Bam! It was Matuszak. He shot a hole in the ceiling to honor the entrance of the guys going to the Super Bowl."

In 1975, for the Chiefs, he'd started all 14 games, recovering three fumbles. But his erratic behavior (showing up drunk for a team meeting) led Wiggin to put him on the block. Allen gave up seventh- and eighth-round draft picks to acquire the Tooz. In his first exhibition game, he came through with a sack. Two games later, though, after another sack, he forgot to take the field on special teams. He'd never played special teams. He was celebrating his sack.

A few days before the season opener in 1976, abruptly, Allen released him. According to Matuszak, Allen said, "I just can't fit you into our plans." Later, Allen expanded. He chalked up his release of the giant to "vodka and Valium, the breakfast of champions."

But now, with the defensive line in such tenuous shape, "we had so many injuries we couldn't even practice," Vella recalls—Madden and Davis both wanted to take the chance. Matuszak was big, and he came free. If any team could turn him back into the player he had once promised to be, it was the Raiders.

Madden knew the man's on-field style well. In one Chief-Raider game, a late Matuszak hit on Clarence Davis prompted

Madden to explode; Matuszak offered the finger to the Raider bench. In the final game of the 1975 season, Matuszak had sacked Blanda, in George's last appearance as a quarterback. The bloodied Blanda had to be helped off the field.

"I hadn't phoned Allen or the coaches in Kansas City and Houston for his report card," Madden later said of this particular acquisition. " [If] you knew too much about a guy, you tend to pre-judge him, to hold his past against him. I wasn't a psychiatrist or a psychologist. I was a football coach."

A psychologist would have discovered pretty easy pickings. This was a kid who had lost two brothers to cystic fibrosis: one at two months of age, another at two years. Matuszak's father, a worker at the power plant in a town a dozen miles outside of Mil-waukee, was selective with his infrequent praise of his only son. He was openly disdainful of Matuszak's love of sports—a love born of the self-esteem it had given an ungainly (6'1" as a 12-year-old), poor student.

When Matuszak began to excel in sports, he found himself, but not his father's approval. His father, Matuszak would later write, humiliated him over bad grades, mocked his love of sports, and used a strap on his butt—the seeds of what Matuszak himself described as his "anger and meanness."

"All that talk about my failings made me feel incompetent and humiliated," he wrote. "My father's admiration never came. . . . There was a terrible void in my life, one I feared I would never be able to fill. I think my father's absence affected me later when I became a young man. It left me angry, frustrated, maybe a little mean. It put a chip on my shoulder that would be difficult for me to lose."

The elder Matuszak, from a severely broken family, was a for-mer Marine who, the big man wrote, "could project a serious sense of menace. He was 6'1" and 180 pounds, not all that big, but he had a temper that could frighten people much larger . . . he would explode so suddenly, it was like watching another person"—words eerily reminiscent of Stabler's own descriptions of his dad in his own book.

The major difference here was that Stabler knew how to rein it all in, and survive. Matuszak would never be able to sublimate the demons.

When word arrived that Matuszak might join the team, Madden asked Hendricks, "Do you think he'll fit in here?" The linebacker answered, "Look around you, John. What's one more going to hurt?"

According to Atkinson, "Matuszak's first visit to us, he was in the training room with his girlfriend in the hot tub. The guys said, 'Well, you fit right in.'"

But more telling was Matuszak's first one-on-ones with his new owner and his new coach. Both welcomed him into the fold. When Davis summoned him for an interview, Matuszak wore a black suit and a silver shirt. Davis sat behind his desk, also dressed in black. Matuszak expected a lecture and instead got a nonjudgmental welcome, a warm handshake. Soon after his arrival, Matuszak was being continually pressed by reporters about his controversial past. Monte Johnson addressed the newsmen. "John's a Raider now," he said. "He's going to stay a Raider, and he's going to be just fine. You guys just leave him alone."

Madden knew from the start that Matuszak's success as a Raider would depend on his teammates' acceptance of the man, and understanding of the ways of Raider family. So Madden enlisted the help of the men he trusted. Madden always involved the veterans—Upshaw, Willie Brown—when the Raiders welcomed a questionable guy, reputation-wise, into the fold. With Matuszak, Madden talked to several of the vets: We need him. Let him know how important he is. Let him know we don't give a damn about his reputation. Just abide by the three rules and do your thing on the field.

Today, teammates insist that Matuszak could be the gentlest giant of them all—as evidenced by that night when Monte Johnson and his wife invited both Stabler and Matuszak to dine at their home: while Stabler and Phyllis Johnson were in the kitchen, Tooz was in the family room with Johnson's youngest daughter on his knee, reading a Sesame Street book and imitating the Cookie Monster. "And he sounds just like Cookie Monster sounds," Johnson recalls.

"I said, 'John, how do you know what Cookie Monster sounds like?' He says, 'I watch him on TV.' That's how John was. Really just an everyday Joe. But put him in the limelight and public, maybe he had this image he thought he needed to live up to."

Bob Moore laughs at a mention of the Tooz. "John was, if he was without any alcohol or drugs, one of the nicest human beings alive. He met my mother one time, and after that he'd always ask about my mother. Get a couple of drinks in him—or something else? It was 'Katie, bar the door.' . . . He clearly had an addictive personality."

According to Matuszak's own book, Johnson was right on the mark in his assessment of the big man's psyche. "It's strange," the Tooz wrote. "When people expect you to be wild, talk about you being wild, encourage you to be wild, you begin to *be* wild. It's almost as if you *become* your image. There were times when I tried to live up to other peoples' expectations, be the life of other peoples' parties. And I wound up getting hurt for it.

"But I don't want that misconstrued. Ultimately, anything I did was my decision."

What he did was abuse his enormous, athletic body. One Buehler anecdote provides as apt an emblem of Matuszak's excesses as you're ever going to find. One day at practice Madden made Matuszak leave the field. "I didn't notice anything. Madden got all pissed off and told him to get out of there. So I asked someone, 'What's going on?' 'He's high on drugs,' someone tells me. I'm thinking, 'This is on Tuesday. Is he still coming down?' I didn't realize he was on his way up."

Matuszak asked Buehler for a ride home. Buehler agreed but told the big man that he had to get a haircut first. "John said, 'That's fine, I need a haircut, too.' We go over to the local Alameda barber who cuts everyone's hair. The barber has an older gentleman there. Tooz jumps over in this old man's chair when the guy is done, and now Tooz is getting a little glazed."

Matuszak told the man to cut his hair short. "The gentleman finished, and the Tooz puts his nose to the mirror. 'Fuck!' he yelled. 'Motherfuck! What happened to my hair?'

"The little barber is working his way out the door now. I go over and get John by the arm and say, 'OK, Tooz, let's go,' and all he's saying is 'Fuck! My hair! You goddamn fucking . . .'" Buehler and his fiancée dragged Matuszak out of the shop, then had to keep him from walking straight into traffic. "By the time I got him home he was passed out in the backseat."

That was the first of exactly two times Buehler had Matuszak in his car. The second ride produced a somewhat calmer confrontation. "We were riding together in my car on the way to a booster-club event in Sacramento, with my fiancée and John's girlfriend. So he pulls out this marijuana cigarette and starts smoking it, and I say, 'Nope, not in my car.' He goes, 'Oh, man, what the hell?' Again, I said, 'Not in my car,' so I drove him back.

"At least it was marijuana. You're not going to OD on marijuana. Whereas the other stuff . . ."

Matuszak would die in 1989 from heart failure, reportedly brought on by an accidental overdose of Darvon. He was 38 years old.

"John was a tender heart," Buehler says now. "He just had a problem. It was sad."

After beating the Chiefs at home to go to 2–0, the Raiders traveled to Houston. "Large Charles" Philyaw, returning to his college town, responded with the game of his life: two sacks, four passes batted down. Despite five starters missing the game due to injuries, including Stabler, who was out with a bad knee, the Raiders eked out a 14–13 win behind two Mike Rae–to–Cliff Branch touchdowns, in a game that featured the requisite Atkinson blow to the head, this time on receiver Kenny Burrough, in the end zone. The penalty gave Houston the ball on the one, but Matuszak, seeing his first action, led a goal-line stand against his old team, and the Oilers had to settle for a field goal.

But the following week, the Raiders uncharacteristically collapsed in New England. Behind a rushing game that amassed an astounding 296 yards, the Patriots tossed the Raiders aside. The final was a stunning 48–17. Had the Raiders been taking too much for granted? The Patriots, running behind Pro Bowlers John Hannah and Leon Gray, were a ground-game powerhouse in 1976. But a 31-point margin? Against the Badasses?

"The hardest games always seemed to be against the Patriots," Villapiano says now. "We just never matched up well against their offensive line. That one just got out of hand."

"I think we were a little overconfident," Buehler says. "We'd beaten the Steelers, and I think we might have thought we were pretty hot stuff. And when our team bus had pulled up to the hotel the day before, all the fans were asking us not to hurt their guys. We took them a little too lightly."

In the rout, Steve Grogan was called on to throw just 17 times—three of the passes for touchdowns. The Raiders tried to compensate with typical bravado. Tatum was penalized for a late hit, and Atkinson outdid him with an unnecessary-roughness call and another penalty for arguing the call. Both were fined. The only upside to the game was Casper's dozen receptions. The Snake–to–the Ghost was by now not only an integral part of the everyday arsenal; the combination was driving the offense. Casper was just too quick, big, and savvy for linebackers to cover.

The one-sidedness of the defeat was too much for a couple of the Raiders to tolerate. The week after the Patriot game, Upshaw and Willie Brown held a players-only meeting with the team. Brown sensed that the team was off-kilter; the Raiders *never* lost games by lopsided margins. The Badass edge was blunted. Something was missing.

"We just told them we needed more," says Brown now. "We wanted to go for it all. We *had* to go for it all. When we asked for more commitment, players didn't even complain about it. They said, 'Yeah. We'll do whatever it takes.'"

Otis Sistrunk recalls the meeting vividly. "They said, 'If you want to win the Super Bowl, we are not losing any more games.' After that, we were rocking and rolling."

"We just knew getting ready for that year we had the team, we had the players to get us over the top," Brown says now. "With all we'd been through, we knew that we knew how to win."

The next opponent was divisional rival San Diego. The Chargers, coming off a 2–12 season, had hired Walsh as their new offensive coordinator. They were a surprising 3–1, and QB Dan Fouts, now in his fourth season, was growing into a star. Their defense now included lanky end Fred Dean, the sack master, and the huge tackle Louie Kelcher—6'5", 300 pounds, size-17 shoes.

For this game, Upshaw's demand for new commitment included his decision to fire up the man who would be facing Kelcher—Buehler—in a most unorthodox fashion. Of course, given the man involved, the remote-control king, it's not a surprise that Upshaw felt the need to bond George with a machine. This one didn't move, though. Upshaw taped the number of the Chargers' enormous tackle, 74, onto a Coke machine in the Raider locker room and told Buehler to practice ramming against it.

"Louis was a load," says Buehler, who somewhat sheepishly admits that he followed his captain's directive. "I think they'd been talking about him being as big as a Coke machine or something. 'There he is,' Gene said, and pointed to the Coke machine. I didn't spend a lot of timing banging on it. I wasn't actually continually attacking it. But I had to bump it around a little bit to make Upshaw happy." If he'd had more time, Buehler probably would have wired the thing to fly.

The night before the game, Stabler eschewed the Coke and partied hard. Then he went out and proved his dictum: "I knew what I could do in the pregame hours and still perform at a peak on the field."

The Chargers had sold out Jack Murphy Stadium for the first time in four years, and their fans were treated to a seesaw contest in which the Raiders trailed, 17–14, with under 11 minutes to play. But as had so often been the case, in the waning minutes Stabler cooled out and swayed the game. He hit Branch for a 41-yard touchdown pass—he'd already hooked up with Branch for 72 yards on an earlier score—and finished the day by completing 20 of 26 passes for 343 yards. The final was 27–17. The Raiders had scored 13 unanswered fourth-quarter points.

Not unexpectedly, the post-game comments on the other side included the mandatory accusations about the Badass style of play. "It's hard to beat them when they can hold like that," said coach Tommy Prothro. "For us to beat them we'd have to hold on every play."

"They gotta protect Snake" was Madden's response. "I'm not saying they don't take a grab here and there."

At the time, this was a game that seemed to signal nothing more than the Raiders getting back on track. In retrospect, Brown and Upshaw had effectively driven home their point in the players-only meeting. The Chargers would win just three more games. The Raiders would not lose again in 1976. The impetus had not been a coach's rant. It had been a plea from two men from within the family.

By now, Matuszak had cracked the starting lineup and had been embraced by his defensive comrades, putting his stamp on the Raiders' style in myriad ways: at practice, and after it.

"Tuesdays are the first days back after a day of licking your wounds on Monday," Monte Johnson relates. "With us, every Tuesday at practice, warming up, Vella would yell out, 'John, what day is it?' Matuszak would answer, 'It's *Toooz*-day.' After that, no matter what day it was, we'd go into practice and Otis and Hendricks would be yelling from the start of practice, 'Right side! Right side!' Then Villapiano and Matuszak would start yelling, 'Left side! Left side!' It was this hoopla of a circus." If Atkinson would try and horn in on the left-side, right-side ranting, Villapiano says, "we'd have to say, 'Get out of here! You're a safety!'"

Naturally, the competition between the left and right sides spilled over into the post-workout activities. "We would go to the Hilton after practice, have a couple of pops, get started," says Foo. "Every night. It was 'Right side,' 'Left side' all over again." Now it was Sistrunk and Hendricks drinking Crown Royal versus Matuszak and Villapiano drinking Chivas Regal.

"Every night," Villapiano says, now with a shake of the head.

"Night after night after night. All the time. That's pretty heavy. It was big glasses. With ice. Freezing cold. It was good.

"But sometimes I wonder: How the fuck did I survive?"

Kicker Fred Steinfort didn't. He pulled a groin, and Davis and Madden brought in Errol Mann, cut by the Lions. Mann would hit 4 of 11 field goals for the Raiders that season—worse than Blanda's numbers the year before. But at this point he seemed to be their only perceptible flaw.

After victories at Denver and Green Bay, the team was 6–1. In week eight, the Broncos came to Oakland, and the Raider defense held them to two field goals in a 19–6 victory. The following week, they just slipped past the Bears. Stabler was knocked nearly unconscious but returned to hit Branch on a tipped-ball, 49-yard winning touchdown in the fourth quarter, giving the Raiders a dramatic, come-from-behind 28–27 victory.

Two games later, they clinched the division with a victory over the Eagles. But the Raiders couldn't let up, for a very specific reason: after a 1–4 start, which included close losses to both the Patriots and the Vikings, Pittsburgh was putting together its own nine-game winning streak.

It was easy for the Raiders to stay focused the following week—or, perhaps, to not have to worry about focus at all: they'd be playing the hapless expansion Bucs. The tangerine-clad Buccaneers were proving to be easy fodder for any and all opponents (and would finish the season without a single win). The Raiders' 49–16 demolition of the new guys included a great day for Stabler (317 yards, three touchdowns), a 110-yard game for Branch, and five sacks of the luckless Steve Spurrier, who, after nine years in San Francisco, with a Heisman trophy in his den, was now quarterbacking the worst team (at that point) in league history.

But in Raider lore—at least, in Junior Board lore—the Buc game proved secondary to the main Badass performance event of the week. Bob Moore, now wearing the pastel orange of the Bucs, was coming home, and his old friends wanted to treat his return to town in style. When the Bucs flew into Oakland the day before the game, Thoms revved up the limo, gathered his Board comrades, and brought out the red carpet. Literally.

"This is before terrorists, so we talked to some people at the airport, and they agreed to let us drive onto the runway," King Arthur remembers. "Well, not the actual runway but the apron. So the Tampa charter plane pulls up. They bring out those stairs they used to have to get off a plane, and right then we pull the limo up.

"Moore came out, walked down the stairs, and walked across the red carpet. We all hugged him, he got in, and we pulled away. John McKay [the Buc coach], I think, wasn't real happy about that."

"McKay had no idea what the hell was going on," Moore recalls, delighted to relive the day. "In fact, at first, *I* had no idea what the hell was going on. Or how they got to the tarmac. The doors open up and Phil and Dalby and Sistrunk all pour out to welcome me."

Raiders being Raiders, and Moore being Moore, the celebration had actually just begun. Moore still owned a condo in Alameda at the time, and they decided to hold a reunion party. "We go somewhere and have a couple of beers. Then we go to my house."

A local television station got wind of the festivity (following the Raiders with a camera was a guaranteed ratings-grabber) and showed up at Moore's condo.

"We have this party going on. And a couple of Tampa teammates are with me. So girls are going in and out, and the television station shows up at about nine. It gets on the 11 o'clock news."

When he got back to the team hotel the next day, "John [McKay] is really pissed off. He said he was watching the 11 o'clock news, and there I am drinking with the guys we're playing the next day. At the same time, actually, I think Spurrier went over to the other side of the bay and had the same kind of party with his guys. We had a team that was not in very good shape that day." Or, actually, on any Sunday.

For the Raiders, the Saturday fete was just another pregame workout.

With two games left, and an 11–1 record, the Raiders' Monday-night match against Cincinnati carried a huge plot twist: the Steelers had won nine in a row, including a defeat of the Bengals the week before, but if the Bengals were to beat the Raiders on national television, the Steelers would be finished. In other words, if the Raiders lost, the Bengals would win their division, and the Steelers would be out of the playoffs. This was a story line the media could hardly ignore. If Madden rested his starters, which would be understandable under modern circumstances, or if his players let down, they could avoid playing their nemesis in the postseason.

This, of course, was not bloody likely, and all the talk helped fuel the Raider determination. "Madden talked to us about it," Vella remembers. "He said, 'We're going to do it the right way. It's not just what you want; it's how you get it.' Anyway, it's not like we feared the Steelers. They were good, but *we* were good. We thought we could beat them. So we went out and played one of our best games of the year against Cincinnati."

The final was 35–20. The offensive line was impregnable. Stabler threw 20 times, completing 16, including four touchdowns: twice to Casper, one to Branch, and for the clincher in the fourth quarter, a seven-yarder to Biletnikoff. Garrett, van Eeghen, and Clarence Davis ran for nearly 200 yards, and the defense picked off three Ken Anderson passes, two by Monte Johnson. They held the Bengals, who had rushed for 269 yards against the Chiefs two weeks earlier, to under 100 yards on the ground.

"That was really big to me," Madden told me. "Of all the games we played, I have as much pride in what we did to Cincinnati as any game I coached, because we had everything clinched. People were saying we were going to lose because we didn't want to play Pittsburgh. And whoever said that said the right thing to get me pissed off."

Atkinson puts it all in a more Atkinsonian perspective today: "That was us telling Pittsburgh, 'No, we're going through these motherfuckers. We're going to do you a favor first, then we're going to fuck you up next.' The thing that was so beautiful about that Monday-night game was the way we were calling Pittsburgh out: 'Come on, guys, you're not going to stop us this year.'"

## CHAPTER SEVENTEEN

# Reaching the Promised Land

Going into the playoffs with a 13–1 record, the Raiders were not considered to be the favorites in the AFC, despite Stabler's unquestioned supremacy: he'd finished the season as the NFL's top-ranked passer in the league, with an astounding .667 completion average, second in league history to Sammy Baugh. Baugh, who completed 70 percent of his throws in 1945, had thrown 182 passes. Stabler had thrown 291. But the team he led was saddled with the weight of too many postseason disappointments.

Pittsburgh was still considered the team to beat, and with good reason: the Steelers had won those last nine games, a streak during which Pittsburgh's defense truly earned its nickname. The Steel Curtain had given up fewer than three points per game. You read that right. Five of the victories were shutouts. On top of which, the Steelers had a chance to be the first team in history to win three Super Bowls in a row. After recovering from neck and wrist injuries early in the season, Bradshaw had completed fewer than 50 percent of his passes, but his run-oriented offense more than compensated: both Harris and Bleier had gained more than 1,000 yards.

And the Raiders? Still widely perceived to lack the mettle to make it to the top. "Having won their division title for the ninth time in 10 years . . . they start over in the postseason tournament carrying a burden of past frustration," wrote *The New York Times*. "In the last three years they have won their first-round games, only to lose to Miami and then the Steelers twice . . . to the Raiders, the playoffs are the opponent."

But their first playoff foe would be the team that had humiliated them during the regular season. The pesky Patriots had won their last six games and finished at 11–3, including a victory over the Steelers.

"The team that won this game," Dave Rowe says now, "was going to win the Super Bowl."

The Patriot offense was predicated on short, game-control passes and the running of Sam ("Bam") Cunningham, one of three Patriot running backs to gain 700 yards or more. The Raiders were favorites by a touchdown, riding that 10-game winning streak that featured every conceivable Raider strength, from the running game to Stabler's marksmanship, and the 3-4 defense that had held opponents to under 13 points a game after the early-season Patriot decimation. The Raiders stood near the top of the league in all categories—including, of course, penalties.

The Patriot game was a messy and rough affair, featuring no fewer than 21 penalties, seven of which gave the Patriots first downs—including the early Atkinson smash that broke Russ Francis's nose, a blow that one writer called "a right hand that Muhammad Ali would have been proud of." But he had help from Villapiano, a man who never met a tight end he didn't want to flatten. Pregame, Madden had instructed his defense to neutralize the all-world Francis. "On every team there was a guy you wanted to take out of the offense," says Foo. "O.J. with the Bills, Floyd Little with the Broncos, Swann with the Steelers. With the Patriots it was Russ Francis.

"So [on that play] I grab him, I shove him to the side. Atkinson just rams him right in the nose, comes in with the elbow, his nose goes off to the side."

With the game still scoreless, the Patriots got the ball down to the one-yard line, where they lined up against the Raider goal-line defense—a configuration that called for Large Charles Philyaw to be inserted into the left side of the line.

"It was the greatest Philyaw moment on the field—ever," Monte Johnson recalls. Grogan was calling two plays back-to-back in the huddle, in case they didn't score on the first. As always, Johnson instructed Villapiano to tell Philyaw what to do.

"Now Grogan's barking the signals," Johnson recalls. "They snap the ball. We hold them. So they jump up real quick and line up again. I gotta call a new defense, because they've only got a foot or two to score. As Grogan is barking out the signals again, Philyaw is down in his four-point stance. All of a sudden, he drops to one knee and almost sits up, with his head up above everybody else, rotating back and forth, and he goes, 'Hey, Phil, what do I do?'

"Rowe hears this and he's laughing so hard he's bouncing up and down in his stance. I'm going to myself, 'You have got to be kidding.'"

The Patriots ran right at Philyaw, double-teaming him. "But he's not ready; he's on one knee looking around like a chicken," says Johnson. "They hit Charlie so hard the back of Charlie's helmet hits me right in the chest, and now I'm lying on my back, and Andy Johnson runs into the end zone, right across my chest."

The Patriots had taken the lead. Madden was livid. "He's beside himself," says Johnson. "He's walking around ranting and raving. Hands going every which way. Anyway, he turns, and we were still giggling. He goes, 'Laughing! What are you two laughing about? And what is so blankety funny?' Rowe, cowardly, walks away. I said, 'John, right now you won't think it's funny. But if we win I'll tell you.'"

After a Mann field goal, Stabler hit Biletnikoff for a 31-yard touchdown pass, a juggling snatch in the end zone with a defender draped all over him. The Raiders led, 10–7, at the half, but they weren't playing well against the Patriot defensive alignment, anchored by tackle "Sugar Bear" Hamilton.

And Francis, despite the Atkinson blow, was back on the field, with a bandaged nose. "When he comes back in the game," recalls Villapiano, "I look at Atkinson and say, 'Oh, my God, we're in for a war now.' By then, Francis is looking for me. By the end of the game, the line judge is just watching us on every play. I think we had three or four penalties on each other. We were going at it every play. We were warped," Villapiano says, with a grin. "It was just too ridiculous."

Francis managed to grab a 26-yard Grogan pass for a third-quarter touchdown, giving the Pats a 14–10 lead. Now a three-yard run by Jess Phillips made it 21–10 going into the fourth quarter. The Raider ground game had been woeful. They'd gained just 81 yards, with van Eeghen leading all runners with 39 yards. And now the Pats were driving for another score that would put the game virtually out of reach.

The Raider defense was nearing exhaustion. Somehow, the bleeding had to be stanched. "They were at our 35 or 40," Monte Johnson recalls, "and we were all tired, and I looked at the DBs, and they were like, 'Please don't call man-to-man. Call a zone.' I mean, we were beat."

Monte Johnson called a time-out. Madden was angry: "Who called time-out? Time-outs are for the offense!" But Johnson insisted that, without a break, the defense would have given up another touchdown.

"They start the game back up," Johnson says, "and New England tries something really stupid. They try a tight-end reverse, and Francis tries to throw the ball, pressured by Sistrunk. Skip Thomas picked it off."

This was the turning point. Stabler drove the Raiders the length of the field for a van Eeghen one-yard plunge: 21–17. On the next possession, Johnson recovered a fumble. But the Pats got it back. No one panicked. They'd been here before. "In the defensive huddle," Rowe recalls, "everyone said, 'Just stop 'em. Snake will take us back.'" The defense stopped the Patriots on the 32; John Smith missed a 47-yard field goal. The Raiders took over with 4:32 to go on their own 32.

"This is it," Stabler told his huddle. "This could be the last time we have the ball all season if we don't get it done." He completed four out of five passes to move the team to the 19, with 1:24 remaining. Then an incompletion and a sack left them with third and 18.

Stabler threw an incompletion, with tackle Sugar Bear in his face. If what had happened in the next few seconds had occurred in the modern era, the replay would have been featured as often on *SportsCenter* clips as the infamous Tuck Rule call. As it is, the play lives on only in the haunted memories of Patriot fans. A flag appeared in the backfield: referee Ben Dreith called a roughing-the-passer penalty on Hamilton, who had barely swiped Stabler's helmet with his forearm. Sugar Bear would claim he'd tipped the ball. But no official thought so.

"[The hit] was somewhere close to his head," says John Vella now. "But it wasn't a very violent hit." By Stabler's own admission, it was just Hamilton's hand hitting him in the face.

"Hey," says Rowe, "it was a rules violation. Sugar Bear hit him in the head. If I'd been with the Pats, I'd never have forgotten it, either."

Now it was first and 10 on the 13. Two plays later, on a third and one, a Banaszak run came close to the first down. But Hamilton had yapped at the officials and earned another penalty. With 14 seconds to go, from the one, Stabler called an option to Casper, who was covered. Stabler rolled left and, with Upshaw leading the way, scrambled into the end zone.

"He acted like it was nothing," Rowe remembers. "He was that cool." The final was 24–21, Raiders.

When the Raider locker room had almost cleaned out, and the happy fog of the come-from-behind victory had subsided, Monte Johnson got his chance to explain the first-quarter hilarity: "Suddenly I get the sense that someone's sitting next to me. It's John. Still got on his blue shirt. He's drinking a Tab and smoking a cigarette. I get the sense he wants me to tell him something. I'd completely forgotten about the play. He goes, 'So you gonna tell me what was so blanking funny?'" Johnson recounted Philyaw's goal-line bafflement. "He starts laughing so hard he almost falls off the stool. Then he says, 'You're right. It wouldn't have been funny then, but it sure is now.'"

The Patriot locker room had a decidedly different vibe. The Raider style of play had obviously left more of an impression than a broken nose for their tight end. To the Patriot way of thinking, alley brawls did not constitute playoff football. "If they're going to go all the way," said a livid Darryl Stingley, "they'd better clean up their act and start playing some football. That's why they can't win the big game. Their method catches up with them. If they continue taking cheap shots and stuff, they're going to have a lot more penalties called on them than they did today."

But the Badass style had provided a winning formula, and today Villapiano savors the memory of that revenge victory, which, he says, provided the impetus for the games to follow.

"We attacked them, held them, grabbed them, smashed them. They were complaining. We were complaining. That's a playoff atmosphere. That time, we gave them a little Raider-style football."

They had to wait one more day to see if they'd earned a shot at the one opponent they wanted to meet—*had* to meet. Pittsburgh did not let them down. The Steelers routed the Colts, the team with the number one offense in the conference, 40–14. Pittsburgh compiled an astounding 526 yards in total offense, including 132 yards for Franco. Bradshaw was sharp, completing 19 of 26 passes, and Swann had two touchdown receptions as the Steelers virtually neutralized Baltimore's vaunted "Sack Pack."

The Raiders, of course, were more than pleased at the outcome. If they were going to go all the way, it had to be through the Steelers. "I wanted to play Pittsburgh all along," said Atkinson. "Baltimore made the Steelers look better than they are. The Colts were intimidated. That won't happen to us. We have a team that can't be intimidated."

In a strange postscript to the Steeler game, a small plane crashed into the upper deck of Memorial Stadium's horseshoe a few minutes after the crowd had dispersed. No one was hurt in the crash. The injuries had happened on the field, where Bleier aggravated his toe and Harris had bruised his ribs. They would be questionable for one of the most highly anticipated rematches in league history: a defense that no one could score upon against an offense that could score upon everyone—in the fourth quarter, anyway.

The Raiders had won 11 in a row. The Steelers had won 10 in a row. But Pittsburgh's defense had been so dominating, with Greene, Holmes, White, and Greenwood on the line, that the Steelers were still seen as holding the upper hand, at least in the impartial New York press, which had no dog in this fight.

"The Steelers, who were being counted out of the playoffs after only five games of the season," wrote Michael Katz in the *Times*, "showed that once again they should be considered the No. 1 team in football." Katz also felt moved to note that "some Raiders talk to some Steelers only through their attorneys. The two teams lead the league in lawsuits against each other."

His colleague William Wallace put it more succinctly: "Perhaps they should call out the National Guard and station troops around the field."

"I guarantee," Joe Greene said, "that if Atkinson starts pulling that stuff, I'll come off the bench to get him, if I have to."

For Stabler, clearly speaking for the whole team, questions of physical decorum were, by now, taking a backseat to the story line that didn't even have to be addressed. The Steelers were two-time Super Bowl champs. The Raiders were no-time nothings. Being the all-time almost absolute best counted for zip. "I'm getting tired of hearing the same question every year," he told a reporter. "'Why can't the Raiders win the big one?' It would be great not having to hear that again the next six months."

The league named Tommy Bell, arguably the most respected official in the game, to head the officiating crew. Not only was Bell known for making quick, sound decisions; he was an attorney. Hopefully, he wouldn't have to litigate on-field. Dwight White publicly thanked the league for tapping the level-leaded Kentuckian.

"This might be the first game," said an NFL official, "where a penalty flag is thrown in the parking lot."

And then there was the matter of Bleier and Harris, who was taking injections for his ribs but still had trouble breathing. "They'll play," said Madden.

But he was preparing his team for the possibility that they wouldn't, Villapiano recalls. "The Friday before the game, we go in after practice, and then Madden calls us all back out. The word came out that the Steelers might use a formation we hadn't practiced: two tight ends and a fullback. Two tight ends is pretty effective. We were laughing, because we figured they were trying to surprise us. We didn't realize Rocky and Franco weren't playing until game day."

"I vividly remember the introductions to that game," Buehler told me. "The Steelers had been introduced before us, and they were all over there on their sideline jumping up and down like high-school kids. I thought that was kind of amusing. I was thinking, 'That kind of thing can disappear pretty quickly in a game.' We were calm. Besides, they had snuffed our hopes too many times. This was something we wanted to close the book on."

For once in the Badass era, it would turn out that no intimidation was needed on this day. Even Swann admitted that it was the cleanest game the teams had ever played. No one was hurt. No one was clobbered. No one on the Raiders wanted anything to get out of hand, and it didn't have to: the Raiders made their statement with a day of simple football dominance. They controlled the line of scrimmage all afternoon. And they collected just 34 yards of penalties—none of the roughing kind.

It was close for only a quarter and a half. After a Mann field goal and a Clarence Davis one-yard run, Reggie Harrison's three-yard run made it 10–7, Raiders, in the second quarter, but the Raiders went ahead 17–7 on a Stabler-to-Bankston four-yard pass just before the end of the half. A 12-play, 63-yard drive in the third quarter, with Stabler effectively mixing the run and the pass, ended with a five-yard Banaszak reception that made it 24–7, which held up as the final.

At the game's end, Swann caught a meaningless completion, and Atkinson, after cleanly defending four passes to Swann, now rushed him—to retrieve the ball.

Without Harris and Bleier—2,164 yards of rushing offense during the season—the Steelers were down to Harrison and Fuqua, and ran out of the tight-end-heavy formation much of the game, but managed just 72 yards on the ground—and not just because the Steelers were lacking their two horses. Because Madden had decided to use Kick 'Em to throw a wrench into the game plan.

"They liked to use a lot of running plays where the offside guard pulled," Dave Rowe recalls. So on that day Madden and Zeman decided to put Hendricks up on the line, right opposite the guard. In Pittsburgh's scheme, if the guard was covered, he wouldn't pull, because whoever was on him would just follow him and take everybody right to the play.

"So Hendricks would line up as a lineman, the guard wouldn't pull, and their running back—that day, Fuqua or Harrison—would be out there alone. I heard—I'm not going to call it dissension, but more like discord—from them that day on the field. 'It was 28-lead! You were supposed to pull!' 'But I had a guy covering me!' Stuff like that. And then Hendricks, of course, would just drop back into the linebacker spot and go to the play."

Fuqua gained 24 yards that day, Harrison 44. The Raider triumvirate of van Eeghen, Davis, and Banaszak churned out 166.

"We didn't care who was back there," Villapiano says now. "We were ready, man. We nullified absolutely everything they did. And we were in the Super Bowl."

"Critics said we couldn't make it to the Super Bowl and that we were a dirty team," Atkinson told reporters after the game. "I say to them, 'Eat your words.'"

"We played without 50 percent of our offense," said Noll afterward. "I'm sorry we didn't have more weapons."

Today, none of the Raiders want to hear about the excuses. This rivalry went beyond personnel. A Raider-Steeler game came down to nothing more than *will*. "That was our time," Madden says now, scoffing at the notion that the Steelers lost because they were undermanned. "They weren't going to stop us that day. They could have had Franco and Bleier and the whole thing, and it wouldn't have made any goddamned difference. That was our day. That was our year."

"Come on—the game was a blowout," says Rowe. "We beat them in every aspect of the game. You're talking about two players. That game was not won or lost on offense or defense. That game was the Oakland Raiders going through the Pittsburgh Steelers. You're talking about scoring 24 points against an incredible defense. And it wasn't like we scored by intercepting a pass or recovering a fumble and getting the ball on the 10 or something. We put some drives together. We drove the football on a great defense. We scored 24 points on them pretty easily."

"When you lose, you always need an excuse, I guess," Stabler says today.

Two years earlier, the Steelers had dominated the line of scrimmage. This time, it was the other way around. The vaunted Steeler defense was on the field two-thirds of the game. "Hey, we were a good running team," says Buehler, who had a typically good day against Joe Greene. "We wanted to show our strength as a running team, to show that it could defeat the run-stopping team."

Moments after the clock ran out, the Raiders tossed Madden, cigar and all, into the showers. Art Shell had advised Madden to bring an extra set of clothes. He hadn't listened. When he made it to the postgame press conference, the water from his face was still patting against the mike. "We've lived with the fact that we haven't been able to win the big one for a long time," he said. "And we felt it was time to disprove that."

In the locker room, Stabler put a grander perspective on the victory. "I'm especially glad for this team," he said. "This may be the closest group we've had, because we've overcome adversity. We had all those injuries and had to rebuild our defense, and then we pulled out one close game after another. Sometimes that can make you better. Maybe in the past we had too many things come too easy to us and then couldn't handle it when they didn't come easy. So maybe these players have done the hardest work and developed the closest feeling we've ever had."

The Raiders had won the game that, for them, counted most. But it wouldn't be a complete victory without one more. For the first time in nearly a decade, they were in the big one. And if they were to lose, the win over the Steelers would surely be relegated to history's scrap heap.

By late that afternoon, the Raiders knew who their opponent would be. In the NFC, the Vikings had beaten the Rams, 24–13, in large part because of their vaunted special teams: they had blocked three kicks, including a short Tom Dempsey field goal, which resulted in a 90-yard touchdown return by Bobby Bryant in the first quarter. In retrospect, one statistic from that day stands out as telling. The Vikings had given up 168 yards rushing.

The stage was set for one team to get a monkey off its back. The Vikings had appeared in three Super Bowls, two in the previous three years, and lost all three. But they'd put together a 13–2–1 season. In one way, the Vikings held a distinct advantage; 22 of their players had played in the last two Super Bowls, and in the big one, it always helps to have been there before. Only four of the Raiders—Willie Brown, Banaszak, Upshaw, and Biletnikoff—had been around for their one-sided loss in the second Super Bowl.

On the other hand, the game would be played in the Raiders' home state, in Pasadena's Rose Bowl. The weather would likely be pleasant. A significant number of the fans would be rooting for the team from upstate. The Badasses had been waiting for this chance since time immemorial.

And once you're past Pittsburgh, Franco or no Franco, who's to be feared? "When you have to go through the Steelers, you feel pretty good about playing Minnesota," says Stabler now. "We felt good about the matchup. We felt a little bit stronger."

## CHAPTER EIGHTEEN

# "I Felt as Confident as I've Ever Felt"

For the nation at large, the Super Bowl by now had blossomed into an event, having emerged from the shadow of the national pastime into the carnival lights of a broadcast extravaganza capable of bringing the nation to a standstill. Streets were deserted, cities seemingly abandoned. "The annual electronic communion," *The New York Times* predicted, would bring "commerce to a national standstill." Befitting the Raiders' vibe and Oakland's reputation as a lowly town far removed from the national cosmopolitan map, the commerce the *Times* chose to feature in Oakland was an adult-movie theater near Jack London Square. "Seems people who come to porno flicks also like football," a young woman told the newspaper's reporter, whose source preferred to remain anonymous, lest her mother back in New York learn of "the circumstances of her employment."

The week of the game, *Time* gave over its cover story to an in-depth examination of "The Great American Spectacle." The statistics that the magazine cited with wide-eyed fascination (165 miles of video cables!) would merit a yawn today, but in January of 1977, the fact that one of every three American citizens would see at least part of the game was deemed newsworthy. The TV audience would be larger than the populations of all but nine nations in the world.

The most obvious barometer of the game's having shifted from field to stage was Pete Rozelle's assertion, when asked by *Time*'s Roger Kahn, if the game had become "show biz." "Sure," answered Rozelle, " . . . but we prefer the word 'entertainment.' . . . Entertainment is all we are." No mention of the game as sport.

Kahn's piece bemoaned the current evolution of athletes into entertainers, with its implicit assumption that the accomplishments of a sports team were increasingly taking a backseat to the exploits of the individual. His thesis didn't apply to the Raiders, who featured no cover boys. But their opponents did have one, which explains why, while the bulk of the magazine's coverage went to outside-football facts, the game analysis lathered more ink on the Vikings—specifically, on Fran Tarkenton. Tarkenton, who had published his own book two months earlier, merited a full page of photographs and his own sidebar. The loquacious quarterback was by now such a reliable interview that before the game the network had constructed transmission towers outside of his Minneapolis home for interviews before the teams traveled to Southern California. It wasn't as if he were a mere performer, though. At that point, the man with the "choir boy" face had amassed the most impressive quarterback numbers in league history, holding records in total yards passing, touchdowns, and completions.

His game was hardly as dramatic or exciting as it had been in the days of yore; at the age of 36, Tarkenton's years of scrambling had come to an end. In the first eight years of his career, he'd averaged more than 300 yards rushing per season: 1976 marked the first year in his career he'd run for fewer than 100 yards in a season, but by now he didn't have to scramble. He was still an All-Pro selection, completing more than 60 percent of his passes, nearly as many to his backs as to his wideouts. Rookie receiver Sammy White was breaking out as a threat, to complement Ahmad Rashad, but versatile, quiet running back Chuck Foreman, the NFC's MVP, was still Tarkenton's favorite receiver. The workmanlike Foreman could forever turn a short pass into a long gain.

The running quarterback was also becoming known as a businessman and inspirational speaker, one of the first athletes to use his football fame in the business world. Tarkenton was articulate, opinionated, and confident, especially when it came to detractors of his game.

But who remembers his guarantee? "We are going to go there January 9th," he told *Time*, "[and] we are going to win." Maybe his words held no traction because so much time had passed since Joe Namath's famous guarantee, seven years earlier. But it was quite the boast: the NFC was by far the weaker conference, and in their own woeful division, no other team finished above .500.

The magazine's coverage of the Raiders? Well, the bearded Stabler earned a small photograph. But the first Raider player mentioned in the magazine's story was Ray Guy. For the most part, Oakland's contingent was cited for its image. The designated "Bad Boys of pro football," who had left behind "a host of battered, angry opponents," were "led by Al Davis"—"master schemer"—certainly the first time the national press had given an owner, not a head coach, credit for leading his team.

With the 3-4 defensive alignment, the Raider defense seemed well suited to face the Viking offense. More linebackers meant more men ready to cover Tarkenton's short passes. The most noteworthy aspect of the Viking game was their remarkable ability to block kicks; the distinct concern going into this game, Tom Flores re-calls, was the Vikings' special-team play.

Excellence in an area that's commonly overlooked fit the Vi-kings' image of a largely emotionless group of automatons, led by Bud Grant, who was famed for his even-keeled, expressionless demeanor. If the Raider coach's natural facial expression ran the rubbery-faced spectrum from raging scream to glowing smile, the Viking coach was as stoic as if he'd been carved out of stone, and his team, following suit, played a distinctly non-Hollywood style of ball. As the immortal Jim Murray of the *Los Angeles Times* put it, "The Vikings play football like a guy laying carpet. The Raiders play like a guy jumping through a skylight with a machine gun."

The Vikings had won the NFC convincingly but not over-poweringly. They *had* beaten the Steelers, in Minnesota. But after finishing first in run defense in the conference the year before, they'd slipped to 17th in 1976. The Viking defensive line, which had gained considerable fame as "the Purple People Eaters," was not constructed to face the Raiders' left-handed offense. The Raiders' two most famous offensive linemen, Upshaw and Shell, would be going up against a couple of Vikings who were severely outweighed.

The Vikings' right defensive tackle, Alan Page, a true great, was a wise, gifted athlete who'd graduated from Notre Dame, was a few years shy of his law degree, and would go on to serve on the Minnesota Supreme Court. But Page weighed all of 236 pounds, and he'd be going up against guard Upshaw, who outweighed him by at least 30 pounds. Not counting the weight of his arm-clubs.

Equally mismatched were the Vikings' right defensive end, Jim Marshall, and left tackle Art Shell. Marshall was fast, and he was sharp; he beat opponents with strategy more often than strength. But he had turned 39 the week before, and he weighed all of 217 pounds at game time. Behind Page and Marshall stood outside linebacker Wally Hilgenberg, 35, who'd been in the league since 1964.

⤬

Madden devised a simple offensive strategy for his Super Bowl play calling: keep the Vikings off-guard.

"You never want to be predictable," he told me, "because offenses and defenses are based in predictability. They were the type of team that was fundamentally disciplined and organized. Just by doing something a little different, it was better than doing the things they focused in on."

But his first challenge was to figure out a way to avoid having the two-week buildup to the game freak out his squad of Super Bowl virgins. So for the first week he concentrated his energy on disposing of any and all distractions. Come Super Sunday, he wanted his team in the regular-season mind-set, clearheaded enough to treat this one as just another game, if that were possible.

"From coaching [four] Pro Bowl teams [where he could tap the brains of myriad Super Bowl–winning players], and observing the Super Bowls," he told me, "I always figured that the team with the fewest complaints always won the game. The team that was complaining about extra tickets, extra people, the practice facility, usually lost. So the first week, I said, 'We're going to get everything out of the way.' I got all the players' tickets right off the bat and told them to get rid of them before we flew down to L.A.

"I made sure that everyone would have an extra room at the hotel. Other teams complain, 'You take wives down; how about if you don't have a wife? A girlfriend? A mother?' Those things could become issues. So I made sure everyone had an extra room for whoever they wanted. Then I made sure everyone had an extra seat on the airplane. I wanted all the extracurriculars out of the way."

And, in a stroke of reverse-psychological wisdom, he told his players not to fear the hoopla but to embrace the publicity as much as possible. This was their moment. They'd earned the spotlight. It might never come again. The pressure, Madden figured, was intense enough; he would do everything he could to defuse it. As Dave Rowe recalls it, the practices up in Oakland were loose: "We played touch football one day." The real stuff would come the following week.

"We did some football work that first week," Madden said, "but we watched a lot of film so we could get acquainted with what they looked like. If you practice the game plan the first week, if you have something done early, you just have to go over it again, and the next thing, I figured boredom would set in.

"And my team wasn't a team that handled boredom well."

He liked what he saw on film. The Viking defensive backfield looked vulnerable. "We really thought we were going to be able to do damage to them in the passing game, because they played a zone, a cover three, and the corners were off. I knew Biletnikoff was going to have a big day. We did very little short stuff anyway, more intermediate and deep. Deep was hard against them, but intermediate would be there: ins, outs, crosses, comebacks, hooks."

For at least one player, linebacker Monte Johnson, this game merited extra homework. Johnson had his own projector and studied at home. "And during my prep for the Super Bowl, I noticed their offense had a tendency in the goal line, how they lined the backs up, how they determined which side of the center they'd run the ball. At one point we were practicing short-yardage defense, and I went to Zeman and Shinnick, and I said, 'Guys, trust me and allow me to call the defense on the line of scrimmage in short-yardage.'

"They said, 'Why would we ever do that?' I said, 'Let me tell you what I've seen.'

"They watched a number of reels. They went to Madden and

said, 'This is what we want to do.' John says, 'Sure.'" It would prove
to be a wise decision.

In the days leading to the game, Davis was nowhere to be seen. It
was said that he was down in Mobile, scouting the Senior Bowl, as
he always did. He'd be back, of course, but he'd be staying at the
Beverly Hills Hotel, not with the team at the Newport Beach Marriott. But even when he returned, he managed to keep a low profile.
"Aw, you know me," he would explain to writer Dan Jenkins. "If I
come around, I say something controversial, and the commissioner
doesn't get the headlines."

In fact, leading up to the game, no one on the Raiders said a single
thing that might inspire the opponent. "We were always careful in
how we approached it from a publicity standpoint," says Flores now.
"We didn't want to put out any fodder verbally." The only somewhat
inflammatory words came from the future judge Page, discussing
Upshaw: "Gene's a great player. But he holds me a lot. He's such a
great player he really shouldn't have to do that. If you want to get
around him you have to go all the way to East Los Angeles."

Upshaw's response was muted. "No offensive lineman likes to
talk about holding—nor do defensive linemen like to talk about
things like late hits or flying elbows."

A more intriguing quote from Page was this measured response
when asked how he'd feel if the Vikings were to lose: "It's a football
game. To win will be nice, but to lose will not be the end of the
world."

It was difficult to envision a Raider thinking that way, given
Madden's annual training-camp emphasis on winning it all—a
striking contrast to an almost baffling Bud Grant quote from one
interview, in which he spoke of how good all of the playoff teams
had been: "The important part is to be one of the eight."

Game week began like any other: no curfews Monday, Tuesday, or Wednesday night. This gave Stabler and Biletnikoff the opportunity to descend upon the Playboy Mansion Monday night, which stretched into Tuesday morning. The partying ended Wednesday night, when Snake, Rooster, and Freddy, who had adjoining rooms at the hotel, sampled the local taverns. After that, it was strictly business.

To Dave Rowe, Madden's approach to their second week of practice made all the difference come game time. Once they got down south, the coach stuck entirely to their season-long workout routine. No sudden two-a-days. No extra meetings. No sense that this was anything but another game. "We didn't change a thing," Rowe recalls. "Tuesday was going over the game plan, Wednesday was defense day, Thursday was offense day, Friday was short-yardage and goal-line, and Saturday was special teams, like it'd been all year."

"He told us to treat it just like a business trip," says Stabler. "And that we were going to go down there to take care of business."

"Yeah, our week was normal," says Madden. "Our football was normal. Our meetings were normal. Other than the press conferences, everything was a normal workweek. No distractions. The only thing that's a distraction is if it's something that isn't planned. I had everything planned."

You didn't say, "Guys, you're about to play the biggest game of your life. This is special"?

"Shit, they knew that," Madden says. "That's the last thing I'd say."

After so many years of flirting with greatness, no Badass needed any motivational prompting. As had always been the case, the team took it on themselves to ensure there'd be no letdowns. Thursday's practice, despite uncharacteristic Southern California rain, featured what several players recall as the single best practice they could ever remember.

"We were fine-tuned, you know?" Atkinson says now. "That practice was like, man, no other. We were crisp, we were sharp. No mistakes. No balls hit the ground. Receivers didn't drop a ball that week, come to think of it."

Saturday's practice lasted, by Banaszak's estimation, about 20 minutes, under the first sun they'd seen in days. This time it wasn't just the sharp execution that buoyed the team. It was the feeling from Madden, and all the way down, that they were as finely tuned as they'd ever been.

"The day before a game," remembers Banaszak, "we'd always just have a 45-minute practice. Just light stuff. We'd work on special trick plays, but of course we'd never call them. Madden always worked on them, but he'd always say, 'You live by the trick, you die by the trick.'

"So after about 20 minutes, Madden calls us in. He says, 'Let's stop right now. Go on in. If we play like we just practiced, it won't be a game. We play like this, we're going to kill them.'"

After the practice, some of the players made a ball out of tape and played softball.

No one is certain which practice a contingent of Chinese reporters attended. But when one of the writers told the team that, on the Chinese calendar, 1977 was the Year of the Snake, it was taken as a pretty beneficent omen.

Tapping their brains today, it's impossible to tell whether the Raiders' insistence that they were supremely confident is partly a by-product of the ultimate outcome. But to a man, they'll tell you they had few doubts, if any at all.

"The most important thing that happened that week before the week of the Super Bowl was that we knew the Vikings didn't have a chance," says Willie Brown. "We knew exactly what we were doing, how we were doing it. The coaches had us well prepared. We just couldn't do enough in practice. At Thursday practice, we knew, 'Hey, it's done. It's over. The game is won. The score is on the scoreboard already. The celebration has already been done.'"

"With the type of game they played, the offenses they ran, there was no question in our mind," Atkinson says now. "When we caught the Vikings, it was just like a dream come true, basically: going in and knowing you were going to win. Not cocky, but confident because of the fact that we were a veteran championship-game team. It was just a matter of how bad we were going to beat them. It wasn't disrespect. We just knew from years of playing tough teams every year in those championships. The teams we played in the championship games normally won the Super Bowl. So we had no doubt about winning it."

The night before the game, Madden gave his own uncharacteristic guarantee, in private, to his owner, on the phone. "I said to him, 'We're going to get these guys. This might not even be close.' He said, 'Don't talk like that!' Like I'm gonna jinx it.

"I wasn't that type of guy, normally. Even if I had those feelings, I wouldn't normally say it. It was just I had a feeling, after the way we practiced that second week. The way Stabler was so sharp in that last offensive practice. I just knew that I liked the matchup. I liked the way we were prepared. I liked the game plan. I felt as confident as I've ever felt."

On Saturday night the team moved into a new hotel, closer to the Rose Bowl, so as to avoid getting stuck in a traffic jam on the way to the game. Davis had found a Hilton with extra rooms in downtown Los Angeles. But the Raiders weren't going to be moving up to more luxurious lodging. The new hotel turned out to be smack downtown, and back in the '70s, downtown Los Angeles offered up a deserted urban wasteland.

"There wasn't one person out on the street the night we were there," says Banaszak. "I mean, we're talking no-man's-zone. The football players were the only ones in the coffee shop. It was kind of a dump. There wasn't a bed big enough for Matuszak. Sistrunk's bed, the middle was falling in. Madden kind of zinged us there." No wonder there'd been available space.

But there was an upshot to the downgrade: no way was anyone going out to break curfew on the night before the biggest game of their lives.

"Not down there," says Rooster. "There was nowhere to go."

If the Super Bowl show had taken its place on the national stage, the game still didn't have enough cachet to go to prime time; kickoff was scheduled for 12:30 PST. And Madden was terrified that they wouldn't get to the Rose Bowl on time. He'd gone out of his way to try to envision any and all things that might go wrong, and that homework had included a call to his old friend John Robinson, with whom he'd grown up in Daly City. Robinson had briefly been a Raider assistant in 1975 before taking over the head job at USC. Robinson warned him against the traffic on the small city streets leading to the stadium in Pasadena. Madden went so far as to hire a helicopter to lead his buses to the stadium.

But even that tactic wasn't enough to stem the coach's anxiety about being late to the game. At breakfast that morning, he changed the 10 o'clock departure time to 9:15. Then he herded everyone on to the buses at 10 after nine.

"He was so worried that morning about getting there," says Banaszak, "he left half the guys back [at the hotel]. That morning you couldn't get a toothpick in his rear end with an air hammer."

Only a handful of players missed the buses. Biletnikoff and Clarence Davis took a cab. Matuszak found his own ride to the stadium. He flagged down a fan outside the hotel dressed in a pirate costume, waving a sword.

Befitting his unconventional coaching methods, Madden tended to avoid game-strategy specifics in his speeches, addressing more elemental perspectives. All week, his overall message to the team had been more philosophic than strategic, as Steve Sylvester recalls. "I remember one thing he said: 'They can take your ring away, they can take your money away, but they can never take the memories of this game away.'"

Now, minutes before kickoff, he gave the shortest speech of his career. "He looks around the room," Villapiano remembers, "and all he says is, 'Guys, this will be the single biggest event of your lives—as long as you win. Let's go.' That's it. Now, I'm an emotional guy. I'm thinking, 'Give me more! Tell me to knock someone's helmet off!' But he wasn't giving us anymore. It's probably a good thing. Who knows? If he tells me to knock someone's helmet off, maybe I get a penalty, it changes the game."

"Pregame speeches are overrated," Madden told me. "Those are very overrated. If you have two weeks to get ready, and you're with your team for those full two weeks, there isn't a lot you haven't said.

"Besides, everyone wants to burst out of there. They want to hit the light of the day, get out of the tunnel, and start playing. *I* just wanted to get the hell out of there—bust down those doors and get on the field."

So Villapiano's memory is more or less correct? "That was the essence of it," Madden says. "I was telling them, 'This is going to be the greatest day of your lives. Act like it and play like it.' You don't remember losing. It had to be a win to be the greatest day of your life. Make a memory."

And was it the best day of your life?

"*Hell*, yeah."

## CHAPTER NINETEEN

# The Game

Under a sunny sky, with the temperature near 60 and 103,438 fans packing the Rose Bowl—and nearly 75 million watching at home—the Raiders won the toss, received the kick, and immediately started to roll. Sticking to the intermediate-pass game, they put together a 54-yard drive, highlighted by a 25-yard Casper reception, only to watch Mann's 29-yard field-goal attempt boing off the left upright.

But Stabler was not dismayed. "We'd moved the ball well," he says now. "We felt good."

But neither team could sustain anything on offense for the next few drives. Five of the Vikings' first seven plays involved Chuck Foreman, producing only one first down in Minnesota's first two series. Tarkenton's only pass to a receiver, Sammy White, was knocked down by Dr. Death, who would have one of the best games of his career.

With five minutes left in the first quarter, on Oakland's third possession, after Viking linebacker Jeff Siemon stopped Clarence Davis two yards short of the first down, the Raiders were forced to punt from deep in their own end. Ray Guy lined up at the nine. Guy had never had a punt blocked in his four years in the league, but he was now facing the best punt-blocking legion in the league. And even though the Vikings were set up in a return formation, not a punt-block formation, linebacker Fred McNeill blew in from the right side and blocked Guy's kick, recovering the ball on the Raider three-yard line.

"What was I thinking when it was blocked? It's not something you can print," says Guy now. "I was mad. God, was I mad."

"I can hear the thud to this day," says van Eeghen, who was blocking in the backfield. "It was all my responsibility. The Vikings were loaded in the middle, [Charlie] Phillips was the cover guy on the right. He was supposed to deliver a hand jab to the chest to the end guy on the line, and I was supposed to step up and secure the center. But I got over to the right too late. I remember that thump to this day."

"But up until that point," Guys says now, "the game was back and forth, each team feeling the other out. It was like we were in a lull. When we heard that sound, I think that lit a fire under us. Because then things began to happen. I don't know whether something went off in us or what. But the clock started up right about then."

On the Raider three, the Vikings went into their short-yardage goal-line offensive formation—the very situation that Monte Johnson had studied for. "So as we're about to run on the field for that defensive series," Johnson recalls, "Madden looks at me and says, 'Don't let me down.' I get out there and say to the team in the huddle, 'Check with me on the ball.' I'm screaming out assignments. We'd practiced this. The Vikings snapped the ball, gave it to Foreman. Three or four of us hit him." Philyaw and Rowe were credited with the tackle that had held Foreman to a yard.

Then Villapiano took over. This was the moment Foo had been preparing for, for five long years. "It was like I knew what was going to happen before it happened. I was so prepared—*so* fucking prepared," he says now, eager to race back through the wormhole and revisit the moment. "I knew that in that situation the Vikings liked to pull out their wide receivers and put in two offensive tackles—load up the line, drill you off so some back would come runnin' through. We called it their Jumbo formation. I'd studied the film. I knew that they only had two plays all year out of that formation: 46 and 48, runs to my side. I said to myself, 'Hey, fuck you. You got two plays? I can stop any two plays.'"

As Johnson stood with his back to the Vikings, calling the defensive formation, Villapiano had his eye on the Viking huddle, and he saw White and Rashad leave the field: "Jumbo! When they went to Jumbo, I'd go inside the offensive tackle. The idea was we'd jam the holes, we'd pinch. We called it Jumbo Pinch. I say to Matzoh Ball [Johnson]: 'Jumbo! Jumbo! We got 'em where we want 'em! We got 'em right where we want 'em!'

"So I get on that big fuck from USC, Ron Yary, and I fuckin' shot right in there, and I saw Tarkenton putting the ball in Brent McClanahan's hands, and I fuckin' drove my head right through there. My helmet hit right on the ball. I could feel the ball pop out as I was rammin' my head down. Then I kept pushing McClanahan back, because I knew the ball was somewhere, and I couldn't get it, so I pushed his hands away from it."

Willie Hall recovered McClanahan's fumble on the two. The statement play of Villapiano's career may have been the turning point of Super Bowl XI. "That set the tone," says Rowe, "for the entire game."

"After that play, on the sideline," Foo says, "Tatum went over to Madden and said, 'You better check out Foo. He's fucked up.' Madden comes over and says, 'Foo, you all right?' I say, 'Of course I'm all right.' He says, 'Well, Tate says you were screamin' in the huddle, "We got 'em where we want 'em."'

"I said, 'Coach, we *did* have 'em where we wanted 'em.' He

fucking laughed. He knew exactly what I was saying. And there's
Raider mentality for you. We were all totally on the same wave-
length. With guys who thought like that, how could we lose?"

The Raiders had the ball on their own three. On first down, Banaszak ran up the middle, but safety Paul Krause blew him up. On
second down, Banaszak probed the left side, and Page made the
tackle for just a two-yard gain. The Vikings appeared to have the
Raiders pinned. Without a long third-down conversion, they'd be
punting from the back of the end zone this time.

But if Villapiano had given his team some emotion, the next
play, in many ways, presaged the eventual victory, at least tacti-
cally. On an apparent passing down, third and seven, Stabler called
the play designed to probe the right side of the Vikings' line, an
overload called 17 Bob Trey-O: "17" was the hole, off left tackle;
"Bob" meant that the fullback would be keyed on the outside linebacker, Hilgenberg; "Trey" meant that Casper would be lining up
on Shell's left shoulder, to the outside, to double-team the slight
Marshall; and "O" meant that Buehler, the offside guard, would
pull from his right-guard spot and help clear out the gap, looking
for the middle linebacker, Siemon.

Clarence Davis didn't just get the first down; he juked and
sprinted through a wide-open hole for 35 yards before Krause
dragged him down. They'd probed the spot that had looked so
advantageous on paper, and the play had come off just the way
it had been drawn up. The Raiders would run the same play all
day long, and Davis would amass 137 yards. (Marshall, Art Shell's
man, would register not a single tackle, nor a single assisted tackle,
in the game.)

"Bob Trey-O," laughs Madden. "That play there was a lot bigger play than we expected. To be honest with you, we were backed

up, and we were just trying to get out of there, get away from the goal line to give Guy some room for comfort. And to get the first down if we could.

"But that whole series was a big turning point," says Madden. "We had the disaster. Then, not only stopping them but getting the ball back? The whole combination—the hit, the fumble, the recovery, Bob Trey-O—it was all right there. We got our shorts straightened out after that."

Two plays later, Casper beat linebacker Matt Blair for 25 yards, to the Viking 23. Just as Madden had foreseen, the intermediate pass plays were working. Four running plays brought the ball to the Viking seven, but after two incompletions to Casper in the end zone, Oakland had to settle for a Mann field goal of 24 yards. It wasn't enough for Madden, in his game uniform of blue short-sleeved shirt, light-blue pants, and blond hair about two weeks due for a haircut. He was gesticulating madly, frustrated despite the 90-yard drive that had exposed the Viking weakness against both the Raiders' passing and running games.

"The offense came off, and I was really pissed," Madden remembers. "My thought process was immediate: 'Gotta get seven, goddamnit. Don't want too many threes.' I believed in finishing, and I'm thinking, 'Fuck it, we got to get that ball in the end zone, goddamnit!' So Stabler put his hand on my shoulder and said, 'John, don't worry. There's plenty more where that came from.' He was like a little kid. It kind of calmed me down. I thought, 'Shit, we *are* moving the ball, and he *is* right, and there *is* plenty more where that came from.'"

On the ensuing possession, Matuszak stuffed Foreman on a third and four for no gain, and the Raiders took it back on their own 36. On a third and two from the Viking 45, Stabler looked, again, to his favorite receiver of the season: Casper, covered by Siemon. It was good for 19 yards, down to the Minnesota 26, and now, for a change of pace, the shifty Garrett, the reclamation project, ran three straight times, down to the Minnesota six. On third and three, Stabler hit Biletnikoff for five yards on a sideline pattern, to the one, Freddy stretching high to make a tough catch before running out of bounds. Then Stabler called an option, rolled out, and again found the open Casper for a one-yard touchdown pass: 10–0.

On the next series, Willie Brown broke up a bomb down the left side to Rashad, the Vikings punted from inside their 10, and Neil Colzie's 25-yard return put the Raiders on the Viking 35. After three running plays, a 17-yard completion to Biletnikoff across the middle put the ball on the one. Now logic called for Madden to let Stabler hand it off to van Eeghen, the workhorse, who would run for 73 yards in this game. Instead, he put in the veteran Banaszak, in his eleventh year, who had carried the ball just 19 times in the first two playoff games.

"When John took me out," van Eeghen remembers, "he said to me, 'Mark, listen, I want you to know. Pete's winding down. He's almost done. He's been with me for a while. You'll get another shot. I want Pete to have a touchdown.' I said, 'I'm with you.' It was personal with John, and I more than understood it."

It made the Rooster feel pretty good, too. Banaszak took it in from the one, over the backs of Vella and Buehler, and despite Mann's missed extra point the Raiders had a 16–0 lead.

The Vikings had one more shot before halftime, getting the ball back with just over three minutes to go. They drove to the Raider 48, but Dr. Death broke up a third-and-two pass to Sammy White, and the Vikings had to punt for the fifth time in the half.

The rout appeared to be on. The Raiders had thoroughly dominated the half, especially on the ground. The defense had limited the Vikings to 27 yards running. The Raiders had already rushed for 166, including 102 in the first quarter alone.

As the team left for the locker room, where Biletnikoff could light up again and reapply the Stickum in preparation for an impressive second half, the players were replaced on the field by a halftime show put together by Disney, featuring the New Mickey Mouse Club. Rebels were winning the day, but Walt World could still hold out for fairy-tale glitter in the sun.

In the beginning of the third quarter, the Raiders sustained the momentum, and picked up right where they'd left off, dominating the line of scrimmage. Matuszak stuffed Foreman again on a third and one, deep in Viking territory. The Raiders took over at their 46, and another Davis scamper on 17 Bob Trey-O was good for 18, setting up Mann's 40-yard field goal: 19–0. On the ensuing drive, the Raiders held again, but a roughing-the-kicker call on Kick 'Em, going for one of his patented blocks, gave the Purple a new life. Now Tarkenton began to click. He hit tight end Stu Voigt for 15, and Rashad caught another pass for a 21-yard gain. Tarkenton's eight-yard touchdown pass to White made it 19–7 at the end of the third quarter. The Vikings were back in the game.

And so it was time for the Soul Patrol to take control. They did so, on, of all things, a Tarkenton–to–Sammy White completion. White beat Thomas on a square-in and caught the ball across the middle. As Tatum came over from his free-safety spot, he lowered his helmet into White's chest, just as Thomas, behind the receiver, threw his right arm into White's head. As White was falling from Tatum's hit, Thomas's forearm tore White's helmet off and sent it flying. It was a chillingly violent collision but entirely legal; Thomas's forearm would have corralled White's shoulder pads if the receiver had still been upright. It just happened to catch his head as the receiver crumpled from the Tatum blow.

Somehow, White held on to the ball as he fell to the ground, bareheaded. As his helmet bounced away, two officials bent over to see if White was, well, alive.

"That hit," says Atkinson now, "let me know from that point

on this is our game. It was all timing, angles, like I always said. It was just the culmination of what you talk about when you talk about what we were perceived as. That was our signature on the deal. We played good, solid, aggressive, fundamentally sound football all day."

Three plays later, facing a blitz from Hendricks, Tarkenton threw to White on the left side, and linebacker Willie Hall intercepted the ball, returning it 16 yards. Two running plays set up a third and six at the Oakland 47, and then Stabler and his old buddy hooked up for the offensive play of the day: a 16-yard pass to Biletnikoff, who cut around his defender and ran another 32 yards, finally getting hauled down on the two.

Then it was Banaszak time again, running over Buehler and Vella on the right side again for the touchdown. For Banaszak, this one was the most memorable moment of all. "In the end zone," Rooster remembers, "Upshaw picked me up and said, 'Throw that son of a bitch into the stands.' I said, 'I don't know if I can throw it that far.' But it turned out to be a pretty good spiral. You know how that turned out? A bartender from Buffalo caught the ball. Some time later, he sent me the ball, with a letter, asking me to sign it. When I saw that ball, I wanted to go to bed with it."

But he signed it and sent it back and swears that, to this day, the ball still hangs in a Buffalo bar.

Now it was 26–7, with less than eight minutes left. In the defensive huddle, players were discussing who should win the MVP, the game seemingly sewn up. But the Vikings rallied again. A 28-yard pass to Rashad put the ball on the Raider 28, with six minutes left. A Viking touchdown would keep them in striking distance, if barely. On first down, Tarkenton faded back.

"I called the coverage," Johnson remembers. "Willie was supposed to be deep. But Willie said to me in the huddle, 'If he runs what I think he's going to, I'm going to jump the route.'" Brown suspected a pass in the flat to Sammy White, whom Tarkenton had been targeting all day, with only mixed success. "I said, 'Willie, this is the Super Bowl. I'm not about to tell you you can't do it, but you better be right.' I said to Tate, 'Shade to the backside if Willie runs an up.'

"Sure enough, Tarkenton does exactly what Willie thought he was going to do. You could read Tarkenton like the backside of a cheap five-dollar novel. Willie jumps the route."

The captain stepped in front of White, gathered the ball in, and ran 75 yards, untouched down the sideline, the swell of the crowd increasing with each stride.

"I knew what was going on," Willie says now. "The way the Vikings had done things in the past, it was like reading an open book, to me, what they were trying to do. I just faked like I was going one way and went back the other way. Because I knew the play was coming. After I intercepted, I knew it was a touchdown. I knew if I could get to the end zone the game was over. They wouldn't have a chance."

"Once Willie scored," says Johnson, "the celebration started. We knew. It was all over. Put out the fire and call in the dogs. The hunt's over." It was 32–7 (Mann missed the extra point again), and as van Eeghen puts it, "After that, it was just kind of a matter of putting them out of their misery."

"It was after Willie Brown's interception that it hit me," says Madden now. "There's a point in the game when you know you've won it, and that was when I started celebrating with my players."

With 25 seconds remaining, Minnesota scored another meaningless touchdown, thrown by backup Bob Lee. Madden never saw it. He was too busy hugging, shaking hands with each and every Badass he'd coddled, cajoled, befriended, and bonded with through the years. He was lost in the joyous scrum of his football family. "To this day I haven't seen that touchdown. I don't know how they scored. I don't know what the hell they were doing. I was celebrating. The whole thing was over before it was over."

The final was 32–14. The one-sidedness of the contest may have dismayed NBC officials, but it was more than sweet to the players; it had certified their might, and emphatically erased their reputations as perennial runners-up. "The average football fans may like the close ones," says Buehler. "We don't. We liked to show the killer instinct: grind them when they're down. And we had."

The Raiders had amassed a Super Bowl–record 429 yards on offense, including a remarkable 266 on the ground. Stabler had to pass only 19 times, completing 12, for 180 yards—an impressive 15 yards per catch. Tarkenton had completed fewer than half his passes. The Raiders had nullified the Viking ground attack. In both of the Vikings' playoff victories, over the Redskins and Rams, Foreman had rushed for more than 100 yards. In this one, he'd been held to 44—less than three yards per carry.

Matuszak had had an outstanding day, as had Sistrunk. Rowe, lined up against Mick Tingelhoff, neutralized the six-time Pro Bowl selectee. "That defensive line that day," says Rowe, "was just like three stumps. We funneled [Foreman] to the linebackers." The defense that had played as a unit for less than a year had allowed the Vikings just 71 yards on the ground—and sacked Tarkenton twice.

To the universal delight of Badass fans, Fred Biletnikoff's selection as the game's MVP couldn't have been more appropriate. He hadn't simply earned just a lifetime-achievement award, either. (Well, maybe just a little; certainly, with his 137 yards rushing, Clarence Davis was a close runner-up.) Not that Biletnikoff didn't deserve it, after 12 years of those after-practice practices, those juggling catches, the quiet leadership-by-example. Biletnikoff had caught just four passes for 79 yards, but those catches had set up three of the touchdowns, and the 48-yarder had been the longest offensive play of the day, setting up the score that had, for all practical purposes, put the game out of reach.

The award could have gone to the entire team. Madden had clearly outcoached his adversary. The entire offensive line had pushed the Vikings back on their heels all day. The team had shown a killer instinct, responding to the Vikings' one brief challenge with a classic Badass display of physical football.

As far as Super Bowls go, this was hardly an all-time memorable contest. Super Bowl XI would take its place in the annals of the countless Super Bowls whose hype had dwarfed the game. But to relegate it to such routine status is to ignore its true significance: Super Bowl XI's very one-sidedness had finally certified the Badass version of the game of professional football. The long climb was over. The rebels now officially ruled the game.

In the pre-Gatorade-bucket days, the routine celebration called for the players to carry the coach off on their shoulders. Hendricks and Philyaw hefted Madden's substantial physique . . . and then, since the Raiders could never do anything in conventional fashion, they dropped him. "They tried to pick him up," remembers Monte Johnson. And they did, sort of. "They got him on their shoulders, for four or five steps. Then he sort of tumbled off. They couldn't carry him."

Madden begs to clarify. "We tripped over a photographer. It was a photographer on the ground, down there on one knee, shooting upward. He didn't move. I saw the trip coming."

He quickly recovered his feet and, as he walked into the tunnel,

Madden held high a sign that had been handed to Upshaw from the stands, which he'd passed on to Madden. Befitting the rough-hewn style of the team it celebrated, this was no carefully lettered signboard. The frayed piece of cardboard's punctuation was a little off-kilter, too, but it told the truth: "We're No 1 #."

In the meantime, while most of the players headed inside for the network-choreographed ceremony, several lingered outside to savor the moment, bathed in the late-afternoon sun. Johnson and van Eeghen found themselves standing side by side at midfield. "It was the first time I felt ecstasy on a football field," says van Eeghen. "Athletic ecstasy—a floating feeling that stayed with me, tangibly, as long as I was out there. I didn't want to go in."

Banaszak finally went over to the stands, to hug the fans, and, having covered himself in Stickum that day, stuck to several of them. Some of them may still be wearing the stuff.

Inside the locker room, bedlam reigned: screams, hollers, and hugs signaled the end of all of the pent-up frustration. After knocking on the door for so many years, they'd finally crossed the threshold by bursting the damned thing open, and nothing was going to rein in the unbridled joy.

"John's face was lit up like a Christmas tree, like a jack-o'-lantern, like a big Howdy Doody, happy as hell," Banaszak remembers. "He was hugging everyone. We were all hugging each other. Even Al was hugging us. First time I ever saw Al hug anyone."

"It was euphoric," says Atkinson. "Pure euphoria. It was joy, pure joy. There was a feeling and an energy that if you could capture and put it in a bottle and share it, it would be worth its weight in gold. You'd be a millionaire. I mean, it was a matter of closure, and I looked around at these faces of joy, these faces of happiness that understood we'd finally done it."

While a fictitious account of the celebration would depict the team chugging from bottles of various size and shape, the truth is that the Raiders didn't have champagne. That would flow later. At the moment, for once, they had no need of liquid celebration. This high was natural.

For Banaszak, who had worn the uniform since 1966, the true delight came in seeing the delirium of his teammates: "The looks on everyone's faces, all these guys, all your friends, all your family. We were so happy for one another. At that moment, it was just the consummate team feeling, not an individual thing.

"We just wanted to sit and savor the feeling. I think I must have sat in my uniform for half an hour before I ripped my tape off. I was numb."

As Rozelle handed Davis the trophy, everyone wondered if they'd talk to each other. But Davis's elation outweighed any desire to play up a petty feud. "And I'll never forget the smile on Al's face," says Foo. "It was the most beautiful smile I'd ever seen. He took that trophy in his hands and he just shook it."

Madden can't remember if they threw him into the showers: "I was so damned happy I could have walked in there myself. I was so goofy, I may have walked in there with my clothes on."

Madden, of course, didn't feel the need to give any pompous post-game speeches. At that moment, more than ever before, he was just one of the guys. "I wasn't one to say, 'All the hard work you put in,' and all that bullshit. It was just, 'Goddamnit, we did it! We're the world champions! We did it, and it's forever. They can never take it away from you.' I get shivers when I think about it to this day."

One tableau sticks out in everyone's mind: Biletnikoff, the man of rote superstition and ritual, was doing something no one had ever seen him do. He was weeping like a baby, with his son between his legs.

"Well, sure, I was crying," says Biletnikoff now. "I mean, think of all the work you've done, all the years you've put in, all the stuff you've done together as a team. You get close, you get close, you get close. And then it finally fell into place for you. It finally went the way it was supposed to."

One unit of the team did enjoy its own private celebration, deservedly so, over in their own corner of the locker room. Upshaw grabbed the trophy from Davis, gathered the offensive line together, and the woolly, scuffed, grinning quintet encircled the glistening prize in various states of undress, helmets and pads piled at their feet, for a photographer. Four of them sported beards. Only Buehler, of course, was shaven. Only Upshaw was still in uniform. They looked like a group of grinning mountain men who had reached the summit, at last.

But as Madden says now, "It's not like someone walks in and tells you you've won the lottery." The glistening sensation of winning it all had been a long time coming, and for many of them, for all of the sweetness of the moment, it would be long time before the power of the achievement would reach their hearts.

"You know when it finally sank in for me?" says Monte Johnson. "I was carpooling back across the country with van Eeghen and Rowe a few days later, and we had a CB radio. That was back when everyone had CBs. We were talking about the Super Bowl, talking about what a great team the Raiders were. People began to talk back and forth on their CBs about the game. Stuff like 'I hate the Raiders' and 'I love them, they're great, glad to finally see them win it.'

"So Rowe starts saying to people, 'That guy who was just talking? That's Monte Johnson, the linebacker. And that other guy was Mark van Eeghen, the running back.' Nobody believed us. 'That can't be him!'

"And that's when it really started to hit you. That's when you really began to realize you're the world champion—when you hear people talking about it on their CBs."

The moments following the victory signified only the beginning of the emotions that would swell over their lifetimes. "The funny thing about the feeling of winning it? It doesn't hit you then," says Vella. "When you're programmed to play the way you do in the NFL, when you're so focused to win every game, on what you have to do, it just didn't hit you then. Yeah, you're happy, but it's bigger when you're a year out. Two years out, 10 years out. For me, it's bigger now than it's ever been. I've enjoyed that Super Bowl the last 30 years more than I did that day."

"The jubilation really comes with the passing of years," says George Buehler. "It grows. I used to say that after we beat the Steelers, the Super Bowl was kind of anticlimactic. But as I've grown older, I realize that's bullshit. Today, I can't imagine my life without having won that Super Bowl."

For the de facto leader of the team, the architect of the offense that had reduced the People Eaters to herbivores, the jubilation was more of the quiet kind. "I just felt a great sense of relief, a great sense of accomplishment," says Ken Stabler. "You'd accomplished what you'd always done everything for, everything you've been trying to do for all of those years: be the best in the world. I was happy for the team. I was happy for the city. I was happy for John.

"And 'You can't win the big one'? We shut that up."

✕

They didn't return to the ragged downtown Hilton that night. They went back to the Newport Beach Marriott, for what Mike Siani calls "the best party I've ever been to in my life."

Davis made sure of that. Every player and coach had his own table for friends and family. For some of them, the liquid libations flowed all night. "I mean *all* night," says Siani. "I remember Matuszak throwing a football with a buddy of mine. Someone from the hotel came over and said, 'You can't do that.' The next thing I saw was the hotel guy running away.

"The next day we were supposed to fly back to Oakland. I think out of the entire team, 13 guys made the plane. The rest of us couldn't get up."

And, yes, it would be tempting to assume that the evening ended with Raiders swinging from chandeliers, pillaging their way through the hotel as they hoisted waitresses under their arms. But the truth is that civility ruled this evening. The presence of family and friends tended to mute the Badass wild side.

On top of which, the post-adrenaline fatigue was overwhelming: for this team, not the release of adrenaline of winning just one big game, but the release of years and years of adrenaline. The culmination of emotions that had been mounting for seasons was almost too much to comprehend.

"I was so tired after that game, so mentally washed out, I was in bed before 12," says Banaszak, which tells you that it was hardly like a night at Big Al's. "But I made good use of my time while I was down there."

"It was more about, you just sit and try and figure it all out," says Stabler. "Let it all sink in. It wasn't a hell-raise night. It was about appreciating what you did.

"After that, later, I did some celebrating. And I'm still celebrating it."

# Epilogue

When did the Badass era end? When did the age of the barbed warriors recede into legend, and the league began to morph into a collection of interchangeable, faceless corporate entertainers?

Perhaps, following a by now all-too-familiar blueprint, the curtain fell 12 months after their Super Bowl triumph, when the gods called down the Fumble in yet another championship-game loss, and America's Team went on to claim its second Super Bowl a few weeks later.

If the Badass days began with Franco's miracle, then perhaps the beginning of the unraveling came with Bronco running back Rob Lytle's cough-up in the old Mile High Stadium. It was a single play that seemed to confirm that the deities had it in for my guys; that They had begrudgingly granted the Badasses a ring, because they simply *had* to, because my Raiders were too special, and too overwhelmingly, inarguably excellent at their game, not to endow them with a title.

But one ring, apparently, was the cosmic limit. Turn the Badasses into a dynasty, elevate them to numeric greatness, and the next thing you know, well, football would be . . . fun. Brotherly. Authentic. Inspiring. Lovable.

The Raiders had finished second to the Broncos in the regular season in 1977. In the opening round of the playoffs, they beat the Colts, 37–31, in the famed double-overtime game in Memorial Stadium that featured the Ghost to the Post: a stunning 42-yard Stabler-to-Casper pass that the tight end gathered in over his head, Willie Mays style, to set up the tying field goal in the game's last minute of regulation. Another Casper touchdown, at the beginning of the sixth quarter, won the game. The Colt game was a marathon of a contest, with eight lead changes. Emotionally, maybe the Badasses had once again left it on the field in the penultimate game, as they had in so many also-ran previous seasons.

In Denver, they couldn't overcome the fates. They couldn't recover from yet another call that the refs got wrong. The Broncos held a 7–3 lead in the third quarter and, driving for another score, had the ball on the Raider two-yard line. Rickety old Craig Morton handed the ball to Lytle, who dove into the scrum near the goal line. Once again, it was Tatum who launched himself into the fray. The ball popped out. Mike McCoy, brought over to Oakland in a trade with the Packers, was playing tackle in the goal-line defense. He burrowed beneath the Bronco offensive line, then looked up from the ground to see the ball. He picked it up on the four. He heard no whistle.

Unimpeded, McCoy sprinted the other way—until he saw Madden "do one of his famed double pumps to the forehead." He began to slow at the 40. Ed Marion, the head linesman, never saw the ball come out. He ruled that there had been no fumble. The officials never huddled to discuss this fateful play. Footage showed the ball to have clearly come loose, but five years after the Deception, the officials still called games without instant replay. Marion's call of "no fumble" stood. The Broncos scored on the next play, and would go on to win it, 20–17. Later, Art McNally would admit the official was wrong on the call.

"If they'd called that fumble . . ." McCoy says now, but this is a big "if." Plenty of time remained in the game. Nor were the Badasses necessarily the better team that day, fumble or no fumble. Sure, they might have played a different style of game had they taken that second-quarter lead, but they rushed for just 94 yards, and Stabler (who had put together another Pro Bowl season) completed fewer than half his passes that afternoon. The Raiders had lost to the Broncos 30–7 earlier in the season. On that day, perhaps the Broncos *were* the better team.

On the other hand, I prefer to see the larger hands of Mount Olympus at work. "When you think about the games we lost," Mark van Eeghen says now. "The Rob Lytle fumble, the Immaculate Reception . . . if Mother Luck is on our side, the team might have won more Super Bowls." But, of course, Mother Luck is one of the gods. Why would she smile on the Raiders?

Or maybe the era came to an end during the second game of that 1977 season, when the gods of the Three Rivers crippled Foo, the truest Badass, for the year, ending his season and delivering a blow to the gut of the team. "If there's one day when our little world started crumbling," says Phil Villapiano now, "it was that day."

On the scoreboard, this was a day of triumph. With both Harris and Bleier healthy, the Raiders beat the Steelers in a supremely defensive battle, 16–7. Harris and Bleier didn't gain 100 yards between them. But it all came at a steep cost—thanks to the Three

Rivers turf. This time it wasn't frozen. This time it featured a brand-new surface, as Foo recalls it: fresh, unforgiving plastic. Call the play that took out Foo for the season the Trip.

"It was just a fluke," he says. The Steelers gave the ball to Bleier, running to Villapiano's side. Foo was in perfect position. But the pulling guard tripped and rolled directly at him. "I try to slide my leg away, but it's stuck. My foot is planted on the turf. The guy goes right through and lands right on my knee. Snapped the knee. Tore the ligament on the inside—just tore it in half.

"We lost four starters that day—Vella for the season, too—and I guarantee the turf had something to do, one way or the other, with all of them. This new field was as sticky as Velcro. You know how with Velcro you gotta pull it straight up, you can't go side to side? That's what this stuff was like.

"And that was the end of me."

And how could there be a team of Badasses without Foo?

Record-wise, the Badass era officially came to an end in 1978, when the Raiders went 9–7, and became, for the first time since 1964, a truly mediocre team. They lost three of their last four and missed out on the playoffs for the first time in nine years. That year, Biletnikoff, now 34, was replaced in the starting lineup by Morris Bradshaw. In 1978, Biletnikoff started just two games and caught just 20 passes. A Raider team without a Biletnikoff was a team without a heart. The 1978 season would be his last in the NFL.

Branch, after being named to four consecutive Pro Bowls, would catch a single touchdown pass that year. Siani had been traded to the Colts. Skip Thomas was gone, replaced by Lester Hayes. Willie Brown was in his final year. Ten players from Super Bowl XI were either off the roster or not starting.

And Stabler's luster was beginning to dim. Four games into the season, he had completed fewer than 50 percent of his passes and averaged three interceptions per game. Stung by growing criticism, the man who had always been one of the most thoughtful and articulate channels to the media stopped talking to the press. That season, his interceptions (30) doubled his TDs (16). Madden came to the defense of his man, pointing out that many of the interceptions weren't Stabler's fault, but when the season ended Al Davis singled out Stabler for the sorry (by Raider standards) season: "You've got to point to someone, so blame Stabler. . . . He makes the most money [$342,000 in 1978]. He gets paid to take the pressure. . . . It all starts with the left-hander."

It was rumored that Davis was shopping his quarterback. (He'd eventually send the Snake to Houston for the 1980 season.) The rumblings of dissension were ominous, and they included an anonymous teammate criticizing Stabler for his off-the-field habits: in essence, decrying an essential element of not only the man but the Badasses as a legion. To criticize a Badass lifestyle was to rip at its gut. The team was losing its class. They had never sniped at each other.

Maybe they'd started taking themselves for granted. Or maybe finally winning one, after the excruciating years of almosts, represented a feat that would have been diminished, in a weird way, if there'd been another trophy for the likes of Snake and Foo and Rooster and Freddy. Maybe the Badasses weren't ever meant to be just another football dynasty, but a cast of characters whose theatrical story line transcended football, with a universal plot about an epic journey of brothers culminating in a singular, riveting climax on the grand stage of the largest stadium to ever host a Super Bowl. How could you top that?

This much we do know: by 1978, the Badass vibe no longer carried over onto the football field. They'd lost their singularity, receded into the faceless pack.

"In 1978," Villapiano says, "we didn't play like Raiders. We took shit for it, and we deserved the shit."

But the Badasses weren't ever about the rings, the records, the yards gained, as impressive as those totems might be. They were about tribal bonding, being a member of a band led by one particular kind of guy, and so this much is inarguable: the true end of the era came on the day that Pinky decided to hang up the shoelace-less sneakers, take the towel off his shoulder, walk away from the sacred turf, and put the bottle of Maalox back in the medicine cabinet, after the 1978 season.

There could be no real Badasses without the man who let them be as bad as they could be. There could be no lovable Raiders without the big man flailing and smiling and laughing on the sidelines, drawing us all into his embrace. Inviting us all into the Badass family.

It's not that Tom Flores wasn't a terrific head coach. He'd collect twice as many rings as his predecessor. But he was just a football coach, like any other coach on every other sideline: efficient, likable enough, but not a . . . *guy.* Not larger than life. He didn't lead with his personality, or his hands. He didn't discuss the headlines before morning practice with his players. Or care for each eccentric one of them as if they were his own kids. He didn't exude joy. Without John Madden the Raiders were just a football team— a very good one, of course. The team would achieve statistical and diamond-encrusted glory behind quarterback Jim Plunkett, a quiet legend himself—but hardly a Snake. An anti-Badass.

Madden remembers speaking of his uncertainty about coming back to the team to no one but his wife. But Stabler insists that his coach told him that he was thinking of hanging up the sneakers during the 1978 season. "Halfway through his last year, after a quarterback meeting, he told me he wasn't coming back. I hated hearing that. He was the perfect coach for me. The perfect coach for all of us. We'd never know another coach who gave us the room he gave us."

No one would. He'd broken the mold. Madden's lifelong appeal as a commentator derived from more than his ability to dissect a play for a television audience. John Madden in the booth spoke of the last public connection with a lost time and a lost joy and a lost playfulness. The All-Madden team wasn't about star-making skill. It was about football. And when he announced that he'd had enough, the news was met with disbelief. The best coach in football doesn't just *resign*.

"It was a *blow*," says Atkinson. "I sure didn't see it coming."

"It was a surprise decision from everyone's standpoint," Steve Sylvester says. "He did state that he started to see things he didn't like. Drugs were coming in. Steroids. There was probably a cocaine problem in the NFL. He hated that stuff. He didn't understand it. Free agency was coming. The game was changing to a bigger platform. And Al probably wore him down."

"He went out too early," says Foo. "I said, 'Forty-three years old? Gimme a break!' I felt very, very bad when he quit, because we were so loyal to him. Hey, maybe John lost it, in some way. Like we lost it as players."

Under Flores, they'd win it all in 1980 and then in 1983, by which time they were playing in a borrowed stadium, in a borrowed city: Los Angeles, home to countless routine endings—and always fictitious ones. They'd win their Super Bowls in a decade when rebellion was not only uncool but downright heretical—as was Davis's move to Los Angeles, at least for the true Badass fan. Search high and low and you'll find no less Badass a town than Los Angeles. When Al Davis decided to go for the money, which the move to Los Angeles represented, the family was officially disbanded forever.

But after John Madden crossed over to the other side of the camera, there was something sweetly reassuring that he started to ride the train in his pre-bus era: the perfect travel medium for the man who had been wound up for so long that he had to decompress. The railroad was an apt emblem for the contrarian feel to the Madden Raiders. Here was a man en route to gaining icon status as a talking head in a second-to-second, instantaneous medium, traveling from city to city in a nineteenth-century mode of transportation where people of all shape and stripe and class could interact. What other network announcer would kick back and spend three days getting to his next assignment? Only a former Raider, going against all conceivable form.

One day in the '80s, I saw John Madden queued up with a cluster of other passengers waiting to board a cross-country train at 30th Street Station, in Philadelphia. He was smiling and talking. That was the day I knew the man had found his bliss—ready to join and befriend the cooks and porters, and trade stories in the observation car like some real-life George Babbitt, only 60 years later than Sinclair Lewis's novel. The time could finally pass slowly for him, the landscape could unscroll, and the Maalox was no longer necessary. Maybe the Badass era finally receded on those vanishing rail tracks.

Of course, much of Madden's preference for on-ground travel stemmed from his intense dislike of flying. One night in 1960, when Madden was getting his masters at Cal-Poly, the Cal-Poly football team's chartered plane crashed taking off after a loss to Bowling Green. Twenty-two of the 44 passengers on board died, including sixteen players and an assistant manager, among them several good friends of Madden's. Madden has admitted that the crash had a "subconscious" effect on his fear of flying.

Whatever its roots, Madden's aversion to being up in that cramped tube was obvious to any and all. Cuniberti recalls flight attendants sponging him off. Stabler recalls him vomiting. (Madden insists he never threw up.)

"It was all claustrophobia," Madden says now. "I was never a good flier. It was just a matter of control. Having to sit there, and not being able to get out. I didn't fear that the plane was going to crash. It wasn't that type of thing. It was the anxiety buildup of having to sit there for so long.

"It got easier when we got charters, because the captain would leave the door open and you could go up there and they'd be talking about the college game they'd seen that day."

According to Steve Sylvester, the exchanges weren't always that civil. "On the way back from Miami one year, our flight path took us over Texas, and there were tornadoes or a hurricane or something, and there was a lot of turbulence. He absolutely went ballistic on Captain Hank, our charter pilot: 'Take the sonofabitch around the storm, not through it!'"

"Well, yeah," says Madden. "I used to tell the pilot, 'We don't need any heroes around here. If there's a storm with lightning in it, and you can see it, fly around the sonofabitch. You can see it's there. Don't go right through it! I don't need an extra fifteen minutes that bad.'"

The most rational explanation for Madden's premature exit from the game could be that once he'd climbed the ultimate mountain, in decisive fashion, and the 100 victories had been achieved in a decade, no thrill could equal the first championship. He was still a young man, he'd achieved all he'd set out to do, from those first Lombardi seminars, through the college years, through the countless might-have-been championship games, and other frontiers beckoned. He'd made his name, he'd honchoed an historic family, and his mind and body were telling him that the epic had reached its final stanzas.

"After I won the Super Bowl," Madden told me, "I knew I wasn't going to be coaching for long after that. I didn't think about retiring then, but I knew that once you've won every game all you can do is win them again. I'd done that, so the end was near.

"Then I got an ulcer, and it would act up on me. I said to the doctor, 'What do I do to get rid of it?' The doctor said, 'The only thing you can do to get rid of it is to get rid of what's causing it. And you're going to have an ulcer until you get out of coaching.'"

"I know he was having problems," Stabler says. "He was always taking something for those ulcers. You could tell he didn't feel good. Before each game I can remember him chug-a-lugging out of the bottle of Maalox." And not just before games. "He'd have a bottle of Maalox in his back pocket," Ted Kwalick remembers, "and he used to drink the whole damned thing during practice. This was *practice*. That's got to be one of the reasons he got out."

There's no question that Darryl Stingley's paralysis in 1978 had something to do with his decision, too. The day an opponent lost the use of his limbs was a day that will live with Madden forever: a landmark day when the fun and games of the Badasses had lost a whole lot of their glow, especially for an empathetic man who understood football players to be actual people.

"That was a factor," Madden says now, "but it wasn't the reason."

Psychologically, outside of Stingley's family and friends, Madden took the receiver's paralysis as hard as anyone, and in retrospect, it's not hard to understand why. Football players were never meat to John Madden, and tragedy and finality had never been part of the Badass catalogue. My Raiders were in the game to get *away* from real life, not to be jarred into it. "Not many people seemed to care enough," Madden would write of the incident. "I started wondering if football people really care about a player, or if football people just care about what a player does."

After the game when Stingley broke his neck, Madden immediately went to Eden Hospital in Castro Valley, where Stingley had been taken, managed to procure a doctor's smock, and entered the operating room. "Everything's going to be all right," he told Stingley. Bothered that no Patriot physicians or representatives of any kind had come to the hospital, he called the Oakland airport.

"I got [Patriot coach] Chuck Fairbanks on the phone," he told me. "I told him it was pretty serious. They didn't come back to the hospital."

A Patriot business manager disembarked and the plane took off—and had an engine malfunction. It had to return, making an emergency landing in San Francisco. "It's like this cosmic boil," Toomay says, "that had to be lanced. Then on another visit, he goes into Stingley's room and something, a ventilator, isn't functioning properly, and John gets help. He possibly saves Stingley's life."

In the ensuing weeks, Stingley's wife would be a frequent visitor at Madden's house for dinner, playing backyard basketball with Madden's kids.

Some of the players sensed a change in the man in 1978. "Was he a different guy?" says Raymond Chester, who returned to the team in that final year, to back up Casper, himself in his last full season as a Raider. "Yeah, yeah, I think so. There were a couple of things. I think he was more relaxed with respect to his pursuit for a championship. He had accomplished that. And at the same time I could tell he was worn. The flights were taking more out of him. The stress of trying to maintain the superlative record he had was beginning to wear on him."

"I think John was just tired," says Banaszak, who called it quits at the same time. "But a lot of us were tired. Sure, we'd have all liked for it to go on. But we did what we wanted. We did what we wanted, and that was it."

So why, then, did he ultimately walk away?

"I had had enough," Madden says now, matter-of-factly. "I just thought, 'Ten years is good.' Lombardi coached 10 years. That's what most people did.

"Had I not had enough, I would have gone back. I had a number of contacts, but I said 'no' before it ever got to the next step. I never went in and interviewed with anyone, or talked with anyone. I never went through the courting process. I was a little afraid to, to be honest. I was afraid they'd talk me into it."

So were you simply burned out?

"I don't think I ever used that term," he says. "It's a term other people used. . . . What I did feel was that my type of personality— A or B or whatever the hell it is—isn't in it for the long run."

"I think there were some real issues for him," says Bob Moore. "He was working way too hard; he was unhealthy. If he had 20 years or 25 years in this business there'd have been no one like him. But I'm not sure anyone can keep up that intensity. He had a wonderful career in broadcasting—and it probably saved his life."

Madden ended up spending three times as many years in the broadcast booth as he did on the sidelines.

"But when I think about that era, it's there forever," Madden told me. "It's never gone away. I mean, it's just *there all the time*."

The aura of true, wildly gleeful Badass football? No traces remain on the professional football landscape. It's still the game of football, but it's not Badass football, and it will never be again, because free agency and the high-stakes bucks and the star-making machinery have conspired to make it impossible to produce a team that plays for the pure, unadulterated joy of it, a team that can coalesce into a brotherly force whose sum is so much grander than its individual parts. Rosters are overfull of Raymond Chester's "independent contractors." They play for themselves, and their own individual fame, and the incomprehensible and illogical wealth that it brings them, as they change uniforms from year to year, as they enjoy the fruits of the curse that ended the innocence of professional football: the absorption of sport into the world of American High Televised Entertainment.

Somewhere along the line, professional football had gone from being the perfect big-backyard distraction to an economic driving wheel. Somewhere along the line, we stopped seeing the players as the everyday overachieving men they once were—athletes whose annual salaries were no more than our own fathers', men who possessed outsize ambition and skill but were, in the end, just people. We started to worship them, and not in a healthy way. We turned the football games into a multibillion-dollar spectacle to fill the void we sensed behind the meaningless "me first" culture.

The evolution from football as football to football as a replay-laden, prancing, self-celebratory, commercially bloated frame for halftime extravaganzas happened because we've lost the perspective the Raiders always carried in those Badass years: that the game is no bigger than the effort you give for the man on each side of you. Fame never once entered the Badass mind. None of them was playing for individual glory. Now the pros are just another group of showmen dancing with the stars.

No trace remains of the innocent Badass in football now. The outlaws of the modern game are true and ugly outlaws, tripwired in all of the wrong ways. Some thump their chests, do their elaborate dances, point to a god above, but always leave you feeling that they're really pointing at themselves. And when guns are owned by players in the modern game, they're actually pointed at someone.

"We seemed to thrive off our own craziness. Everybody in the league wanted to be the Raiders. How we acted, how we dressed. It was so perfect, what we had, and everybody knew it," says the man with the silvering hair, wearing the suit with perfect creases, his shoes buffed so cleanly they reflect the arc lights of the parking lot outside the Jersey hotel lounge where we've met. He props his leg horizontally on the empty chair to his side, to lessen the pain from a recent knee replacement, a legacy from the plastic turf and all the years of playing the part of the on-field wild man, the years that fueled his life. The pain he feels on this night is a black-and-silver badge of courage.

He's just finished a business meeting. He sells space on transatlantic container ships, and makes a good living at it. His handsome, tanned, deceptively young face speaks of a love of life, a love of the moment. He smiles just for the sake of smiling. His entire demeanor reflects something between wealth and privilege. He looks like a CEO. There is no trace in this salesman of the linebacker of legend, to look at him from afar.

It's only after a beer that the bullet intensity in his eyes reveals Foo, as he starts going right back in time, in a microsecond, to try to put it all in perspective.

"God equals out the bodies. Someone's bigger, someone's quicker. Some do more curls, some more bench presses. But the thing that makes you win is your brain. The Raiders? We were guys who could think football. That was the key. You know what? No one's ever talked about that. 'Hey, this guy got out of jail. This guy did this. This guy did that. They're all fucked up. They got thrown off other teams. They were wild.'

"Well, we *were* wild. We all lived on the edge. Well, yeah. In a certain way. . . . But we thought like football players. Like fucking winners."

He orders another beer, rubs the knee, smiles the smile that starts with the wild eyes.

"I had a certain way of playing football, and it was exactly the way I wanted to play football. It was exactly rough enough and nasty enough. And now my work life is terrific. What else could you ask for? You couldn't ask for anything else. So sometimes I try to become the new Phil, and a day later, I say, 'Fuck it. I'm just Phil the fucking Raider.' It doesn't work for me to become the new Phil. I want to be a fucking Raider *right now.*"

"Why do people still remember us? Why do people still talk about us?" Rooster ponders the question. "It was the cast of characters. But that cuckoo's nest was pretty disciplined, when you get down to it. We had mental toughness. What is mental toughness? I define it as all the feelings we had for each other as a group. The amazing thing is how we blended together. Black, white, misfits, college grads, guys out of the Continental League . . . We *loved* each other—the type of love you have for a guy you line up with week in and week out and beat your brains out for 60 minutes. That's the kind of love it was.

"I wish I could do it over 100 times again. There isn't a day that goes by I don't think of it. I guarantee that if you talk to any player on that team they'll tell you the same thing. And you know what the greatest thing in the world is? It stayed with me. It stayed with all of us."

The team stays intact, of course; the bonds were too strong to ever be broken. They gather at charity events, tournaments—golf, not air hockey—and at unofficial reunions in Davis's box at the coliseum. They seize any chance to cross paths with their brothers. "This will typify everything for you," Mike Siani told me. "Some of us went to see the Raiders play the Jets a few years ago. The game ends at four in the afternoon. We go back to the Hilton. And at about two thirty the following morning, I'm leaving the bar. And keep in mind this started at four in the afternoon. This has been going on for eight to ten hours. Stabler, Hendricks, and Phil were still sitting in the bar holding court. 'I can't drink anymore,' I said. 'You guys are out of your minds.'"

The Badass tradition lives on. We just don't get to see it anymore. We get to see self-celebrating, linoleum-haircutted talking heads calling the games. We get to see confetti at the Super Bowl and graying halftime rock bands who have no more to do with professional entertainment than Plato does. We get to watch mini-corporations. We get to watch The Show.

The Badasses get to relive history, every day. Like so many of his teammates, on his travels, with his current friends, at high-school reunions, Pete Banaszak is always pressed to tell the stories of the Badasses, and he is always eager to comply.

"I got the best story of all," he says. "It's a true one."

"It was a glorious time," George Atkinson told me the last time I saw him, in his tree-lined backyard. He was wearing a shirt emblazoned with the Raider emblem. "It was collectively about us. It brought about a feeling that people can achieve things together, regardless of race, regardless of age.

"And I'm proud of that legacy that has withstood time. Could it ever be re-created? Never. It was once in a lifetime. It was supreme, and you can't re-create that. It's not going to come again."

"It's hard to translate the feelings into words, you know what I'm saying? I think about it all the time." Ken Stabler pauses, and says it again for emphasis, lest I miss what he's said: "I think about it *all the time.*

"It was a great time, and we'll always have it. It was the greatest team to play for. There was a love for each other. Everything fit from top to bottom. A great bunch of characters. A great band of personalities. A fun-loving band of rogues. You played for John. You played for Al. You played for a city. You played for each other. You played for a great, big-hearted football team. What else can a football player ask for? It always stays with you. I loved being part of it then, and I love it now.

"I tell my girls Raider stories. They think I was a badass. They say, 'Dad, you were a badass.' I say, 'I was part of a Badass *team.*'"

# Acknowledgments

David Hirshey at HarperCollins mentored and guided this book with an editing expertise of which few others—as any of his writers will attest—are capable. Much appreciation for his tolerance and patience during the rocky parts. Special thanks, also, to Assistant Editor George Quraishi, who worked tirelessly and skillfully on the manuscript, as well as to Barry Harbaugh, whose contributions are much appreciated. Thanks to Rob Fleder, my old editor at *The National,* for his assistance with the cover image of the book. And, as always, many thanks to Esther Newberg at ICM.

John Herrera of the Oakland Raiders was more than patient with my endless requests, and for this I am grateful. Special thanks to the staff of the Oakland Public Library, the Edsel Ford Memorial Library at the Hotchkiss School, and the New York Public Library. And special thanks to Carl Francis at the National Football League Players Association.

I am, of course, endlessly grateful to all the Oakland Raiders who were willing to participate in this project. In particular, Phil

Villapiano and George Atkinson went out of their way to accommodate my requests for their time, and deserve special mention for their kindness and indulgence.

A shout-out to Ken Lauber for all the moral support. Lastly, I am endlessly grateful to my wife, Melissa Davis, for putting up with all the craziness.

Readers who are interested in further exploring the Raiders and their history will find titles in this book worth pursuing. I especially recommend Mark Ribowsky's entertaining and definitive biography of Al Davis, *Slick: The Silver-and-Black Life of Al Davis*.

And one more caveat: the passage of time has a way of producing permutations in the memories of men who are recalling events of a lost era. While *Badasses* intends to be a definitive history, it is also an oral history of a long-gone time, and it is hoped that the reader will approach this work with the full knowledge that history, as retold by several different voices, is an elastic thing. This is a work comprising tales told by distant warriors, each with a different perspective and different memories of their glorious shared past. Someone once said that the truth isn't to be found in the various details. The details simply record the event, like measurements in a file. The truth is something larger. In this case, it's that the mythic legend of the Badasses told the singular story of the game we once knew of as football.

# Selected Sources

## Books

*America's Game*, Michael MacCambridge, Anchor Books, 2004.

*Better to Reign in Hell*, Jim Miller and Kelly Mayhew, The New Press, 2005.

*Cruisin' with the Tooz*, John Matuszak with Steve Delsohn, Franklin Watts, 1987.

*The Good, the Bad & the Ugly*, Steven Travers, Triumph Books, 2008.

*Hey, Wait a Minute (I Wrote a Book!)*, John Madden with Dave Anderson, Villard, 1984.

*Jim Otto: The Pain of Glory*, Jim Otto with Dave Newhouse, Sports Publishing Inc., 1999.

*Just Win, Baby*, Glenn Dickey, Harcourt Brace Jovanovich, 1991.

*Namath: A Biography*, Mark Kriegel, Penguin Books, 2004.

*One Knee Equals Two Feet*, John Madden with Dave Anderson, Villard, 1986.

*One Size Doesn't Fit All*, John Madden with Dave Anderson, Villard, 1988.

*Raiders Forever*, John Lombardo, Contemporary Books, 2001.

*Slick: The Silver-and-Black Life of Al Davis*, Mark Ribowsky, Macmillan, 1991.

*Snake*, Ken Stabler and Berry Stainback, Doubleday, 1986.

*Sports and the Racial Divide,* Michael Lomax, editor, University of Mississippi Press, 2008.

*Stadium Stories: Oakland Raiders,* Tom LaMarre, Globe Pequot Press, 2003.

## Periodicals

"Al Davis Isn't as Bad as He Thinks He Is," Gary Smith, *Inside Sports*, May 31, 1981.

"Bad to the Bone," Kevin Cook, *Playboy* magazine, October 2009.

"Emperors and Clowns," Roger Kahn, *Time* magazine, January 10, 1977.

"The House That the Immaculate Reception Built," Chuck Finder, *The Sporting News*, December 2000.

"Just Live, Baby," Bryan Curtis, *Play* magazine, August 19, 2007.

"The Most Hated Winner in Football," Leonard Schecter, *Look* magazine, November 1969.

"Raider Nation," Pat Toomay, ESPN.com.

"The Super Show," B. J. Phillips, *Time* magazine, January 10, 1977.

"A Walk on the Sordid Side," William Oscar Johnson, *Sports Illustrated*, August 1, 1977.

"Who Is This Mad Hatter?," Paul Zimmerman, *Sports Illustrated*, October 17, 1983.

## Newspapers

*The New York Times*

*The Oakland Tribune*

*The San Francisco Chronicle*

## Videos

*Raiders: The Complete History*, NFL Productions, 2004.

*Rebels of Oakland: The A's, The Raiders, The '70s*, HBO Studio Productions, 2003.